IFMBE Proceedings 102

Series Editor

Ratko Magjarević, *Faculty of Electrical Engineering and Computing, ZESOI, University of Zagreb, Zagreb, Croatia*

Associate Editors

Piotr Ładyżyński, *Warsaw, Poland*
Fatimah Ibrahim, *Department of Biomedical Engineering, Faculty of Engineering, Universiti Malaya, Kuala Lumpur, Malaysia*
Igor Lackovic, *Faculty of Electrical Engineering and Computing, University of Zagreb, Zagreb, Croatia*
Emilio Sacristan Rock, *Mexico DF, Mexico*

The IFMBE Proceedings Book Series is an official publication of *the International Federation for Medical and Biological Engineering* (IFMBE). The series gathers the proceedings of various international conferences, which are either organized or endorsed by the Federation. Books published in this series report on cutting-edge findings and provide an informative survey on the most challenging topics and advances in the fields of medicine, biology, clinical engineering, and biophysics.

The series aims at disseminating high quality scientific information, encouraging both basic and applied research, and promoting world-wide collaboration between researchers and practitioners in the field of Medical and Biological Engineering.

Topics include, but are not limited to:

- Diagnostic Imaging, Image Processing, Biomedical Signal Processing
- Modeling and Simulation, Biomechanics
- Biomaterials, Cellular and Tissue Engineering
- Information and Communication in Medicine, Telemedicine and e-Health
- Instrumentation and Clinical Engineering
- Surgery, Minimal Invasive Interventions, Endoscopy and Image Guided Therapy
- Audiology, Ophthalmology, Emergency and Dental Medicine Applications
- Radiology, Radiation Oncology and Biological Effects of Radiation
- Drug Delivery and Pharmaceutical Engineering
- Neuroengineering, and Artificial Intelligence in Healthcare

IFMBE proceedings are indexed by SCOPUS, EI Compendex, Japanese Science and Technology Agency (JST), SCImago. They are also submitted for consideration by WoS.

Proposals can be submitted by contacting the Springer responsible editor shown on the series webpage (see "Contacts"), or by getting in touch with the series editor Ratko Magjarevic.

Simona Vlad · Nicolae Marius Roman
Editors

8th International Conference on Advancements of Medicine and Health Care Through Technology

Proceedings of MEDITECH 2022
October 20–22, 2022
Cluj-Napoca, Romania

Springer

Editors
Simona Vlad
Faculty of Electrical Engineering
Technical University of Cluj-Napoca
Cluj-Napoca, Romania

Nicolae Marius Roman
Faculty of Electrical Engineering
Technical University of Cluj-Napoca
Cluj-Napoca, Romania

ISSN 1680-0737 ISSN 1433-9277 (electronic)
IFMBE Proceedings
ISBN 978-3-031-51119-6 ISBN 978-3-031-51120-2 (eBook)
https://doi.org/10.1007/978-3-031-51120-2

This Springer imprint is published by the registered company Springer Nature Switzerland AG
The registered company address is: Gewerbestrasse 11, 6330 Cham, Switzerland

Preface

This volume presents the Proceedings of the 8th "Conference on Advancements of Medicine and Health Care Through Technology"—MediTech2022 which took place in Cluj-Napoca, between October 20 and 22, 2022, in online format.

This conference continues a series of MediTech conferences organized by the "Romanian National Society for Medical Engineering and Biological Technology" in collaboration with "International Federation for Medical and Biological Engineering" every two years in Cluj-Napoca Romania.

Two local universities and a hospital were co-opted in the organization of this conference, Technical University of Cluj-Napoca, "Iuliu Haţieganu" University of Medicine and Pharmacy of Cluj-Napoca and "Dr. Constantin Papilian" Military Emergency Hospital Cluj-Napoca, Romania. The possibility of disseminating the results from university research with those from the current practice offered by the hospital was thus created.

At MediTech2022, 90% of the received papers were accepted after a double blind review process, the average number of papers assigned to each reviewer being 3. We would like to thank reviewers from the Scientific Advisory Committee for their efforts and expertise in contributing to reviewing.

A large number of guests from Europe, Asia and Romania participated in the conference as invited speakers or authors of articles. They presented the latest news in the field of biomedicine as well as results obtained in their research activity. The exchange of information was vast and extremely useful for both specialists and young researchers.

We were honored by the presence of specialists from the IFMBE board such as Prof. Ratko Magjarević—IFMBE President, Prof. Kang Ping Lin—IFMBE Vice President, as well as Dr. Christoph Baumann—Springer Editorial Director.

In his opening speech of the conference, Prof. Ratko Magjarević—IFMBE President said:

"On behalf of IFMBE and my own, I am honored to be invited to speak at the 8th International Conference on Advancements of Medicine and Health Care through Technology to be held in Cluj-Napoca, Romania. As a member and current President of the **International Federation for Medical and Biological Engineering** (IFMBE), I am glad to see that there is a will and enthusiasm to organize such an important Conference which aims to provide opportunities for Romanian and foreign experts and professionals to exchange their research results, experiences and know-how and in addition to build up collaboration in one of the most complex fields of science and technology-biomedical engineering.

Let me convey my appreciation and support to the Romanian National Society for Medical Engineering and Biological Technology for succeeding in creating a series of Conferences over the past years, for recognizing the importance of Biomedical engineering in the present time and for inviting the biomedical engineering community to be part of this scientific adventure. The research results presented at this conference are being repeatedly published in the IFMBE Proceedings Series. The Proceedings of the MediTech2022 Conference will contribute to the body of knowledge in biomedical engineering which we all are building for a number of decades."

Finally, we would like to thank all the participants, invited speakers, academics, researchers, medical specialists, sponsors, media partners and members of the Scientific and Organizing Committee for their contribution and dedication to the success of the conference.

Cluj-Napoca, Romania
October 2022

Prof. dr. sc. Ratko Magjarević
IFMBE President

Prof. Nicolae Marius Roman
MediTech 2020 Conference Chair

Organization

Organizers

Romanian National Society for Medical Engineering and Biological Technology
Technical University of Cluj-Napoca, Romania
"Iuliu Haţieganu" University of Medicine and Pharmacy Cluj-Napoca, Romania

Partner

"Dr. Constantin Papilian" Military Emergency Hospital, Cluj-Napoca, Romania

Conference Chair

Nicolae Marius Roman—*Romanian National Society for Medical Engineering and Biological Technology*

Honorary Chair

Radu Vasile Ciupa—*Romanian National Society for Medical Engineering and Biological Technology*

Scientific Advisory Committee

Ancuta-Coca Abrudan (RO)
Laura Bacali (RO)
Doina Baltaru (RO)
Radu Ciorap (RO)
Paul Farago (RO)
Stefan Gergely (RO)
Zoltan German-Sallo (RO)
Laura Grindei (RO)
Rodica Holonec (RO)
Ioan Jivet (RO)
Mihaela-Ruxandra Lascu (RO)
Marius Muji (RO)
Calin Munteanu (RO)
Mihai S. Munteanu (RO)
Radu A. Munteanu (RO)
Anca I. Nicu (RO)
Maria Olt (RO)
Tudor Palade (RO)
Doina Pisla (RO)
Sever Pasca (RO)
Alessandro Pepino (IT)
Dan V. Rafiroiu (RO)

Mircea Leabu (RO)
Kang-Ping Lin (TW)
Angela Lungu (RO)
Eugen Lupu (RO)
Dan Mandru (RO)
Winfried Mayr (A)
Bogdan Micu (RO)
L. Dan Milici (RO)
Nicolae-Marius Roman (RO)
Corneliu Rusu (RO)
Adrian Samuila (RO)
Marina Topa (RO)
Doru Ursutiu (RO)
Radu C. Vlad (RO)
Simona Vlad (RO)

Local Organizing Committee

Ancuta-Coca Abrudan
Mihaela F. Baciut
Doina Baltaru
Radu V. Ciupa
Levente Czumbil
Rodica Holonec
Angela Lungu
Dan S. Mandru
Bogdan Micu
Calin Munteanu
Anca I. Nicu
Razvan Nicu
Maria Olt
Sever Pasca
Doina Pisla
Nicolae Marius Roman
Adrian Samuila
Marina Topa
Vasile Topa
Simona Vlad

Speakers at the Opening Ceremony

Prof. Ratko Magjarević, President of the International Federation for Medical and Biological Engineering (IFMBE)
Prof. Kang-Ping Lin, Vice-President of the International Federation for Medical and Biological Engineering (IFMBE)
Prof. Radu Vasile Ciupa, Honorary President of the Romanian National Society for Medical Engineering and Biological Technology, Romania
Dr. Christoph Baumann, Editorial Director, Springer Nature, The Netherlands
Prof. Mihaela Băciuţ, Vice-Rector "Iuliu Haţieganu" University of Medicine and Pharmacy, Cluj-Napoca, Romania
Prof. Doina Pîslă, Director of Council for University Doctoral Studies within the Technical University of Cluj-Napoca, Romania
Med.Col. Doina Baltaru, Commander of the "Dr. Constantin Papilian" Emergency Military Hospital Cluj-Napoca, Romania
Prof. Nicolae Marius Roman, President of the Romanian National Society for Medical Engineering and Biological Technology, Romania

Invited Speakers

Ratko Magjarević, President of the IFMBE; Department for Electronic Systems and Information Processing, Faculty of Electrical Engineering and Computing, University of Zagreb, Croatia
Biomedical engineering—building International networks for growth of health care and well-being
Kang-Ping Lin, Vice-president of the IFMBE; Department of Electrical Engineering, Chung-Yuan Christian University, Taiwan
Prospects of AI/ML Medical Devices
Helmut Hutten, Institute of Medical Engineering, University of Technology, Graz, Austria
How can Medical and Biological Engineering and Science (MBES) contribute to the Development of the Humanistic Society (Society 5.0)?
Alessandro Pepino, Department of Biomedical Engineering, University of Naples "Federico II", Italy
How the Post COVID-19 University will be more inclusive and more accessible for student with disabilities and learning disabilities and even more effective for all the students.
Lenka Lhotská, Czech Institute of Informatics, Robotics and Cybernetics, Czech Technical University in Prague, Czechia
Artificial Intelligence in Health and Social Care: Ethical and Legal Issues
Doina Pîslă, Research Center of Robots Simulation and Testing, Technical University of Cluj-Napoca, Romania
Innovations in Medical Robotics
Winfried Mayr, Center of Medical Physics and Biomedical Engineering, Medical University of Vienna, Austria
Spinal cord stimulation after spinal cord injury—encouraging accomplishments, but problematic public relations
Doina Baltaru, "Dr. Constantin Papilian" Emergency Military Hospital of Cluj-Napoca, Romania
Artificial Intelligence in Military Medicine Diagnostic and Caregiving Services. Review of the Literature
Tony Ward, Department of Electronic Engineering, University of York, England
Is Higher Education changing in a positive direction to meet the requirements industry has in graduates?
Timo Jämsä, Research Unit of Health Sciences and Technology, University of Oulu, Finland
Interpretation of physical activity data collected with accelerometers
Magdalena Stoeva, Department of Diagnostic Imaging, Medical University of Plovdiv, Bulgaria; Secretary General IOMP, Secretary General IUPESM
Educational strategies for capacity building in medical physics and technology
Piotr Ladyzynski, Nalecz Institute of Biocybernetics and Biomedical Engineering, Polish Academy of Sciences, Warsaw, Poland
The digital ecosystem facilitating treatment of people with diabetes

L. Dan Milici, Stefan cel Mare University of Suceava, Romania
Technical Creativity in a Knowledge-based Society
Lucio Tommaso De Paolis, Augmented and Virtual Reality Laboratory (AVR Lab), Department of Engineering for Innovation, University of Salento, Italy
Augmented Visualization in Medicine and Surgery
Dan L. Dumitraşcu, Member of the Romanian Academy of Medical Sciences; "Iuliu Haţieganu" University of Medicine and Pharmacy Cluj-Napoca and Cluj County Clinical Emergency Hospital, Romania
Breath tests for digestive diseases: an update
Cristian Dinu, Mihaela Băciuţ, Simion Bran, Florin Onişor, Sergiu Văcăraş, Gabriel Armencea, Ileana Mitre, Sebastian Stoia, Tiberiu Tamaş, Daiana Opriş, Horia Opriş, Avram Manea, Grigore Băciuţ
University of Medicine and Pharmacy, Maxillofacial Surgery Clinic, Cluj-Napoca, Romania
Patient specific therapeutic solutions in cranio-maxillofacial surgery
Horaţiu Rotaru, Department of Cranio-Maxillofacial Surgery, "Iuliu Hatieganu" University of Medicine and Pharmacy, Cluj-Napoca, Romania
Daniel Ostas, Nicolae Balc, Horea Chezan, Cosmin Cosma, Mircea Ciurea, Rares Roman, Dinu Cristian, Dragos Termure, Madalina Moldovan, Horatiu Stan, Stefan Florian, Mihaela Hedesiu
Personalized approaches in cranio-maxillofacial surgery
Thierry Marchal, Ansys, Inc. and Avicenna Alliance
The fundamental role of computer model and simulation (CM&S) and Artificial Intelligence (AI) to digitalize healthcare towards Participatory, Personalized, Preventive and Predictive (P4) medicine.
Irina David, INAS SA—Romania
The important role that software solutions play in the biomedical field. Innovation, precision, accuracy
Thomas Lauwers, Maastricht University Medical Centre, The Netherlands
Han Haitjema, Mechanical Engineering Department, KU Leuven, Belgium
Leonard Cezar Păstrăv, Smart Instrumentation Research Group, K.U. Leuven, Belgium
Kathleen Denis, Smart Instrumentation Research Group, K.U. Leuven, Belgium
Pyrocarbon implants used in hand and wrist surgery. Measurements of the in vivo wear
Thordur Helgason, Reykjavik University and Landspitali-University Hospital, Iceland; President of the Icelandic Society for Biomedical Engineering and Medical Physics (HTFI)
Patellar reflex test, transcutaneous spinal cord stimulation (tSCS), H-reflex analysis, and brain activity analysis in spinal cord injured and brain disorders
Doru Ursuţiu, Cornel Samoilă, Horia Modran
"Transilvania" University of Braşov, Romania
Virtual Instrumentation and Remote Technologies in Biomedical Engineering
Mihaela Ioana Baritz, "Transilvania" University from Braşov, Romania
Experimental optometry—a new paradigm on interdisciplinary procedural investigations correlated with biomechanics
Mircea Gelu Buta, "Babeş-Bolyai" University of Cluj-Napoca, Romania

Economic influences on medical services quality
Mircea Leabu, "Victor Babeş" National Institute of Pathology and Research Center for Applied Ethics, University of Bucharest, Bucharest, Romania
Value sensitive design, an ethical concern of medical engineering and biological technology

Chairmen

Radu Vasile Ciupa
Laura Grindei
Rodica Holonec
Eugen Lupu
Dan Mandru
Anca Iulia Nicu
Tudor Palade
Andra Păstrăv
Nicolae Marius Roman
Adrian Samuila
Marina Topa
Simona Vlad

Sponsors

INAS SA
Farmec SA
Tehno Industrial SA
Laitek Medical Software—Romania HQ
Medical Technologies Infinity SRL
Cefmur SA

Media Partners

TVR Cluj
Radio Romania Cluj

Contents

Biomedical Imaging and Image Processing

Hepatocellular Carcinoma Recognition from Ultrasound Images Through Convolutional Neural Networks and Their Combinations

Delia Mitrea[1](✉), Raluca Brehar[1], Sergiu Nedevschi[1], Mihai Socaciu[2,3], and Radu Badea[2,3]

[1] Faculty of Automation and Computer-Science, Technical University of Cluj-Napoca, Baritiu 26-28, Cluj-Napoca, Romania
{delia.mitrea,Raluca.Brehar,sergiu.nedevschi}@cs.utcluj.ro
[2] I. Hatieganu University of Medicine and Pharmacy, V. Babes 8, Cluj-Napoca, Romania
rbadea@umfcluj.ro
[3] Regional Institute of Gastroenterology and Hepatology, 19-21 Croitorilor Street, Cluj-Napoca, Romania

Abstract. The Hepatocellular Carcinoma (HCC) represents the most frequent malignant liver tumor. It evolves from cirrhosis after a restructuring phase, at the end of which dysplastic nodules result, which can transform into HCC. The needle biopsy is the golden standard for HCC diagnosis, being, however, invasive, dangerous, as it could lead to infections, respectively to the spread of the tumor through the body. Ultrasonography is a medical examination method which is non-invasive, inexpensive, thus safe, and repeatable. In our research, we developed computerized, non-invasive methods for computer aided and automatic diagnosis of HCC, based on ultrasound images. In the current work, we explored the role of representative Convolutional Neural Networks (CNN), respectively of their combinations, to achieve an optimal classification accuracy. The considered CNNs were fused at classifier level, by employing various combination schemes, based on relevant feature selection, respectively on Kernel Principal Component Analysis (KPCA). At the end, a classification accuracy above 95% resulted.

Keywords: Hepatocellular carcinoma (HCC) · Ultrasound images · Convolutional neural networks (CNN) · Classifier-level fusion · Classification performance

1 Introduction

HCC is the most frequent malignant liver tumor, being present in 70% of the liver cancer cases. HCC usually evolves from cirrhosis, after liver parenchyma restructuring, dysplastic nodules resulting, which can evolve into HCC. The golden standard for HCC diagnosis is the needle biopsy, which is invasive, dangerous, as it could generate infections, also the spread of the malignancy through the body [1].

S. Vlad and N. M. Roman (Eds.): MEDITECH 2022, IFMBE Proceedings 102, pp. 3–11, 2024.
https://doi.org/10.1007/978-3-031-51120-2_1

Ultrasonography is a medical examination technique which is non-invasive, inexpensive, undangerous, repeatable, suitable for patient disease monitoring. Other similar techniques, such as the endoscopy, the Computer Tomography (CT), the Magnetic Resonance Imaging (MRI) are irradiating and/or expensive. Within ultrasound images, advanced HCC usually appears hyperechogenic and heterogeneous, due to the interleave of various tissue types, such as active growth tissue, necrosis, fibrosis, and fatty cells [1].

Regarding the state of the art, formerly, the texture analysis methods were widely used in combination with conventional classifiers, to perform disease recognition within medical images [2–4]. More recently, CNNs were successfully employed, for performing the automatic recognition of affections such as fatty liver [5]; cirrhosis [6]; liver [7] and lung cancer [8]. The estimation of the cirrhosis severity grade within 2D shear wave elastography images, for patients affected by chronic, B-type hepatitis was performed in [3], using a CNN containing four convolution layers and a single fully connected layer, a performance larger than 85%, estimated through the Area under ROC (AuC), being obtained. Lately, more complex approaches appeared, involving the fusion of the deep learning features obtained from multiple deep learning architectures [9], respectively the fusion of classical and deep learning features [10]. In [9], the authors combined the deep learning feature maps provided by ResNet50 and DenseNet201, for brain tumor recognition. After feature selection, the relevant features were fused through a serial approach, then a Support Vector Machines (SVM) classifier was employed, yielding an 87.8% accuracy. However, no relevant approach exists to perform a systematic study regarding the role of the recent CNN architectures, respectively the fusion among CNNs, in the context of HCC recognition within ultrasound images.

We developed non-invasive, computerized techniques, for the automatic characterization and diagnosis of HCC within ultrasound images. We defined the textural imagistic model of HCC, by employing various types of textural features [11]. The relevant textural features were provided as input to powerful conventional classifiers and metaclassifiers, providing a classification accuracy above 80% [11]. The CNNs were experimented with the same purpose, considering both standard and original architectures, the latter ones leading to an accuracy above 90% [12].

In the current work, we experimented on a new dataset, various CNN architectures, well known for their performances. These CNNs were combined at classifier level: the feature vectors obtained at the end of the convolutional part of these networks were fused through various combination schemes. As the alternative class, we considered the cirrhotic parenchyma on which HCC evolved (PAR), being known that HCC visually resembles this type of tissue in many situations.

2 The Proposed Solution

2.1 Convolutional Neural Networks (CNN)

CNNs are deep, feed-forward, Artificial Neural Networks (ANN), employed for image recognition [13, 14]. Their structure was inspired from biology, the organization of the connections between the neurons resembling that of the animal visual cortex. Regarding the CNN structure, it combines multilayered perceptron elements that become activated when recognizing a specific input [14]. The main CNN components are the convolutional layers, which compress the input data into recognized patterns, for reducing the data size. CNNs also contain pooling layers, which aggregate the pixel values of the neighborhoods through specific functions, such as maximum or average, this procedure reducing the computational complexity at the superior levels of the CNN, inducing translation invariance. Rectified Linear Unit (ReLU) layers are also part of CNNs, enhancing the non-linear properties of the network. The last section of CNN usually consists of fully connected layers, a distribution over classes being obtained through the *softmax* function. Multiple CNN architectures were conceived during the last decade, for progressively increasing performances. LeNet and AlexNet were firstly designed, followed by SqueezeNet, which employed the "fire modules". GoogLeNet and InceptionV3 appeared thereafter, being based on inception modules, which replaced the sequential convolutions with simultaneous convolutions. For avoiding the gradient vanishing, ResNet and DenseNet implemented residual connections. More recently, EfficientNet was conceived, scaling all the dimensions in an efficient manner, for speed and accuracy improvement [13, 14].

2.2 Dimensionality Reduction Methods

The *feature selection methods* provide a reduced set of relevant features, for removing redundancy and improving class differentiation, by choosing only those features that maximize the selection criterion [15, 16]. Correlation based Feature Selection (CFS) belongs to the category of filters [15], aiming to identify that feature subset which maximizes the feature-class correlations, while minimizing the correlations between the features. CFS is employed with a search algorithm, for exhaustively reaching feature subsets [15].

The *feature extraction methods* perform the projection of the feature vector on a new space, of smaller dimensionality, where properties of interest are emphasized. Principal Component Analysis (PCA) highlights the main variation modes within the data [16], being represented by *the first d eigenvectors*, corresponding to *the highest d eigenvalues* of the covariance matrix. Kernel PCA (KPCA) is the generalization of PCA, assuming the transposition of PCA to a space of larger dimensionality, achieved by applying a kernel function K, which can be linear, Gaussian or polynomial. KPCA derives the eigenvectors of the kernel matrix, the transposition of the original data (X) onto a reduced dimensionality dataspace (Y) being achieved through formula (1), where α_k, $k \in \{1, .., d\}$ are the first d eigenvectors of the kernel matrix, α_k^j being the j-th element of α_k.

$$y_i = \left\{ \sum_{j=1}^{n} \alpha_1^j K(x_i, x_j), .., \sum_{j=1}^{n} \alpha_d^j K(x_i, x_j) \right\} \quad (1)$$

2.3 The Proposed Methodology

In this approach, we chose representative CNN architectures, assessed their classification performance on a new dataset and combined them at classifier level. We experimented the ResNet and InceptionV3 architectures, well-known for their performances. We also experimented EfficientNet, a recently designed architecture, having good scaling properties on large datasets. Each of these networks was separately evaluated on the dataset, classifier-level fusion being performed thereafter, according to Fig. 1. Thus, two CNNs were combined, by extracting the features at the end of the convolutional part of the network, before the fully connected layers and fusing them through the procedures:

(1) The concatenation of the feature vectors.
(2) Feature selection through CFS, on each feature vector, followed by concatenation (*CFS + Concat*).
(3) The concatenation of the two vectors followed by feature selection (*Concat + CFS*).
(4) The application of KPCA on each vector, followed by concatenation (*KPCA + Concat*).
(5) The concatenation of the two vectors followed by KPCA (*Concat + KPCA*).

For KPCA, the Gaussian kernel was employed, which provided the best results.

The combined feature vector was provided as input to a conventional classifier. The following classification techniques, well-known for their performance, were considered: SVM, Random Forest (RF) and AdaBoost with the C4.5 method of Decision Trees [17].

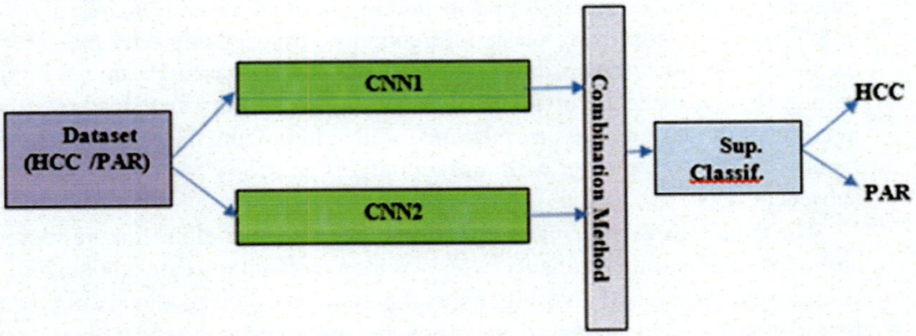

Fig. 1. Classifier-level fusion of two CNNs.

The classification performance was assessed through the recognition rate (accuracy), sensitivity (True Positive Rate), specificity (True Negative Rate) and AuC [17]. The dependencies between the features provided by different CNNs were also studied, employing the Pearson correlation [17].

3 Experiments and Discussions

3.1 The Dataset and Experimental Settings

The dataset contained B-mode ultrasound images of the liver affected by advanced HCC, belonging to 96 patients, biopsied for diagnostic confirmation. The images were acquired by experienced radiologists, at the 3rd Medical Clinic in Cluj-Napoca, with a Logiq9 (GE, USA) ultrasound machine, under the same settings: Frequency 6.0 MHz, gain 58, depth 16 cm, Dynamic Range (DR) 69. For each patient, at least three images were considered, corresponding to various transducer orientations. Inside each image, HCC was manually delimited through a polygon, using the VIA software [18]. Then, rectangular regions of interest(patches), corresponding to the HCC and PAR classes, having 56 × 56 pixels in size, were extracted, using our own algorithm: if the patch was inside the polygon, having an intersection of at most 10% with the region outside the polygon, was considered HCC, otherwise it was considered PAR. Thus, 10000 patches/class resulted, 75% being integrated in the training set, 8% in the validation set, 17% representing the test set.

CNNs were employed in Matlab_R2021b, using the Deep Learning Toolbox [19], ResNet101, InceptionV3 and EfficientNet_b0 being exploited. The Stochastic Gradient Descent (SGD) learning strategy was employed, with a batch size of 30, a learning rate of 0.0001, a momentum of 0.9, and 100 training epochs. The feature selection methods were implemented in Weka 3.8.6 [20], by using the CfsSubsetEval technique with BestFirst search. The conventional supervised classifiers were also implemented in Weka 3.8.6: the Sequential Minimal Optimization (SMO) algorithm for SVM was applied with polynomial kernel of third degree, AdaBoostM1, standing for the AdaBoost metaclassifier, was employed with 100 iterations, the J48 technique, the Weka equivalent of the C4.5 method for decision trees was adopted as well, RandomForest with 100 iterations being also considered. KPCA was implemented in Matlab_R2021b using a specific library [21]. The correlations between the CNN features were computed in Matlab_R2021b, using the *corrcoef* function. These experiments were conducted on a computer with Intel(R) Xeon(R) Gold 6230 CPU, at 2.10 GHz, 128 GB of RAM and NVidia RTX graphical card (CloudUT).

3.2 CNN Assessment

In Table 1, the classification performance parameters for the considered CNNs were depicted. The highest performance was achieved for InceptionV3: accuracy 80.39%, sensitivity 81.36%, specificity 79%, AUC 86%.

Table 1. The classification performance of the CNN architectures

CNN	Accuracy (%)	Sens. (%)	Spec. (%)	AUC (%)
ResNet101	78.4	80.39	75.5	78.75
InceptionV3	**80.39**	**81.63**	**79**	**86**
EfficientNet_b0	74.32	75.22	73.22	74.33

3.3 Assessment of the CNN Combinations

Regarding the classifier level fusion, CNN features were firstly extracted: 2048 features were obtained from ResNet101, respectively InceptionV3, at the output of the *pool5*, respectively *avg_pool* layers, while for EfficientNet_b0, 1280 features were extracted at the end of *GlobAvgPool*. Concerning the classifier level fusion between ResNet101 and InceptionV3, the best accuracy, 97.79%, the highest specificity, 98.9% and the highest AUC, 97.8, resulted for *KPCA + Concat*, for AdaBoost, while the best sensitivity, 97.9%, resulted for the same scheme, for the RF classifier. Regarding the combination between ResNet101 and EfficientNet_b0, the best accuracy, 97.165% the best sensitivity, 97.9%, the best specificity, 97.9% and the best AUC, 97.6%, resulted for *KPCA + Concat*, still for the RF classifier. As for the fusion between EfficientNet_b0 and InceptionV3, the highest accuracy, 97.165%, the highest sensitivity, 97.6%, the best specificity, 97.6% and the best AUC, 97.65%, were obtained for *KPCA + Concat*, in the case of AdaBoost. Within Table 2, the arithmetic mean of the performance parameters is depicted, for each CNN combination, for each fusion method. For *ResNet101 + InceptionV3*, the best average accuracy, 93.46% and the best average specificity, 94.50%, resulted for *KPCA + Concat*, while the best average sensitivity, 93.5% and the best average AUC, 95.1%, resulted for *FS + Concat*. For the fusion between ResNet101 and EfficientNet_b0, the highest average accuracy, 90.14% and the best average specificity, 97.33%, resulted for *KPCA + Concat*, while the best average sensitivity, 87.9% and the highest mean AUC, 88.78%, resulted for *FS + Concat*. For the fusion between EfficientNet_b0 and InceptionV3, the highest average accuracy, 95.05%, the best average sensitivity, 94.17%, the best average specificity, 95,67% and the best mean AUC, 93.95%, resulted for *KPCA + Concat*.

Table 2. The classification performance for CNN combinations at classifier level

Combination	Fusion method	Accuracy	Sens.	Spec.	AUC
ResNet101 + InceptionV3	Concat	83.52	86.5	80.57	88.23
	FS + Concat	90.66	**93.5**	87.93	**95.1**
	Concat + FS	86.09	90.2	82	90.93
	KPCA + Concat	**93.46**	92.50	**94.50**	93.48
	Concat + KPCA	86.61	87.77	85.47	91.63
ResNet101 + EfficientNet_b0	Concat	81.33	87.33	75.37	86.27
	FS + Concat	83.68	**87.90**	79.37	**88.87**
	Concat + FS	83.05	87.80	78.30	85.60
	KPCA + Concat	**90.14**	82.47	**98.33**	88.53
	Concat + KPCA	75.24	85.17	64.93	78.23
EfficientNet_b0 + InceptionV3	Concat	84.05	88.30	79.30	86.63
	FS + Concat	83.39	87.53	79.13	88.43
	Concat + FS	81.30	84.40	77.90	84.83
	KPCA + Concat	**95.05**	**94.17**	**95.67**	**93.95**
	Concat + KPCA	89.69	92.70	86.80	92.28

3.4 Discussions

As we notice from the results above, the best classification performance usually resulted for the *CFS* + *Concat*, respectively *KPCA* + *Concat* fusion schemes, when employing the RF, respectively the AdaBoost metaclassifiers. For providing a more synthetical view upon these results, in Fig. 2, a graphical representation of the average accuracy, for each fusion scheme, for each CNN combination, is provided. Above, the arithmetic mean of the classification accuracies, for each fusion scheme, considering all the CNN combinations, is depicted: the best performance was achieved for *KPCA* + *Concat*, the overall average accuracy being 92.18%, followed by the *FS* + *Concat*, the overall average accuracy being 85.91%. We must observe that performing first feature selection or KPCA, on each CNN feature vector, separately, followed by concatenation, led to better results than the procedures achieving first concatenation, then FS or KPCA. We also notice that the simple concatenation of the CNN features was overpassed by all the other fusion schemes. Regarding the CNN combinations, the best results were provided by *Resnet101* + *InceptionV3*, followed by *InceptionV3* + *EfficientNet_b0*, respectively by *ResNet101* + *EfficientNet_b0*. The currently achieved classification performance overpassed the results formerly obtained in the domain, based on both advanced texture analysis [11], respectively deep learning [10, 12].

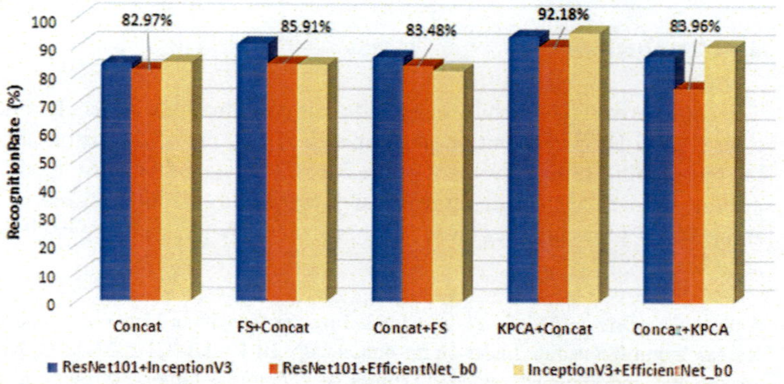

Fig. 2. Comparison of the average classification accuracies for each fusion scheme, for every CNN combination

In Fig. 3 the correlations between the ResNet101 and InceptionV3 features are depicted, the first 2048 features corresponding to ResNet101 and the next 2048 features corresponding to InceptionV3. The correlations are increased among the same type of features, the correlations between features extracted from different CNNs being not that high, having maximum values around 0.5.

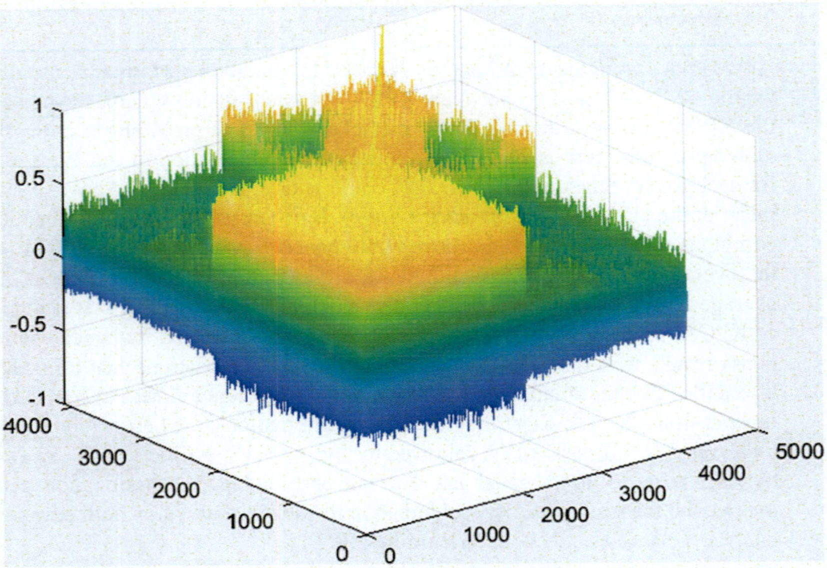

Fig. 3. The correlations between the CNN features extracted from InceptionV3 and ResNet101

4 Conclusions

The considered CNN architectures and their combinations at the classifier level led to a very good HCC recognition performance. Thus, the CNN fusion at classifier level led to a significant improvement of the classification performance, finally providing an accuracy above 95%. In our future research, we aim to also employ Canonical Correlation Analysis [22] for classifier level fusion, respectively to assess the decision level fusion schemes.

Acknowledgement. This work was funded by the Romanian National Authority of Scientific Research and Innovation under Grant number PN-III-P1-1.1-TE-2021-1293, Nr. TE 156/2022, "Automatic and computer aided diagnosis of abdominal tumors, through advanced machine learning, within various types of medical images (ACADTUM)".

Conflicts of Interest The authors declare they have no conflict of interest.

References

1. American Liver Foundation (2022). https://liverfoundation.org/for-patients/about-the-liver/diseases-ofthe-liver/liver-cancer/
2. Yoshida, H., Casalino, D.: Wavelet packet-based texture analysis for differentiation between benign and malignant liver tumors in ultrasound images. Phys. Med. Biol. **48**, 3735–3753 (2003)

3. Sujana, H., Swarnamani, S.: Application of artificial neural networks for the classification of liver lesions by texture parameters. Ultrasound Med. Biol. **22**, 1177–1181 (1996)
4. Duda, D., et al.: Computer aided diagnosis of liver tumors based on multi-image texture analysis of contrast-enhanced CT. Stud. Log. Gramm. Rhetor. **35**, 49–70 (2013)
5. Byra, M., Styczynski, G.: Transfer learning with deep convolutional neural networks for liver steatosis assessment in ultrasound images. Int. J. Comput. Assist. Radiol. Surg. **13**, 1895–1900 (2018)
6. Liu, X., et al.: Learning to diagnose cirrhosis with liver capsule guided ultrasound image classification. Sensors **17**(1), 1–11 (2017)
7. Vivanti, R., Epbrat, A.: Automatic liver tumor segmentation in follow-up CT studies using convolutional neural networks. In: International Workshop on Patch-Based Techniques in Medical Imaging (2015)
8. Li, W., Cao, P.: Pulmonary nodule classification with deep convolutional neural networks on computed tomography images. Comput. Math. Methods Med. (2016). https://pubmed.ncbi.nlm.nih.gov/28070212/
9. Aziz, A., et al.: An ensemble of optimal deep learning features for brain tumor classification. Comput. Mater. Continua **69**(2), 2653–2670 (2021)
10. Paul, R., et al.: Predicting malignant nodules by fusing deep features with classical radiomics features. J. Med. Imaging 5(1), 011021-1–011021-11 (2018)
11. Mitrea, D., et al.: Automatic recognition of the hepatocellular carcinoma from ultrasound images using complex textural microstructure co-occurrence matrices (CTMCM). In: Proceedings of 7th International Conference on Pattern Recognition Applications and Methods (ICPRAM), Scitepress, pp. 178–189 (2018)
12. Brehar, R., Mitrea, D., et al.: Comparison of deep-learning and conventional machine-learning methods for the automatic recognition of the hepatocellular carcinoma areas from ultrasound images. Sensors **20**, 1–22 (2020)
13. Mishkin, D., et al.: Systematic evaluation of CNN advances on the ImageNet, CoRR (2016)
14. Liu, S., et al.: Deep learning in medical ultrasound analysis: a review. Engineering **5**, 261–275 (2019)
15. Hall, M., et al.: The WEKA data mining software: an update. SIGKDD Explor. **11**, 10–18 (2009)
16. Van der Maaten, L., et al.: Dimensionality Reduction: A Comparative Review (2009). https://lvdmaaten.github.io/publications/papers/TR_Dimensionality_Reduction_Review_2009.pdf
17. Meyer-Base, A.: Pattern Recognition for Medical Imaging. Elsevier, Amsterdam (2009)
18. Dutta, A., et al.: VGG Image Annotator (VIA) (2022). http://www.robots.ox.ac.uk/~vgg/software/via/
19. Deep Learning Toolbox for Matlab (2022). https://it.mathworks.com/help/deeplearning/index.html?s_tid=CRUX_lftnav
20. Weka 3 (2022). http://www.cs.waikato.ac.nz/ml/weka/
21. Kitayama, M.: Matlab-Kernel-PCA Toolbox (2017). https://it.mathworks.com/matlabcentral/fileexchange/71647-matlab-kernel-pca
22. Gao, L., et al.: Discriminative multiple canonical correlation analysis for information fusion. IEEE Trans. Image Process. **27**(4), 1951–1965 (2018)

Detecting Polyps in Endoscopic Images with U-Net Based Architectures - A Preliminary Evaluation

Radu Razvan Slavescu[1](✉), Zsófia Fodor[1], and Kinga Cristina Slavescu[2]

[1] Technical University of Cluj-Napoca, Cluj-Napoca, Romania
Radu.Razvan.Slavescu@cs.utcluj.ro, Zsofia.Fodor@campus.utcluj.ro
[2] Iuliu Hatieganu University of Medicine and Pharmacy, Cluj-Napoca, Romania
Cristina.Slavescu@umflcuj.ro

Abstract. This paper aims to explore some proposed solutions for solving the problem of automatic polyp detection in endoscopic images. These solutions rely on four state of the art Convolutional Neural Networks, designed for the medical image segmentation. The four architectures are the U-Net, U-Net++, ResUNet and ResUNet++, which were tuned by changing the values of different hyperparameters with the aim of achieving the best results. Binary image classification was used to make classifications at pixel level, having two classes: polyp and background. The achieved results were compared using some predefined metrics such as Precision, Recall and mean Intersection over Union. The best results were achieved by the ResUnet architecture, with performances close to those of alternative approaches of the problem.

Keywords: Endoscopy · Medical image segmentation · Binary image classification · U-Net · U-Net++ · ResUnet · ResUnet++ · Convolution neural networks

1 Introduction

According to recent studies [1, 2] colorectal cancer is the third deadliest cancer following prostate and lung cancer for the male gender and breast and lung cancer for females. However, it is one of the most preventable form of cancer if found and diagnosed in an early stage. Colorectal cancer begins in the form a polyp which is a benign tissues growth on the lumen of the colon. Using colonoscopy as a screening method, these polyps can be identified. Hence, we need to develop automated polyp detection methods. These must be able to identify polyps with a high rate of precision and accuracy.

Our main goal was to identify and localize the polyps that are small of size, because they have a higher probability of being removed. They are also likely to be missed by the doctor. The predictions were made using some existing image segmentation models.

In this paper we present our findings regarding the use of some of the existing Convolutional Neural Networks (CNN) architectures for the aforementioned task. We aimed to choose and tune them in order to achieve results comparable to the existing

S. Vlad and N. M. Roman (Eds.): MEDITECH 2022, IFMBE Proceedings 102, pp. 12–20, 2024.
https://doi.org/10.1007/978-3-031-51120-2_2

ones and to analyze the pros and cons brought by each of these architectures. The four architectures that were targeted are the U-Net, U-Net++, ResUNet and ResUNet++, each of which brings an enhancement to the first one, the U-Net architecture. After tuning each architecture, the achieved results are discussed.

The paper is structured in the following way: Sect. 2 presents others studied architectures that try to tackle the same problem, Sect. 3 shows with little details the architectures that were chosen for the experiment. In Sect. 4 we describe the experiment setup. Section 5 will show the results achieved and Sect. 6 draws some conclusions and sketches ideas for future improvements.

2 Related Work

Several architectures have been tried on the problem of medical image segmentation of endoscopic images. This section briefly presents some architectures that have achieved good results in this respect.

One such system is DoubleU-Net [3], which consists of two consecutive U-net like architectures. For the first U-Net architecture, a pretrained VGG-19 network was chosen for the encoder part. This first network will provide a binary mask for the input, which then will be fed to the second network after being multiplied with the input. For their experiments, binary cross-entropy was used as the loss function and NAdam optimizer was used. The training was done on 300 epochs with a learning rate equal to 1e-5. Having these parameter values, the achieved results were of a 95% Precision, 86% Recall and 86% mean Intersection over Union (mIoU), outperforming some already existing results presented in [3].

Another system that needs to be mentioned is the MultiResUnet architecture [4], which provides the possibility of analyzing various sized objects due to the fact that it uses repeated lightweight convolutional operations, by gradually increasing its size, instead of one larger one. Another improvement brought by the MultiResUnet is the incorporation of convolutional layers along the shortcut connections to reduce possible semantic gaps. For the training of the model the *binary cross-entropy* loss function was used, together with the *Adam optimizer* with a number of 150 epochs. The performance was measured by analyzing the mIoU value reached by the model, which was of 78%.

3 Explored Solutions

This article explores four known architectures and compares their performances on the problem at hand. In the first phase the U-Net [5] architecture was chosen, which is based on a simple encoder-decoder architecture, presented in Fig. 1. The encoder path has a typical Convolutional Neural Network (CNN) architecture, consisting of repeated *convolution applications*, each followed by a *rectified linear unit* (ReLU) and a *max-pooling* operation that reduces the image size. The decoder or expanding path is made up of an *up sampling* followed by a convolution that has as result halving the feature channels number, a concatenation with the cropped feature from the encoder path and two convolutions followed by a ReLU activation.

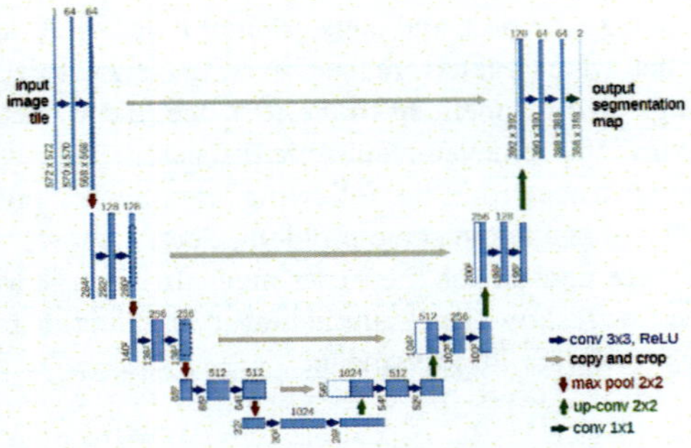

Fig. 1. U-Net architecture [5]

In the second phase of our experiment, the U-Net++ [6] architecture was explored. This aims to improve the U-Net architecture by bringing a *denser skip connection* as an addition, in order to reduce the semantic gap between the subnetworks.

The third phase consisted of further search for other architectures, time in which we came across the ResUNet [7], which also relies on the previously presented U-Net architecture, but brings the power of residual blocks as an addition to the basic U-Net one. The simple unit from the U-Net architecture were replaced by residual units, which aim to solve the problem of degradation. As Fig. 2 shows, what these residual unit bring in addition to the plain unit is *the batch normalization* and the *identity mapping*, to further ensure that relevant data will not be lost.

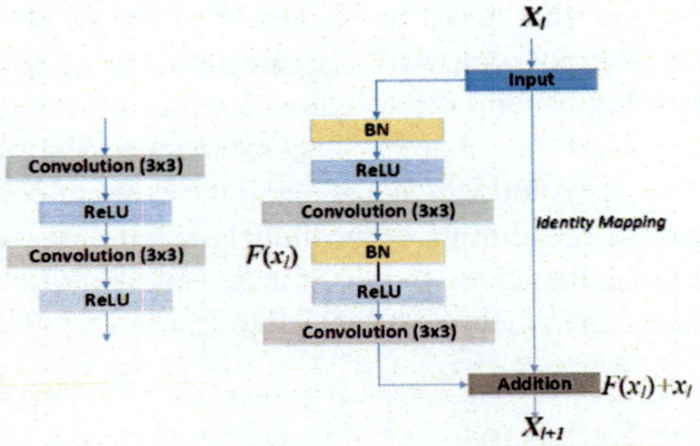

Fig. 2. Traditional plain unit versus residual unit [7]

In the last phase, we chose to experiment with the ResUNet++ architecture, which is a further improvement of the previously presented ResUNet architecture, by introducing the residual blocks in order to create a deeper network. Using residual blocks reduces computational costs, minimizes the information loss and the training phase will be much shorter.

The experiments were performed using the TensorFlow library and consisted of gradually increasing the number of epochs from 20 to 200 epochs. After finding a suitable number of epochs, the other hyperparameters were also tuned in hopes of obtaining better results. All experiments were run on the DGX virtual machine.

4 Experimental Setup

The dataset used was the Kvasir-SEG [9] dataset, which is a publicly available dataset, containing 1000 images and their corresponding binary masks. Being an imbalanced set, we managed to find images that did not contain any polyps and created the binary mask for each of them, thus managing to balance the dataset. Figure 3 shows the polyp distribution among the images from the dataset. This set of images was further split up into training set, testing set, and validation set with a ratio of 80%–10%–10%.

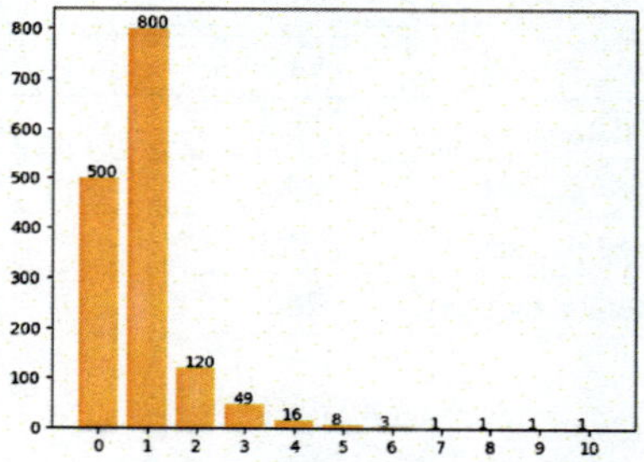

Fig. 3. Distribution of polyps among the images in the Kvasir-SEG dataset

Another possible dataset would have been the CVC-ClinicDB, which is also a widely used dataset, but having a smaller number of images, we chose to stick with the Kvasir-SEG dataset.

For the setup of the experiments the loss function used by us was the binary cross-entropy, which was the most suitable one, considering our task, with the Adam optimizer. The experiments consisted of tuning further hyperparameters besides the number of epochs to achieve greater results.

The performance metrics used to evaluate our models were Precision, Recall and mIoU values.

5 Results and Discussion

Our experimenting consisted of combining different values of the hyperparameters such as the number of epochs mentioned above, which was set to 150/200 for all the models. The batch size, which specifies the number of samples used by the model at each training phase was firstly set to 8, then increased to 16, which actually improved the performance of our models. Another hyperparameter which (not surprisingly) proved important was the learning rate, which specifies how quickly the model adapts to the specific problem. The value of the learning rate varied between 1e-4 and 1e-5, but the *ReduceLROnPlateau* was also activated during the training phase, which reduces the learning rate when a specific metric has stopped improving.

After several rounds of experiments, we managed to achieve promising results in terms of the metrics used for the evaluation of these models. Table 1 presents the highest scores achieved by each of our models. We also performed several rounds of dataset augmentation (rotations, flips and noise adding) in order to have a bigger set of training data.

Table 1. Best results achieved throughout the experiments

Architecture	Precision (%)	Recall (%)	mIoU (%)
U-Net	75.8	58	42.4
U-Net++	79.5	69.7	46
ResUNet	73.7	64.2	42.7
ResUNet++	74.6	51.4	43.1
U-Net, augmented dataset	78.3	61.3	45
U-Net++, augmented dataset	80.8	67	43.4
ResUNet, augmented dataset	77.5	75.7	43.5
ResUNet++, augmented dataset	76.8	59.4	45

The results presented in Table 1 show that, due to the augmentation of the dataset, the performance has increased with a few percentages in case of all the models. The Precision value of the ResUNet architecture increased from 73.7 to 77.5%. For the Recall value, this difference was even more significant, from 64.2 to 75.7%.

Taking these improvements into consideration, we went on to further augment our dataset, in hopes of achieving better results. In case of the augmentation it is important to take into account to create real-life scenarios, that can really appear in during an endoscopic evaluation.

The precision-recall curve shows the relation between the Precision and Recall values, which are of high interest for us. We aim to reach the point (1, 1), which would mean a Precision and a Recall of 100%, representing a 'perfect' prediction model. We aim to have an Area Under the Curve (AUC) equal to 1, meaning that the curve does not slice the area (or to get as close as we can). We analyzed our precision-recall graphs, taking into account several values for a threshold raging between 0.3 and 0.6. Figure 4 shows some Precision-Recall curve examples, where we can see a performance that gets close to the (1, 1) value, while the other one is slightly worse, showing just an average performance.

Table 2 shows the values achieved for each threshold as mentioned above. We can see that as the threshold increases the Precision also increases, but the Recall value tends to decrease in case of some models. By increasing the threshold, we got a Precision as high as 89.5% in case of the ResUNet architecture and a Recall value of 86.9% for the same threshold value.

Compared to the results achieved by other researchers, the results we obtained so far stand really close to the already existing ones with similar architectures. Table 3

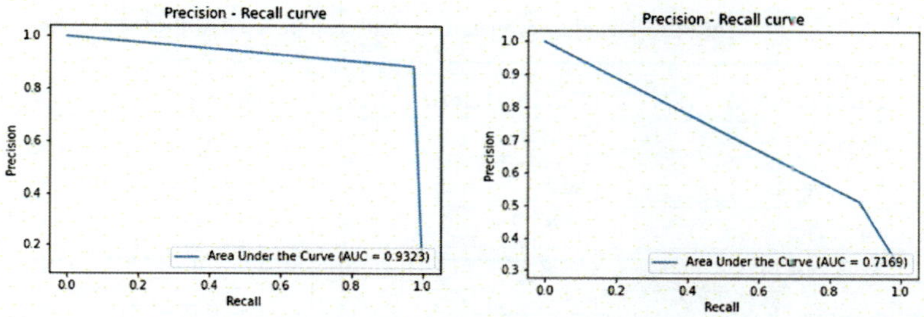

Fig. 4. Examples of precision-recall curves

Table 2. Average scores achieved throughout the test set

Model	Threshold	Average precision (%)	Average recall (%)
U-Net	0.3	67.1	77.7
	0.4	70.1	71.1
	0.5	73.1	63.8
	0.6	76.4	56.4
U-Net++	0.3	63.4	86.6
	0.4	67.6	83.8
	0.5	71.4	80.8
	0.6	74.9	77.3
ResUNet	0.3	85.5	84
	0.4	87.5	89
	0.5	89.1	87.6
	0.6	**89.5**	**86.9**
ResUNet++	0.3	66.5	78.4
	0.4	72.3	71.3
	0.5	76.8	64.5
	0.6	78.9	56.8

compares the results achieved by the authors of the articles presented in Sects. 2 and 3. As we can see the best results were achieved by the Double U-Net architecture having a Precision value of 95% and a Recall value of 84%. In our experiments the U-Net++ performed the best in terms of Precision, achieving a value of 80%, but in terms of Recall, which is of higher interest for us, since we aim to reduce the number of false negatives, the ResUNet architecture performed better, getting a value of 75.7%.

Figure 5 shows the predicted binary masks by each model on some relevant images from the dataset. We tried to select images that contained bigger objects, smaller ones or have lighting disturbances, to see how well our models perform in all these cases.

Table 3. Results compared to results achieved by other researchers

Architecture	Precision (%)	Recall (%)	mIoU
U-Net	78.3	61.3	45
U-Net++	80.8	67	43.4
ResUNet	77.5	75.7	43.5
ResUNet++	76.8	59.4	45
U-Net++ [6]	–	–	92
ResUnet [7]	72	50	43
ResUnet++ [8]	87	70	79
Double-UNet	95.9	84.5	86.1
MultiResUNet	–	–	82.05

Analyzing the results in Fig. 5, it is clearly visible that the ResUNet architecture gives the best results, being the one model that is not so disturbed by lighting conditions.

A characteristic that is present is almost all architectures is the identification of the shiny parts from the images as being polyps. This is the problem we will focus on in the future, because these conditions can arise frequently during the endoscopic procedure since the gastrointestinal tract contains mucus.

Another lesson we learned from our preliminary experiments is that for the task of identifying small polyps, the ResUNet architecture is the most promising one, but there is much room for improvement in this direction.

6 Conclusions and Future Work

We aimed to address the problem of detecting polyps in endoscopic images. To this end, we conducted experiments with four already known network architectures, specifically designed for medical image segmentation, to evaluate how they work and where they perform better: U-Net, U-Net++, ResUNet and ResUNet++. Each of them relied on the basic U-Net architecture, having an encoding and a decoding path connected through skip connections.

By fine tuning the values of different hyperparameters, we managed to achieve promising results that come close to the ones already existing for the same or similar architectures. The best results were achieved by the ResUnet architecture, which combines the strong points of the U-Net architecture with the benefits brought by the Residual blocks, thus managing to achieve a Recall score of 75% and a Precision score of 77%. When integrating our models into a system, we have seen that the predictions were made in a few milliseconds, when run on a GPU enabled computer.

We have also found that the identification of smaller polyps tends to be a challenging, along with the lightning conditions which seem to disturb our models.

For future work we would need to further enlarge our dataset, possibly with images that have lighting disturbance, so that our models could learn from these and tune the

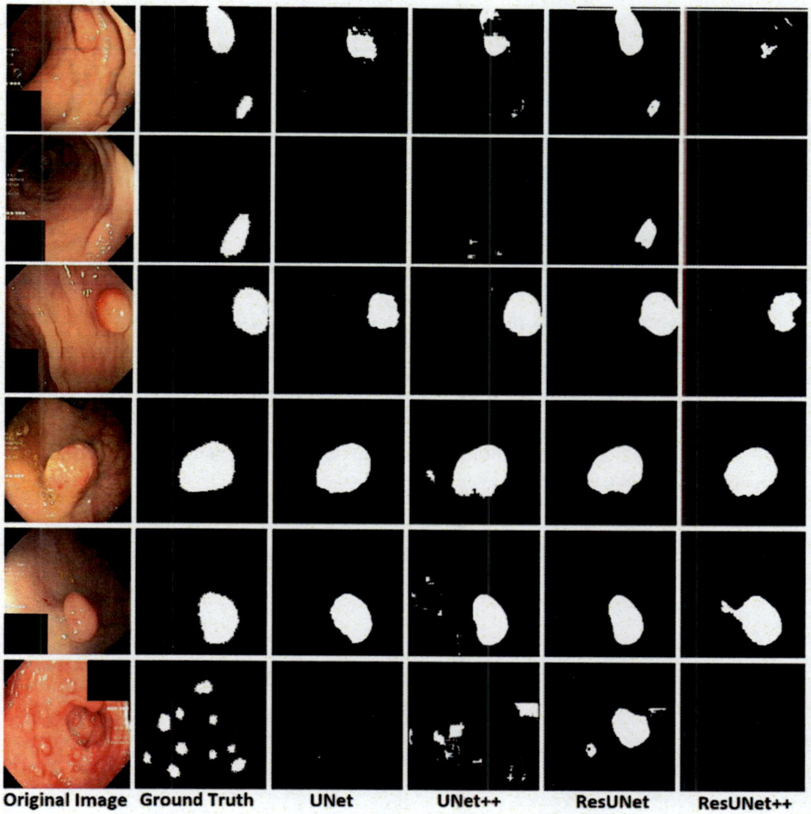

Fig. 5. Predicted binary masks by each model

architectures to be able to identify the differences between an object and a shiny particle of the image.

Acknowledgments. This work was supported by the Technical University of Cluj-Napoca, Romania. The first author was supported in part by UEFISCDI Romania, grant PN-III-P2-2.1-PED2021-2709.

Conflict of Interest The authors declare they have no conflict of interest.

References

1. Huck, M.B., Bohl, J.L.: Colonic polyps: diagnosis and surveillance. Clin. Colon. Rectal. Surg. **29**(04), 296–305 (2016)
2. Marley, A.R., Nan, H.: Epidemiology of colorectal cancer. Int. J. Mol. Epidemiol. Genet. **7**(3), 105 (2016)

3. Jha, D., Riegler, M.A., Johansen, D., Halvorsen, P., Johansen, H.D.: Doubleunet: a deep convolutional neural network for medical image segmentation. In: 2020 IEEE 33rd International Symposium on Computer-Based Medical Systems (CBMS), pp. 558–564. IEEE
4. Ibtehaz, N., Rahman, M.S.: MultiResUnet: rethinking the u-net architecture for multimodal biomedical image segmentation. CoRR, vol. abs/1902.04049 (2019)
5. Ronneberger, O., Fischer, P., Brox, T.: U-net: convolutional networks for biomedical image segmentation. CoRR, vol. abs/1505.04597 (2015)
6. Zhou, Z., Siddiquee, M.M.R., Tajbakhsh, N., Liang, J.: Unet++: a nested u-net architecture for medical image segmentation (2018)
7. Zhang, Z., Liu, Q., Wang, Y.: Road extraction by deep residual u-net. CoRR, vol. abs/1711.10684 (2017)
8. Jha, D., Smedsrud, P.H., Riegler, M.A., Johansen, D., de Lange, T., Halvorsen, P., Johansen, H.D.: ResUNet++: an advanced architecture for medical image segmentation (2019)
9. Pogorelov, K., Randel, K.R., Griwodz, C., Eskeland, S.L., de Lange, T., Johansen, D., Spampinato, C., Dang-Nguyen, D.-T., Lux, M., Schmidt, P.T., Riegler, M., Halvorsen, P.: Kvasir: a multi-class image dataset for computer aided gastrointestinal disease detection. In: Proceedings of the 8th ACM on Multimedia Systems Conference, ser. MMSys'17, pp. 164–169. ACM, New York, NY (2017)

U-net Network Optimization for 3D Reconstruction in Robotic SILS Pre-planning Phase

Doina Pisla[1], Iulia Andras[2], Gabriela Rus[1], Claudia Moldovan[3], Nicolae Crisan[2], Tiberiu Antal[1], Ionut Ulinici[1], and Calin Vaida[1](✉)

[1] CESTER, Technical University of Cluj-Napoca, Cluj-Napoca, Romania
{doina.pisla,Gabriela.Rus,Calin.Vaida}@mep.utcluj.ro,
ionut.ulinici@omt.utlcuj.ro

[2] Iuliu Hatieganu University of Medicine and Pharmacy, Cluj-Napoca, Romania
{Iulia.Andras,Nicolae.Crisan}@umfcluj.ro

[3] Emergency Clinical County Hospital of Cluj-Napoca, Cluj-Napoca, Romania

Abstract. Artificial intelligence has become a powerful and increasingly reliable tool, being implemented in various domains. However, a very difficult task is to correctly identify the information use to train the AI for a specific task. The aim is to offer an in-depth analysis on the semantic segmentation process for kidneys CT data using Convolutional Neural Network, to help surgeons in the pre-planning phase for robotic assisted SILS (Single Incision Laparoscopic Surgery). Different hypermeters and hardware configurations for U-net neural network were used to provide a high-quality solution for CT data segmentation.

Keywords: AI · Machine learning · Deep learning · Semantic segmentation · 3D reconstruction · U-net · Robotic-assisted SILS

1 Introduction

The ability to learn from their own experiences is the most significant feature of Machine Learning algorithms.

In medicine artificial intelligence (AI) is used in: image computing, image interpretation, computer assisted evolution of chest pathology, detection for cardiovascular diseases, breast cancer screening, neurological diseases, drug delivery, clinical trials and assistive medical robotics [1].

Semantic segmentation is a technique for better comprehending images by providing a name to each pixel in the image, allowing organs or anomalies such as tumors or cysts to be highlighted.

Although SILS has been known for a long time, the last two decades have brought significant improvements to these procedures, with the introduction of SILS robotic devices in the operating room. In this field, a series of innovative robots were developed, as can be seen in [2] and [3]. SILS has a few limitations that may hinder the surgeon's ability to perform surgery procedures. Because the instruments are introduced through

S. Vlad and N. M. Roman (Eds.): MEDITECH 2022, IFMBE Proceedings 102, pp. 21–29, 2024.
https://doi.org/10.1007/978-3-031-51120-2_3

a single incision (2.5 cm), the operating field is reduced, limiting surgeon access and the movement of the endoscopic camera, resulting in a poor environment perception. Tumors, blood vessels, and access trajectories are difficult to see in this condition, which could jeopardize the procedure's accuracy and safety [4].

An effective method to manage these constraints is given by the preoperative pre-planning process, in which the clinician has the possibility to plan very detailed the surgery procedure. The preplanning system consists of the visualization and analysis of CT or MRi images to identify regions of interest, the best approach for that operation, and the modeling phase, which was introduced in the last decade and allows the doctor to see the tumor, organs, or blood vessels connected to the target organ in 3D format.

In this way the surgeon has a superior view of the operating field being capable to perform the procedure in better conditions especially if in pre-planning phase is involved an AR (Augmented Reality) system [5].

The recent advancement of AI algorithms led to development of Convolutional Neural Network (CNN).

CNN, also known as Deep Neural Network (DNN), is a multi-layered ANN. It is utilized for image classification, computer vision, and semantic segmentation being able to handle large amount of data. This network typically consists of three layers: a convolutional layer, a pooling layer, and a fully connected layer [6, 7].

In [8] the authors introduced a bilinear squeezing reasoning network for surgical image segmentation, which improved the semantic segmentation process by providing better local features for objects. This study aims to provide a better surgical scene understanding through the semantic segmentation process for surgical robot control and computer-assisted surgery. To increase the precision of robotic surgery, Choi J. and colleagues deployed the U-net and YOLACT networks to conduct the semantic segmentation procedure for anatomical regions. The study's purpose was to gain a better understanding of how different CNNNs can be used to guide the surgeon during a robotic-assisted surgery [9].

As previously illustrated interest in this issue is growing as new approaches are introduced constantly. In this context, finding an adequate optimization for a specific type of segmentation in a short amount of time may be difficult, so this paper aims to synthetize the information for semantic segmentation of CT dataset for kidneys, to highlight the process by which image segmentation is performed and used in the SILS using for validation a dataset of kidneys images.

Following the Introduction section, the paper is structured as follows: Sect. 2 presents a brief description of how AI can be introduced into robotic assisted surgery and Sect. 3 illustrates methodology of semantic segmentation procedure for CT data (tissue characterization). Section 4 shows the analysis of different configuration of U-net neural network followed by the Sect. 5 which contains several conclusions regarding the developed work.

2 AI Module for the Challenge SILS Robotic System

The introduction of the AI module in the robot assisted SILS procedure is widely discussed. The growing number of different artificial intelligence agents has led to the emergence of innovative ideas to improve the environment and increase patient safety during medical procedure [10].

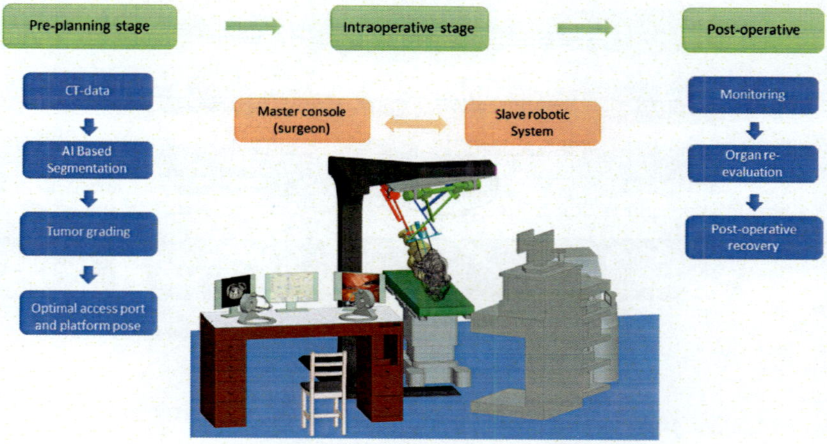

Fig. 1. Robotic-assisted SILS procedure

Figure 1 illustrates the three main stages of the robotic assisted SILS procedure [11] using an innovative parallel robotic system [12]. During the pre-planning stage the doctors are analyzing all available patient data to establish an optimum surgical strategy. Using AI agents, the tumors can be accurately located and interpreted enabling the definition of resection margins, access route and potential areas of interest inside the surgical field. The intraoperative stage is performed using the Challenge robotic system in a Master-Slave architecture, where the surgeon is manipulating highly dexterous haptic devices to control the position of the surgical instruments which are manipulated by the slave robotic system. Using both intraoperative endoscopic images and the data obtained in the pre-planning stage the surgeon can safely perform the surgery. Following the surgical procedure, in the post-operative stage the patient will be monitored to ensure an optimum recovery and possible additional treatments depending on the nature of resected tumor.

3 Methodology

The use of a high-accuracy convolutional neural network for semantic segmentation is critical in the pre-planning phase of robotic-assisted SILS procedure, as shown in medical protocol presented in [13].

Because it deals with medical images utilized in surgical procedures, which require a significant level of attention to detail, this process must be very accurate. The segmentation process was executed in collaboration with certified medical personnel.

Figure 2 illustrates the process of semantic segmentation of CT images datasets.

For this purpose, Matlab programming platform was used including Computer Vision Toolbox, Deep Learning Toolbox and Parallel Computing Toolbox.

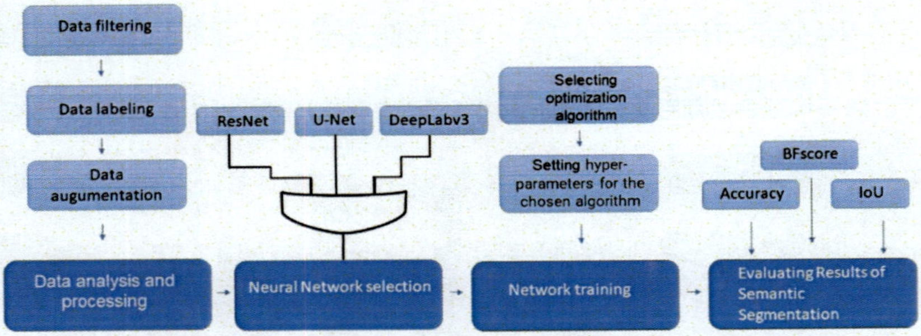

Fig. 2. Process diagram for semantic segmentation of the kidney

A. Data Analysis and Processing

The Institutional Review Board of Clinical Municipal Hospital of Cluj-Napoca, Romania, approved this study (approval code: nr. 15/2020/11-June-2020) and waived the requirement for formal written consent. For this study were used multi-phase abdominal computed tomography (CT) of 250 patients with renal tumors, approximately 10–15 from each patient. Were included just those images where the kidneys are visible. The images were resized to have 512 $\times$ 512 dimensions.

Data filtering is the process where the input data is analyzed in order to keep just useful data. From the total number of images, 70% were selected to be the training set, 15% for validation set and 15% for test set. Images were selected randomly.

Pixel labeling is a required procedure considering that image classification and thus semantic segmentation is part of supervised learning category. In this procedure each pixel on an image is assigned to a class label from a predefined set. The procedure was made in Image Labeler tool (Matlab), which automate labels in ground truth data (Source of ground truth data, Label definitions, Label data for each ROI and scene label).

Data augmentation is a technique used to artificially expand the size of the training test to improve the model performance. It includes a variety of image editing operations such as shifts, flips, zooms, etc.

B. Neural Network Selection

To obtain satisfactory results for CT images segmentation, a variety of algorithms can be used, most popular being: ResNet, DeepLabv3 and U-net. For this paper the U-net model has been studied, which was specially developed for medical segmentation. The architecture is evolved from a traditional convolutional neural network combined with an expansive path which aims to increase the resolution of images [14]

C. Network Training

Optimization algorithms are crucial in machine learning because they are the process of iteratively training a model to identify a minimum and maximum for function evaluation. At each iteration, the results are compared to lower the loss function and improve accuracy. For this network stochastic gradient descent with momentum (SGDM) and Adam, was used to accelerate the optimization process.

Setting hyperparameters stage is important for a satisfactory performance of the chosen optimization algorithm. In an effort to achieve the best performance for this architecture, different configurations of hyperparameters for SGDM and Adam were tested, where the learn rate, epochs and mini batch size have different values. The network is tested against the validation data every epoch.

D. Evaluating Results

An adequate method to evaluate the output of a trained network is to measure the accuracy for multiple test images, where factors like Intersection over union (IoU), the boundary contour matching score (BFscore) and accuracy can help to obtain a better view of trained neural network.

4 Results

An analysis of the neural network is performed at the end of the training phase, measuring the accuracy for multiple test images. Global accuracy, Mean accuracy, Mean IoU, Wheited IoU, and Mean BF score are the data metrics utilized for evaluation and can be seen in Fig. 3.

GlobalAccuracy	MeanAccuracy	MeanIoU	WeightedIoU	MeanBFScore
0.97047	0.97056	0.94001	0.94279	0.92119

Fig. 3. Network analysis on validation set

The results were acquired using two PC hardware configurations in order to provide a more detailed insight of the role of hardware in the computational process. For training, one machine uses an Intel(R) Core(TM) i7-7700 CPU running at 3.60 GHz, while the other uses two NVIDIA Quadro-P4000 graphics cards, with 1792 cores each.

The Mean Accuracy represents an adequate parameter for an initial study of the training network to achieve a quality approximation of the neural network. As shown in Fig. 4, accuracy varies based on the hardware system, the number of images used for training, and the hyperparameters such as "learning-rate" and "mini-batch-size."

Learning rate is one of the most important hyperparameter to set considering that a too-high learning rate can cause the model to converge too rapidly to a suboptimal solution, while a too-low learning rate can cause the process to stall.

To highlight the importance of data inputs, respectively how many images must be used, to obtain a satisfactory accuracy, three sets of data were used, with different number of images. As has been expected the 200 data package obtained poor performance both on CPU and GPU systems, even though the mini batch size value was 2.

Adding 150 images, the accuracy is increased to 95.99% CPU and 96.58% GPU. At the and with 500 datasets has approached the accuracy on 98.69% CPU and 97.17% on GPU.

The computational system has a considerable impact on the training time and, implicitly, on the operation cost, but no negative impact on the network's accuracy. Different values for mini batch size (small batches from training dataset) parameters were evaluated to see how the network behaved, findings revealed that a bigger value for this parameter leads to poorer accuracy but more processing time.

No of images	Computational Hardware	Optimizer	Mini Batch Size	Learning Rate	No of Epochs	Global Accuracy	Time for computation
200	GPU	SGDM	2	0.003	30	0.9508	19'36''
200	GPU	SGDM	10	0.003	30	0.9334	29'25''
200	CPU	SGDM	2	0.003	30	0.9206	685'45''
350	GPU	SGDM	2	0.003	30	0.9658	33'27''
350	GPU	SGDM	10	0.003	30	0.9417	50'25''
350	CPU	SGDM	2	0.003	30	0.9599	813'27''
500	CPU	Adam	2	0.001	30	0.8094	771'30''
500	GPU	SGDM	2	0.003	30	0.9741	71'37''
500	GPU	SGDM	10	0.003	30	0.9717	58'26''
500	GPU	Adam	2	0.003	30	0.9707	45'9''
500	GPU	Adam	8	0.003	30	0.9713	49'13''
500	**CPU**	**SGDM**	**2**	**0.003**	**30**	**0.9869**	**859'30'**
500	GPU	Adam	8	0.001	65	0.9680	50'55''
500	GPU	Adam	2	0.001	65	0.9796	45'17''
500	GPU	Adam	2	0.001	65	0.8709	82'13'
500	**GPU**	**Adam**	**10**	**0.001**	**65**	**0.8003**	**94'22''**
500	GPU	Adam	4	0.001	65	0.8394	87'37''
500	GPU	Adam	4	0.001	65	0.8436	85'32''
500	GPU	SGDM	2	0.001	65	0.8865	80'23''
500	GPU	SGDM	2	0.001	65	0.8735	80'15''

Fig. 4. Most significant result from training phase

The optimizer algorithm is another significant aspect in the training process. It has been proved that SGDM does not perform as well as others for a particular task, and it is frequently compared to Adam optimizer [15]. This network was tested using both SGDM and Adam optimizers, showing that for this particular task of semantic segmentation, Adam obtained a lower accuracy but a less working time too, but just if the network has a 0.003 value for learning rate. If the value is lower e.g. 0.001, SGDM loses considerable accuracy which proves that SGDM works better than Adam with learning rate value set at minimum 0.003, even if the network was trained by a greater number of epochs.

In (Fig. 5 a) it can be observed that SGDM performed better then Adam, both being tested 10 times with different number of epochs but with the same learning rate value. When learning rate value was modified from 0.003 to 0.001, Adam behaved the same way, but SGDM obtained much lower accuracy values (Fig. 5 b).

Another important factor is the loss function, used also for the model optimization. This factor is defined as the value which indicates the difference from the desired target state(s). This function can be used to estimate the model's loss so that the weights can be adjusted in the next evaluation to lower the loss.

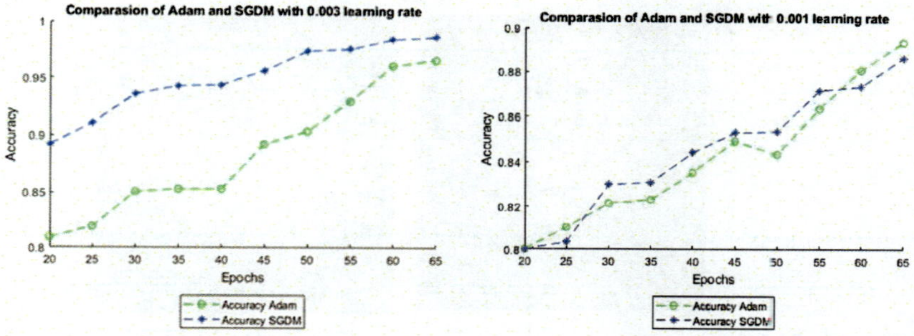

a) b)

Fig. 5 a) Comparison of Adam and GSD using 0.003 value for learning rate b) comparison of Adam and GSD using 0.001 value for learning rate

During training, the Mini-batch Accuracy and Mini-batch Loss can be evaluated to observe how the training phase evolves. It can be seen in Fig. 6 that the initial value for accuracy is quite low, while the number for Mini-batch Loss is significant. This situation will be reversed during the learning process, as shown in the table lines below.

Epoch	Iteration	Time Elapsed (hh:mm:ss)	Mini-batch Accuracy	Validation Accuracy	Mini-batch Loss	Validation Loss	Base Learning Rate
1	1	00:01:20	39.18%	50.06%	7.7207	6.2842	0.0600
1	20	00:02:54	80.38%		2.3959		0.0600
1	40	00:04:34	60.79%		2.4139		0.0600
1	50	00:06:37	57.36%	68.33%	1.6559	1.3490	0.0600
1	60	00:07:27	71.36%		1.3977		0.0600
1	80	00:09:06	91.27%		0.4569		0.0600
1	100	00:12:00	86.12%	88.01%	0.6039	0.5161	0.0600
1	120	00:13:40	92.93%		0.2820		0.0600

Fig. 6. The evolution of the learning process

In Fig. 7 can be observed a CT segmentation executed by networks with 80.94% accuracy compared with a CT segmentation performed by a network with 98.69% accuracy. It can be observed that for this particular case, where the target organs are the kidneys, that even an accuracy of 80% can be considerated poor (the values of the pixels kidneys are too close to values of the pixels for other organs). In that case the accuracy of the segmentation should be over 91%.

a)
b)
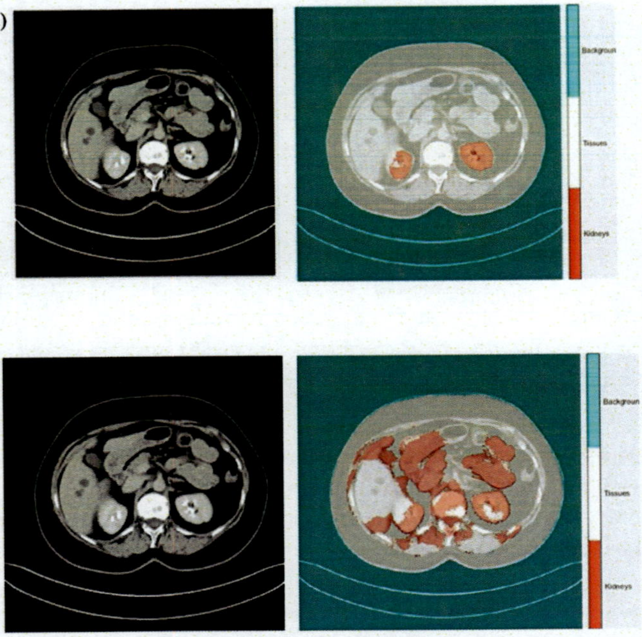

Fig. 7 a) Automated semantic segmentation with U-net Network 98.69% accuracy. b) Automated semantic segmentation with U-net Network 80.94% accuracy

5 Conclusions

Semantic segmentation is one of the most important procedures in the pre-planning stage of complex surgical procedures, being integrated as a compulsory step in our medical protocol for robotic-assisted SILS. With this method of image processing, the surgeon can visualize organs, tumor or blood systems from ROI to make a propriate plan for the surgical procedure.

The paper presented an optimal way to execute the semantic segmentation for CT datasets (kidneys images) intending to obtain the best accuracy for the network discussed. The images were manually labeled, and different parameters for SGDM optimizer and Adam optimizer, were tested in multiple training sessions.

The tests revealed that U-net with SGDM optimizer, for this type of task represent the best option even for a small dataset if learning rate value is over 0.001. Also was demonstrated how important is for a network to have parameters as: learning rate or mini batch sets for a specific task with a specific number of images. From all the training sessions performed, the best result was achieved having value of 2 for mini-batch size and 0.003 for learning rate configuration, with SGDM optimizer where 500 images were used as input where both CPU and GPU training obtained a value over 97%. As can be seen the process is time consuming and with powerful computer architectures the training time is reduced, enabling the use of more data leading to better CNN. Another point that needs to be made is that utilizing the proper optimizer for a certain task is more crucial than employing large number of images.

Acknowledgment. This work was supported by a grant of the Ministry of Research, Innovation and Digitization, CNCS/CCCDI–UEFISCDI, project PCE171/2021-Challenge within PNCDI III, project POCU/380/6/13/123927–ANTREDOC, "Entrepreneurial competencies and excellence research in doctoral and postdoctoral studies programs", project co-funded by the European Social Fund through the Human Capital Operational.

Conflict of Interest The authors declare no conflict of interest.

References

1. Ranschaert, E., et al. (eds.): Artificial Intelligence in Medical Imaging (2019)
2. Pisla, D., et al.: Kinematics and design of a 5-DOF parallel robot used in minimally invasive surgery. In: Advances in Robot Kinematics: Motion in Man and Machine, pp. 99–106 (2010)
3. Pisla, D., et al.: PARASURG hybrid parallel robot for minimally invasive surgery. Chirurgia **106**(5), 619–625 (2011)
4. Penza, V., et al.: Dense soft tissue 3D reconstruction refined with super-pixel segmentation for robotic abdominal surgery. IJCARS **11**(2), 197–206 (2015)
5. Rehder, R., et al.: The role of simulation in neurosurgery. Child's Nerv. Syst. **32**(1), 43–54 (2015)
6. Albawi, S., et al.: Understanding of a convolutional neural network. In: 2017 International Conference on Engineering and Technology (2017)
7. Navab, N., et al. (eds.): Medical Image Computing and Computer-Assisted Intervention—MICCAI 2015. Lecture Notes in Computer Science (2015)
8. Ni, Z.L., et al.: Space squeeze reasoning and low-rank bilinear feature fusion for surgical image segmentation. IEEE J. Biomed. Health Inform.
9. Choi, J., et al.: Video recognition of simple mastoidectomy using convolutional neural networks: detection and segmentation of surgical tools and anatomical regions. Comput. Methods Programs Biomed. **208**, 106251 (2021)
10. Vaida, C., et al.: Preliminary assessment of artificial intelligence agents for a SILS robotic system. In: 2021 International Conference on e-Health and Bioengineering, pp. 1–6 (2021)
11. Pisla, D., et al.: Application oriented modelling and simulation of an innovative parallel robot for single incision laparoscopic surgery. In: Proceedings of the ASME 2022, IDETC/CIE2022 August 14–17, 2022, St. Louis, Missouri (2022)
12. Pisla, D., et al.: Family of modular parallel robots with active translational joints for SILS, OSIM-A00733/03.12.2021
13. Vaida, C., et al.: Preliminary control design of a single-incision laparoscopic surgery robotic system. In: 2021 25th International Conference on System Theory, Control and Computing (ICSTCC), pp. 384–389 (2021)
14. Guo, Y., et al.: A review of semantic segmentation using deep neural networks. Int. J. Multimed. Inf. Retr. **7**(2), 87–93 (2017)
15. Jiang, X., et al.: Fingerspelling identification for Chinese sign language via AlexNet-based transfer learning and Adam optimizer. Sci. Program. **2020**, 1–13 (2020)

Classification of Hemorrhagic Stroke Lesions Based on CT Images and Machine Learning Algorithms. A Study on a Highly Imbalanced Dataset

Madalina Ianovici, Simona Vlad, and Angela Lungu(✉)

Faculty of Electrical Engineering, Technical University of Cluj-Napoca, Cluj-Napoca, Romania
angela.lungu@ethm.utcluj.ro

Abstract. Hemorrhagic stroke is a common disease that has a high mortality rate. The patient's chances of a complete recovery depend on where in the brain the hemorrhage occurred. Automatic classification based on machine learning (ML) techniques is often proposed in clinical applications, depending on the availability of data and computational resources. The traditional ML algorithms, such as Random Forest and Support Vector Machine, are often applied to tabular data requiring smaller datasets and less intensive computational power, while the more advanced, but costly techniques, such as convolutional neural networks, are frequently applied to image data. This paper describes the automatic classification of the 5 subtypes of hemorrhagic stroke, namely Intraparenchymal (IPH), Subarachnoid (SAH), Intraventricular (IVH), Epidural (EDH) and Subdural (SDH), comparing the results after applying traditional machine learning and deep learning (DL) methods, on the same dataset. The detection of the 5 classes had 74% balanced accuracy for the best identified ML algorithm and 90% after applying a DL method.

Keywords: Hemorrhagic stroke classification · Machine learning · Deep learning

1 Introduction

Stroke is the main cause of disability and mortality in the world. It is defined as a neurological and cardiovascular disease which occurs in the central nervous system. Based on the cause of occurrence, there are two types of strokes: ischemic stroke, caused by a clot blocking the blood vessels, and intracerebral hemorrhagic stroke (ICH), caused by bleeding blood vessels within the brain. According to their location in the brain, five types of ICH may be distinguished: Intraparenchymal (IPH), Subarachnoid (SAH), Intraventricular (IVH), Epidural (EDH) and Subdural (SDH). The severity of ICH varies depending on the location and size of bleeding [1]. Pablo et al. [2] show that patients with large EDH, IPH, SDH have a higher mortality risk.

S. Vlad and N. M. Roman (Eds.): MEDITECH 2022, IFMBE Proceedings 102, pp. 30–39, 2024.
https://doi.org/10.1007/978-3-031-51120-2_4

The stroke diagnosis should be set as soon as possible to increase the patient's chance of survival. Computerized Tomography (CT) assists the physician in identifying brain tissue damage and personalizing treatment for each patient [3].

The correct classification of hemorrhagic stroke has predictive value, supporting the correct medical treatment and patient's recovery [4]. The use of AI technology in stroke diagnosis may achieve high precision results [5–7].

The current study investigates the potential of traditional machine learning (ML) algorithms for correct classification of all types of hemorrhagic stroke subsets based on information extracted from CT brain images. The results are compared with the ones obtained after applying a pre-train, publicly available convolutional neural network. One particularity of this work described in the following sections is represented by the high-class imbalance of the dataset.

1.1 Related Works

Several studies [5–7] used artificial intelligence for automatic stroke diagnosis. This disease is a challenge for AI algorithms due to the diversity of shapes, dimensions, and locations, but also due to the limited data available.

A classification of intracranial hemorrhage and subtypes in non-contrast CT images was studied [5] by Hai Ye et al. The proposed method is based on three-dimensional (3D) convolutional and recurrent neural network (CNN-RNN). The performance of multi class classification (five classes) was evaluated on 194 patients and achieved 0.8 for the area under the curve AUC metric for all classes. Among the five subtypes, IPH had the highest percentage of cases and the best sensitivity, higher than 90%, whereas EDH was the minority class and had lower sensitivity, i.e. 69%.

Sundar et al. [8] built a connected convolutional network, called DN-ELM, used for ICH diagnosis. The method involves multiple processes, such as feature extraction, preprocessing, segmentation, and classification. Another method which uses deep convolutional neural networks in ICH detection and classification was described by Lee et al. [9], who developed a new algorithm for artificial neural network and ICH classification into three subtypes (EDH, SDH, SAH).

The research studies referred to above focused mainly on DL algorithms, while, to the best of our knowledge, the studies evaluating the performance of traditional ML algorithms, based on images features, for all hemorrhagic stroke subtypes classification, are scarce. It has been often shown that the classification results obtained using DL techniques have high accuracy, specificity, and sensitivity. However, these require access to large amounts of data, and longer lasting training and computing power. On the other hand, traditional ML algorithm may be implemented even when computational and data resources are modest.

2 Materials and Methods

2.1 Database

The database used in this study was obtained from PhysioNet [6] and contains CT scans of 82 patients. Examples for each subtype of ICH as well as for normal CT are shown in Fig. 1.

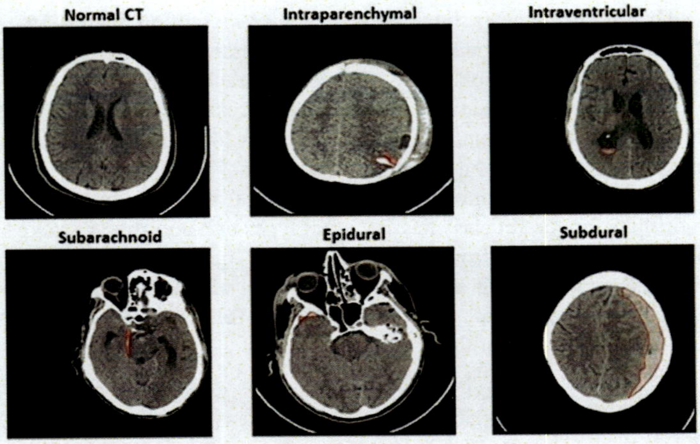

Fig. 1. Examples of CT slices from the database

Each patient record consists of 30 slices, which were evaluated by two radiologists to identify the hemorrhagic area. The total number of images used in this study is listed in Table 1.

Table 1. Number of CT images

Hemorrhagic type	Number of CT images used in this study
Intraventricular IVH	13
Intraparenchymal IPH	52
Subarachnoid SAH	9
Epidural EDH	167
Subdural SDH	52

As one may notice, the used data is characterized by high-class imbalance. Techniques such as oversampling of the minority class, or down sampling of the majority class could be adopted to equilibrate the classes [10]. Each of these methods have advantages and disadvantages, and according to [11], careful consideration is needed when choosing a method or another.

2.2 Traditional Machine Learning Workflow

Feature Extraction

Shape and texture attributes were both extracted from the available dataset. In order to determine shape characteristics, the segmented images from the original dataset were used to isolate the bleeding area. The analysis includes the following shape properties: area, perimeter, minor axis length, major axis length, circularity, object center and orientation. The texture information was extracted using the grey level co-occurrence matrix (GLCM) [12] and included: contrast, energy, homogeneity, and correlation. All the steps described in this paper were implemented in MATLAB (www.mathworks.com).

Model Selection

The dataset was randomly divided into training and testing sets in a 0.8/0.2 ratio. The latter was used to evaluate the performance of the best selected algorithm.

Four ML algorithms, KNN (K-Nearest Neighbor), Random Forest, Binary Trees, and SVM (Support Vector Machine), were evaluated to find the most suitable one for the ICH classification. Considering that the dataset is rather small, 5-fold Cross Validation with stratified sampling was applied on the initially selected training set. Stratified sampling ensures that the proportion between classes is the same as in the original dataset, having the advantage that the validation results are close to the results of a test set [13].

At the model selection stage, the above-mentioned models were characterized by the MATLAB pre-defined parameters listed below:

- Random Forest: 5 learners (trees), 1 for the minimum number of leaf and the indicators for the out-of-bag information and feature importance were set to 'off'.
- Support Vector machine: an SVM template, with standardized predictors, with linear kernel. Since SVM is an ML algorithm frequently used for two classes, it is rather problematic when more classes need to be classified. Therefore, Error Correcting Output Codes (ECOC), multiple classification algorithms with multiple classes, were generated for this study.
- Decision Trees: 1 for the maximum number of splits and Gini split criterion.
- K-Nearest Neighbor: 5 neighbors and Euclidian distance metric.

The classifiers' performance was evaluated using balanced accuracy [14, 15]. The calculation of general accuracy is not suited for imbalanced sets because it depends on the performance achieved on the biggest class. Table 2 shows the values of balanced and general accuracy obtained for each of the tested models, on 5-fold cross-validation.

Table 2. Accuracy for ML algorithms

ML algorithm	Balanced accuracy (%)	Accuracy (%)
Random forest	66	78
Support vector machine	54	69
Decision trees	46	69
K-nearest neighbor	44	62

Random Forest had the highest average balanced accuracy of all 4 tested models and was chosen for further evaluation.

Random Forest Model

One important parameter that influences the performance of a Random Forest model is the number of learners (trees). The model was trained and verified on the cross-validation subsets, with the number of trees ranging from 5 to 200, with a 5 step. The best-balanced accuracy was obtained with 45 trees.

Another parameter used in this step was out-of-bag (OOB) prediction and refers to a prediction made for a feature in the original dataset using only base learners who have not been trained on this specific feature. This information was used to determine the predicted class probabilities for each tree in the ensemble. The latter were used for estimating the values of the applied cost matrix.

Cost Matrix

The main problem when dealing with imbalanced multiclass tasks is the incorrect prediction of the minority class because the model tends to predict the majority class. A cost matrix, C_{RF} with the values shown in Fig. 2 was introduced to reduce the negative effect of imbalanced data on the algorithm. Depending on the class ratio misprediction of minority classes has a significant penalty.

$$
\begin{array}{lcccccl}
 & \text{IVH} & \text{IPH} & \text{SAH} & \text{EDH} & \text{SDH} & \\
 & 0 & 5 & 2.4 & 17 & 5 & \text{IVH} \\
 & 2.1 & 0 & 1.9 & 3.4 & 2.8 & \text{IPH} \\
C_{RF} = & 3.4 & 5 & 0 & 17 & 5 & \text{SAH} \\
 & 1.9 & 2.1 & 1.9 & 0 & 2.1 & \text{EDH} \\
 & 2.1 & 2.8 & 1.9 & 3.4 & 0 & \text{SDH}
\end{array}
$$

Fig. 2. Cost matrix values

2.3 Deep Learning. Pre-Trained Convolutional Neural Network

A pre-trained convolutional neural network, available in MATLAB, AlexNet [16], was used to evaluate the automatic classification potential of ICH bleeding sub-types.

The 0.7–0.1–0.2 ratio was used for splitting the dataset into training, validation and testing. The images included in the sets were randomly selected, the only constraint being to preserve equal ratios of the five classes in the training and test sets.

The network was initially trained without augmenting data with the scope of analyzing the results. Several augmentation techniques were introduced for the data in the training set in order to vary the data, including: rotation [−10, 10], scaling [1, 1.2] and X-axis mirroring. The ADAM optimizer [17] was used for training, with 20 epochs, 10 mini batch size, and a learning rate of 0.001. For the case where the data was augmented, AlexNet was trained with same optimizer and learning rate, but on 100 epochs and a mini batch of 2. The training parameters were chosen for both cases (with/without augmentation) following a selection process, in which the number of epochs, mini batch size and learning rate varied incrementally, having the results checked on the validation set.

3 Results and Discussions

The results in this section were obtained on the test sets. Table 3 shows the results obtained for the traditional ML algorithm. The two cases considered for the Random Forest algorithm with and without applied cost-matrix were marked column wise with C2 and C1.

Table 3. Metrics for Random Forest model: **C1** refers to the model without the cost matrix and **C2** refers to the model with the cost matrix

Class	Testset images number	Sensibility (%)		Specificity (%)		Precision (%)		Balanced acc (%)	
		C1	C 2	C1	C2	C1	C2	C1	C2
Epidural	34	100	91	75	83	85	89	67	74
Intraparenchymal	10	80	60	98	98	89	86		
Intraventricular	2	0	100	100	95	0	40		
Subarachnoid	2	0	50	100	96	0	33		
Subdural	10	90	70	100	98	100	88		

Figure 3 shows the Receiver Operation Characteristics curve (ROC) obtained by applying the Random Forrest algorithm, based on the metrics described in Table 3.

It can be readily seen that, without applying a cost matrix, the majority class, Epidural, shows ideal sensitivity, whereas the sensitivity of the minority classes, i.e. Intraventricular and Subarachnoid, is null. The influence of the majority class is evident in the results presented in Fig. 3 a), in the confusion chart. All EDH instances were correctly classified and most of the incorrect classified cases were also labeled as EDH.

The application of the cost matrix improves the balanced accuracy of the model and the sensitivity and precision of the minority classes. This improvement came with a loss in sensitivity of the other classes. Therefore, one should carefully consider the compromise brought by the penalization of a class to the detriment of another. According to Steven and Thorell [18], the presence of subarachnoid bleeding could quickly worsen the patient's status and its rapid identification is highly desired.

The classification of ICH types using a Random Forest algorithm combined with shape and texture features showed promising results when a cost matrix was applied. However, when comparing these findings with the results reported in literature [8, 9] on other cranial stroke classification problems based on DL algorithm, the current ones are less reliable. A simple, pre-trained neural network available in Matlab, AlexNet, was

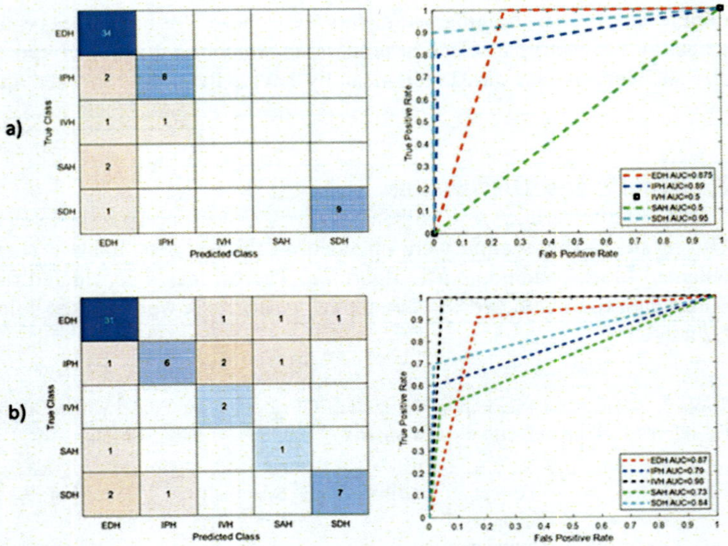

Fig. 3. Confusion matrix and ROC for Random Forest: a) without the cost matrix; b) with the cost matrix

tested on the given dataset in order to compare the results referred to above of traditional ML algorithms with the ones achieved by a DL method.

Table 4. Metrics for AlexNet method. **C3** refers to the initial dataset and **C4** to the augmented training dataset

Class	Testset images number	Sensibility (%)		Specificity (%)		Precision (%)		Balanced acc (%)	
		C1	C 2	C1	C2	C1	C2	C1	C2
Epidural	33	96	100	92	100	94	100	73	90
Intraparenchymal	10	80	100	96	98	80	90		
Intraventricular	3	100	100	100	100	100	100		
Subarachnoid	2	0	50	98	100	0	100		
Subdural	10	90	100	98	100	90	100		

Table 4 lists the results for the AlexNet network trained on dataset without any augmentation (C3), and on the augmentation training set (C4), respectively. Without any prior preparation of the dataset, the method had a balanced accuracy similar to the best Random Forest model, i.e., 73%. Moreover, the intraventricular class, although minority, was correctly identified. Unlike the models using images features, the one using the whole image is less affected by class imbalance. According to Yang. et. al. [19], data augmentation proved almost mandatory when applying DL algorithms. The simple data augmentation techniques employed in this study improved the results considerably, as showed in both Table 4 and Fig. 4.

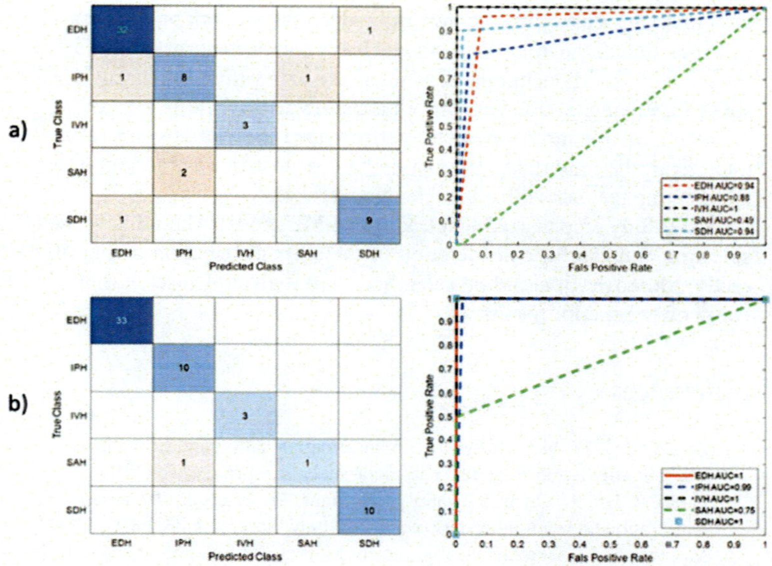

Fig. 4. Confusion matrix and ROC for AlexNet a) initial dataset b) augmented dataset

The AUC values improved after applying data augmentation to all ICH types, having a perfect ROC curve for three classes: EDH, IPH and SDH. Also, the balanced accuracy of the model increased to 90%. The subarachnoid class sensitivity also improved for the augmented case to 50% (one of the two instances of the test set was correctly identified). The correct identification of the subarachnoid class was also considered challenging in previous studies [5, 9] using DL models.

4 Conclusions

The correct automatic classification of the hemorrhagic stroke subtypes could support healthcare professionals during patient recovery since it has been shown to have an important prediction value [4].

Artificial intelligence algorithms are now part of clinical routine, showing great results. The choice of the model depends however on the available data. The most complex models, those based on DL techniques, are usually computationally expensive requiring large amount of data for training, to offer the model enough variability during the training process. The current study analyzed whether traditional ML algorithms, requiring less resources and data, could deliver results similar to DL-based algorithms.

A Random Forest classifier was identified as the model with the best performance on the given dataset when compared to a SVM, K-NN and decision tree model. The results showed that its performance was influenced by the high-class imbalance characterizing the original dataset. The application of a cost-matrix improved the balanced accuracy of the model from 67% to 74%. The results were compared with the ones obtained after applying a pre-trained convolutional neural network on the same data. Without any manipulation of the images, the model had a balanced accuracy of 73%. Data augmentation, a well-known technique used to ensure data variability during the training process, substantially increased the balanced accuracy to 90%.

When analyzing the models' performance individually, on each class, the results underlined the importance of applying a cost-matrix for Random Forest algorithm and augmenting the dataset for the AlexNet network.

This study emphasized that traditional ML models should have adequate parameter selection and careful consideration of the class distribution to classify ICH types correctly. Moreover, it could be seen that, on the given dataset, simple DL-based models could offer superior results.

References

1. Audrey, C.L., et al.: Intracerebral hemorrhage location and functional outcomes of patients: a systematic literature review and meta-analysis. SpringerLink **2016**(05), 384–391 (2016)
2. Pablo, P., Ian, R., Omar, B., Maralyn, W., Jane, M., Fiona, L.: Intracranial bleeding in patients with traumatic brain injury: a prognostic study. SpringerLink **08**, 03 (2009)
3. Marwan, E.-K., Gerhard, S., Caspar, B., Marcel, A.: Imaging of Acute Ischemic Stroke. Eur. Neurol. 309–314 (2014)
4. Ajaya, K., Unnithan, A., Parth, M.: Hemorrhagic stroke. StatPearls Publishing LLC (2021)
5. Ye, H., Gao, F., Yin, Y., Guo, D., Zhao, P., Lu, Y., Wang, X., Bai, J., Cao, K., Song, Q., Zhang, H., Chen, W., Guo, X., Xia, J.: Precise diagnosis of intracranial hemorrhage and subtypes using a three-dimensional joint convolutional and recurrent neural network. Eur. Radiol. 6191–6201 (2019)
6. Hssayeni, M.: Computed Tomography Images for Intracranial Hemorrhage Detection and Segmentation (2020). https://physionet.org/content/ct-ich/1.3.1/. Accessed 15 noiembrie 2021
7. Emily, L., Esther, L.Y.: Computational approaches for acute traumatic brain injury image recognition. Front. Neurol. (2022)
8. Sundar, S., Vijayakumar, V., Gavaskar, S., Jegathesh, A.J., Sumathi, A.: Machine learning model for intracranial hemorrhage diagnosis and classification. Electronics 2574 (2021)
9. Hyunkwang, L., Sehyo, Y., Mohammad, M., et al.: An explainable deep-learning algorithm for the detection of acute intracranial haemorrhage from small datasets. Nat. Biomed. Eng. 173–182 (2019)
10. Lian, Y., Nengfeng, Z.: Survey of imbalanced data methodologies. arxiv 7 (2021)
11. Krawczyk, B.: Learning from imbalanced data: open challenges and future directions. Prog. Artif. Intell. **5**(4), 221–232 (2016). https://doi.org/10.1007/s13748-016-0094-0
12. Mohanaiah, P., Sathyanarayana, P., GuruKumar, L.: Image texture feature extraction using GLCM. Int. J. Sci. Res. Publ. **3**(5) (2013)
13. Diamantidisa, N.A., Karlisb, D., Giakoumakisa, E.A.: Unsupervised stratification of cross-validation. Artif. Intell. **116**, 1–16 (2000)

14. Margherita, G., Enrico, B., Giorgio, V.: Metrics for multi-class classification: an overview. arxiv (2020)
15. Vicente, G., et al.: Index of balanced accuracy: a performance measure for skewed class distributions. In: Conference: Proceedings of the 4th Iberian Conference on Pattern Recognition and Image Analysis (2009)
16. Alex, K., Ilya şi, S., Geoffrey, E.H.: ImageNet classification with deep convolutional neural networks. NIPS 1106–1114 (2012)
17. Diederik, P.K., Jimmy, L.B.: ADAM: a method for stochastic optimization. In: 3rd International Conference for Learning Representations, San Diego (2015)
18. Steven, T., Thorell, W.: Intracranial Hemorrhage. StatPearls Publishing (2022)
19. Suorong, Y., Xiao, W., Mengcheng, Z., Suhan, G., Jian, Z., Furao, S.: Image data augmentation for deep learning: a survey (2022)

Medical Image Data Cleansing for Machine Learning: A Must in the Evidence-Based Medicine?

Mircea-Sebastian Șerbănescu[1,2(✉)], Alexandra-Daniela Rotaru-Zăvăleanu[1], Anca-Maria Istrate-Ofițeru[1,2,3,4], Berbecaru Elena-Iuliana-Ana Maria[3], Iuliana-Alina Enache[3], Rodica Daniela Nagy[3,5], Cristina Maria Comănescu[2,3], Didi Liliana Popa[2], and Dominic-Gabriel Iliescu[1,2,3,5]

[1] University of Medicine and Pharmacy of Craiova, 2-4 Petru Rareş St., 200349 Craiova, Romania
mircea_serbanescu@yahoo.com
[2] University of Craiova, 13 A. I. Cuza St., 200396 Craiova, Romania
[3] University Emergency County Hospital, 2-4 Petru Rareş St., 200642 Craiova, Romania
[4] Research Centre for Microscopic Morphology and Immunology, 1 Tabaci St., 200349 Craiova, Romania
[5] Ginecho Clinic, Medgin, 29 1 Mai Bvd., 200355 Craiova, Romania

Abstract. Preparing the data for machine learning is important, as it has been proven that the quantity and quality of the input data is a strong predictor for the output. In a deep-learning with transfer learning context, an ultrasonography image dataset is cleaned. The performance of the cleaned dataset against the original one is measured using the accuracy and area under the curve metrics running three different network architectures: AlexNet, GoogLeNet, ResNet-18. Both metrics show significantly superior results on the cleaned dataset, though 49.81% of the original dataset has been removed. We conclude that data cleansing must be done before applying any machine learning algorithms, physicians should cope with the machine learning terminology and focus on understanding the models in use, and last but not least, the data cleansing should be driven by computer scientist though they have less understanding of the medical problem itself.

Keywords: Image dataset · Cleansing · Performance · AlexNet · GoogLeNet · ResNet-18

1 Introduction

To conduct a research study, you have to follow three steps that can help you obtain relevant data that can offer valuable scientific conclusions: the first step is to establish your goal, to formulate a hypothesis, in order to know exactly what kind of data you need and how to choose the most efficient material and method that can help you obtain it. The second step is to perform the experiment itself (no matter if you talk about in vitro experiments, in vivo ones or even a combination between the two of them). This step

S. Vlad and N. M. Roman (Eds.): MEDITECH 2022, IFMBE Proceedings 102, pp. 40–50, 2024.
https://doi.org/10.1007/978-3-031-51120-2_5

is crucial because it represents the fundament of our study. The last step is represented by an efficient interpretation of the results. Sometimes the data that we have are not as relevant as we want them, or at least not all of them. It is important to find a way to select the most relevant results and to express them to sustain or even modify our initial hypothesis. Choosing the best results for our study's needs can be a long-lasting process that can waste a lot of time from our scientific team.

Machine learning on medical data has become a common practice [1–6] putting together a team of physicians and a team of computer scientists.

Preparing the data for machine learning is important as it has been proven that the quantity and the quality of the input data is a strong predictor for the output [7, 8] of the model, and it can be resumed: garbage in – garbage out.

Data cleansing (data cleaning) is the process of detecting and correcting (or removing) corrupt or inaccurate data as Kang and Tian defined it [9].

Data cleansing is regarded as a first step, or a preprocessing step and is a necessary precondition for successful knowledge discovery [10].

In general, the physicians only care about the solution's output, not on its implementation details and thus do not provide suitable datasets for proper machine learning.

As [8] states reason for data cleansing is that if we have treated data quality properly, planned from the beginning, then we should not really have to worry about ever cleaning data, since it should already be fit for use by the time the user sees it.

The current paper aims assessing the cleaning results of an ultrasonography image dataset designed for image classification using deep learning classification results as performance measurement, and emphasize current dataset mistakes.

2 Material and Methods

2.1 Original Image Dataset

The dataset consists of 1592 ultrasonography images of fetal morphology sections acquired using Voluson E10, Voluson E8, and Voluson 730 Pro (General Electric System, GE Healthcare, Zipf, Austria), and Philips Elite Epiq (Bothell, USA) ultrasound machines, equipped with a 4–8-MHz curvilinear transducer. The dataset consists of 8 classes of the abdominal plane and the image distribution was: 3 vessels plus bladder (n = 199), gallbladder (n = 103), transverse cord insertion (n = 188), anteroposterior kidney plane (n = 146), biometry plane (n = 365), kidney sagittal plane (n = 274), bladder plane (n = 63), sagittal abdominal plane (n = 254).

All the eligible participants were pregnant women admitted to the Prenatal Unit for the second-trimester morphology within the University Emergency County Hospital Craiova, Romania, and Ginecho Clinic, Craiova, Romania. All participants gave written informed consent for their data to be processed for research purposes.

The images were selected from archived ultrasonographic records and labeled by obstetricians with minimum 2 years of experience. Their labeling task was to add images in 8 folders based on their class membership.

A sample of the original (and cleaned) dataset images can be seen in Fig. 1.

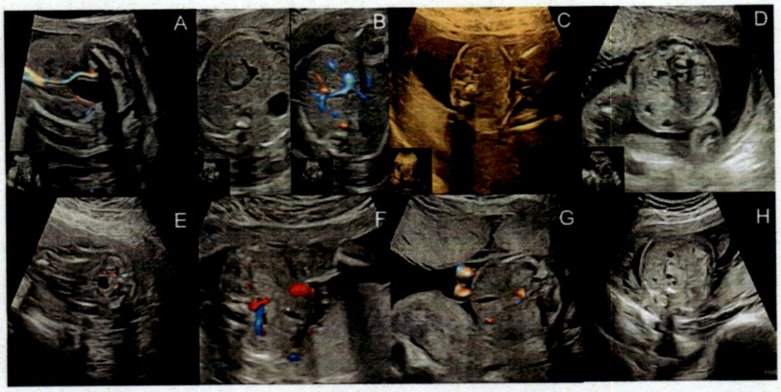

Fig. 1. Dataset sample. Images A, B, C, and D belong only to the original dataset, while images E, F, G, and H belong also to the cleaned dataset.

2.2 Data Cleansing

Trained computer scientists on image process went through the hole dataset and cleaned the data by removing the images that were considered to have information that could alter the classifier's performance.

From the original dataset of 1592 images resulted a new dataset consisting of a total of 793 images distributed as follows: 3 vessels plus bladder (n = 87), gallbladder (n = 43), transverse cord insertion (n = 91), anteroposterior kidney plane (n = 77), biometry plane (n = 152), kidney sagittal plane (n = 155), bladder plane (n = 34), sagittal abdominal plane (n = 154).

The original dataset reduction was 49.81%, with the lowest class reduction size of 41.64% and the highest of 60.62%. The class reduction can be seen in Fig. 2.

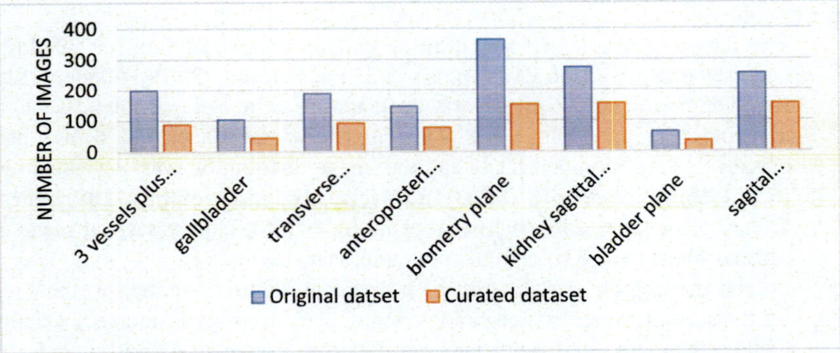

Fig. 2. Dataset cleansing. Original and cleaned dataset sizes on each class.

The resulting dataset will further be called cleaned dataset, while the images that were removed from the original dataset will be called excluded dataset.

2.3 Deep Learning Classification

With a combination of good accuracy (ACC) and prediction time, as shown on the MATLAB website [11] three pre-trained, deep learning, neural networks were selected that proved to offer good results in our previous work [12–17].

The first network we tested was AlexNet [18], a convolution-based with five convolutional layers. AlexNet model is available for free [19], and it has been integrated in MATLAB as a software package. It was introduced in 2012.

The second model we tested is GoogLeNet [20], a non-linear architecture network that has 22 layers, and uses the concept of "inception". GoogLeNet model is available for free [21], and it has been integrated in MATLAB as a software package. It was introduced in 2014.

The last model we tested was ResNet-18 [22], having similar non-linear architecture to GoogLeNet and 18 layers. It was introduced in 2016. The network model has also been integrated in MATLAB as a software package.

All models have been trained on ImageNet [23] and their aim is to classify (label) images in 1000 classes of the real world.

The transfer learning was implemented identically to all three networks. Their final fully connected classification layer was replaced with a new one, having 8 output classes for the new classification task. The new classification layer was designed to have 8 classes to match the labels of our datasets. Next, the new networks went through a re-triaging procedure. We have used the tenfold cross-validation methodology where 10% of the datasets were kept for validation and 90% for the training itself.

All three architectures were trained using the same training hyper-parameters options. The training hyper-parameters were tuned empirically: Mini Batch Size 100, initial learning rate 0.0001 and validation patience 4.

The stochastic gradient descent with momentum was used as optimizer.

The performance was assessed in terms of ACC and area under the curve (AUC).

2.4 Excluded Dataset Evaluation

The best performing architecture of each network type and each dataset were used to predict the classes of the images within the cleaned and excluded dataset. Again, the performance was assessed in terms of mean ACC and AUC.

2.5 Statistical Assessment

The deep learning networks are part of the larger family of stochastic algorithms this means that the weight adjustment is dependent on the way the training data is presented to the network. Aiming for a robust and trustworthy result, the networks have been independently run multiple times. To obtain a suitable statistical power – two-tailed type of null hypothesis with default statistical power goal $p \geq 95\%$ and type I error $\alpha = 0.05$ – level of significance, all three models have been independently run 100 time using the tenfold cross-validation previously described. At each run, input data was randomly selected and splinted in training and validation.

In the end, the networks performance results are presented as mean and standard deviation (SD).

3 Results

Using the described methodology, we obtained 100 trained networks having AlexNet architecture, 100 GoogLeNet, and 100 ResNet-18 on the original dataset and the equivalent on the cleaned dataset. Mean and SD for ACC and AUC for both datasets and for all three networks are presented in Tables 1 and 2.

Table 1. Original dataset performance assessment (mean ± SD).

Network	ACC (%)	AUC
AlexNet	91.58 ± 2.98	0.99981 ± 0.00027
GoogLeNet	82.14 ± 2.61	0.99714 ± 0.00111
ResNet-18	84.92 ± 3.09	0.99881 ± 0.00076

Table 2. Cleaned dataset performance assessment (mean ± SD).

Network	ACC (%)	AUC
AlexNet	95.47 ± 1.5	0.99998 ± 0.00004
GoogLeNet	86.36 ± 2.22	0.99773 ± 0.00100
ResNet-18	88.64 ± 1.73	0.99918 ± 0.0006

Since the sample size corresponds to 100 computer runs, the distribution of data is nearly Gaussian, as the Central Limit Theorem states that the distribution becomes normal on samples larger than 30. This in turn lets us use the parametric tests for mean assessment, namely Student's t test (for two samples) and ANOVA (for multiple samples).

Running One-way ANOVA on the ACC of the original dataset showed SS = 4708.67, with two degrees of freedom, MS = 2354.33, F = 278.00, $F_{crit} = 3.02$ and a p-value < 0.001 meaning there are significant differences between the ACCs of the three architectures. Running Student's t test between the ACCs of the three architectures on the original dataset showed a p-value < 0.001 between each pair, interpreted as significant.

Running One-way ANOVA on the AUC of the original dataset showed SS = 0.00036, with two degrees of freedom, MS = 0.00018, F = 289.31, $F_{crit} = 3.02$ and a p-value < 0.001 meaning there are significant differences between the AUCs of the three architectures. Running Student's t test between the AUCs of the three architectures on the original dataset showed a p-value < 0.001 between each pair, interpreted as significant.

Running One-way ANOVA on the ACC of the cleaned dataset showed SS = 4492.57, with two degrees of freedom, MS = 2246.28, F = 661.06, $F_{crit} = 3.02$ and a p-value < 0.001 meaning there are significant differences between the ACCs of the three architectures. Running Student's t test between the ACCs of the three architectures on the cleaned dataset showed a p-value < 0.001 between each pair, interpreted as significant.

Running One-way ANOVA on the AUC of the cleaned dataset showed SS = 0.00026, with two degrees of freedom, MS = 0.00013, F = 280.14, F_{crit} = 3.02 and a p-value < 0.001 meaning there are significant differences between the AUCs of the three architectures. Running Student's t test between the AUCs of the three architectures on the cleaned dataset showed a p-value < 0.001 between each pair, interpreted as significant.

The above statistical assessment shows that AlexNet statistically outperformed ResNet-18, and, in turn, ResNet-18 statistically outperformed GoogLeNet on all datasets and on all performance measurements (ACC and AUC).

When comparing each architecture on different dataset and on different performance measurement, we obtained Student's t test p-value < 0.001, considered significant. This means that the cleaned dataset statistically outperformed the original dataset on all performance measurements.

Results for the cleaned dataset of the best performing networks are shown in Table 3 and for the excluded dataset in Table 4.

Table 3. Cleaned dataset performance assessment of the best performing networks.

Network	Training dataset	ACC (%)	AUC
AlexNet	Original	95.71	1
GoogLeNet	Original	86.63	0.9980
ResNet-18	Original	92.05	0.9998
AlexNet	Cleaned	97.22	1
GoogLeNet	Cleaned	89.40	0.9981
ResNet-18	Cleaned	91.55	0.9995

Table 4. Excluded dataset performance assessment of the best performing networks.

Network	Training dataset	ACC (%)	AUC
AlexNet	Original	97.24	1
GoogLeNet	Original	87.35	0.9997
ResNet-18	Original	91.36	0.9999
AlexNet	Cleaned	62.82	0.9926
GoogLeNet	Cleaned	60.20	0.9829
ResNet-18	Cleaned	56.19	0.9836

4 Discussion

The explosive growth of medical investigations has resulted in both the accumulation of new data, but also in larger datasets, not necessarily quality datasets. The need for computational tools that can help with all this data analysis has become more and more stringent, not to mention the fact that computational analysis is involved in almost every step of scientific study.

Our study used a dataset obtained from pregnant women admitted to the Prenatal Unit for second-trimester morphology within the University Emergency County Hospital Craiova, Romania, and Ginecho Clinic, Craiova, Romania. We had 1592 ultrasonography images of fetal morphology sections that were cleansed until we obtained a dataset consisting of 793 images.

The cleaned dataset had a statistically better performance than the original dataset, though its size was reduced by 49.81%. The three networks had a constant behavior, AlexNet statistically outperformed ResNet-18, while ResNet-18 statistically outperformed GoogLeNet. Nevertheless, average ACC performance was above 80% for all networks on all datasets.

Important insights stand out from Tables 3 and 4. From Table 3 we can see that the networks that were trained on the original dataset underperform the networks from the cleaned dataset. This is in spite of the fact that the cleaned dataset is included in the original dataset. So, the networks trained on the original dataset found some different features to differentiate between the images. From Table 4 we see that the performance of the networks trained on the original dataset is actually larger than the average performance on the original dataset. This could be, again, due to irrelevant features learned from un-cleaned data. The networks that were trained on the cleaned dataset, this time, have a drop in performance at about 60% ACC. This could be due to the fact that they have never encountered un-cleaned images in the training and validation sequences, or perhaps they themselves have evolved to select irrelevant features.

In general, data quality includes many different issues, for example, questions of completeness, accuracy, consistency, timeliness, duplication, validity, availability, and provenance [24]. We encountered four main image characteristics in our original dataset that disqualified the images that we removed. The first aspect was the overview of the image, present in the bottom-left corner (Fig. 1 A-D). The second aspect that was used for discarding images was the dual view in the same screen – standard versus Doppler – as in Fig. 1 B. The third aspect was a different color of the overall image (Fig. 1 C) resulted by using contrast enhanced ultrasonography. The last aspect was the presence of large shadow cones, possibly generated by the positioning of the probe, as in Fig. 1 A.

The fact that we found more than 49% of the data to be unsuitable for the task is not that astonishing as Fayyad et al. concluded that as much as 40% of the collected data is dirty in one way or another [10].

In the medical field, approaching a slightly different problem from our own - as it did not use images, Brusic et al. [25] conclude that the high accuracy of the models was achieved by data cleansing techniques and by cyclical retraining using the new data. Using the same ten-fold cross-validation methodology, Barakat et al. [26], run several machine learning algorithms on their original dataset, and their results were of moderate quality. Consecutively the clean dataset provided better results and was used for their research. No further cleansing details were offered, as their research goal was different. Rokham et al. [27] show an improvement in the accuracy of the deep learning model even for the first iteration after data cleansing.

Through their experiments, Juak et al. [28] note that neural network and linear regression models performed best for imputation. Koszalinski et al. [28] concluded that the models will likely improve in accuracy with increasingly robust data sets, but their concern was on missing data, and not on the quality of data.

In other fields, data cleansing shows good results. Høverstad et al. treat data cleansing as a correction problem (unlike us where we removed data) and get better results on energy load prediction after applying the process. In the field of human activity recognition, Neira-Rodado et al. [29] used as evaluation metrics the results of k-nearest neighbor, and random forest classifiers the performance of the classifier was improved from 55.9% to 63.59% by data cleansing. In the field of urban bus commercial speed prediction, Lyan et al. [30] conclude that data quality is needed to ensure acceptable data sets statistics and prediction accuracy.

Hara et al. [31] take our approach to the next level. They design a model based on SGD (the optimizer used in our research), that can detect the "influential instances". They demonstrate that machine learning models can be effectively improved by removing the influential instances suggested by the proposed method. Though this might sound great we consider human interaction in data cleansing to be crucial, and would use a predictive system as their proposal just to highlight the cases, not for the final decision.

Ridzuan et al. [32] make a review on data cleansing methods for big data and conclude that the importance of domain experts in the data cleansing process is undeniable as verification and validation are the main concerns of the cleansed data. We argue that the final data cleansing should be done by a non-expert in the field of data, and by an expert in data science. A field expert will always be subjective, and muscle-memory and connections with knowledge outside the dataset will influence their decision. Hosseinzadeh et al. [33] find five categories of data errors: machine learning-based, sample-based, expert-based, rule-based, and framework-based mechanisms. As they identify the expert-based class we would argue that the classes sample-based and rule-based have, at least in part, their origin in the expert.

As mentioned before, it is very important to establish very clear criteria when trying to cleanse a dataset. Also, it is very important, not to allow the software to take control over the cleansing itself, but to guide it thoroughly from the start, according to human chosen criteria. Here, we must mention the idea of defining a standard. Having standard criteria, that the algorithm can use to cleanse the database is useful not only for the relevance of our study's data, but it can also be valuable when it comes to the study's reproducibility. The first step in defining a standard should be to invite all data users to define what they believe to be the standard criteria. The second step consists in defining a simple set of rules that can lead to the final, standard form of the data. The last step involves presenting it to the scientific committee of the study for comments and potential improvements.

Regarding the legal aspects and fundamental rights, The European Union Agency for Fundamental Rights prepared, in 2019, a focus paper: Data quality and artificial intelligence – mitigating bias and error to protect fundamental rights [34] where they make two outstanding observations (1) it is important to increase awareness and knowledge among businesses – both public and private – about how algorithms work; as part of an improved understanding of algorithms, it is important to query what the basis for the development of algorithms is: the data, and (2) the quality of data can give the rise of discriminatory or otherwise erroneous machine learning systems. The observations should apply also to physicians working on medical research projects, as their responsibility is to transfer their knowledge in a correct way. Also, underlining the legal aspects of data cleansing Stöger et al. [35] motivate, demonstrate, and justify why data cleaning is important for the quality and safety of medical AI systems and should not be underestimated from either a technical or legal perspective.

Munappy et al. [36] conclude that deep learning technology has achieved very promising results and that the current focus should be on the field of data management to build high-quality datasets if we ever want to have production-ready deep learning systems.

A future research direction will investigate the integration of various methods to address automated error detection. The ultimate goal of this direction is to design and implement software tools to address the data cleansing problem.

5 Conclusion

As for evidence-based medicine, data cleansing must be applied before applying any machine learning algorithm before the preprocessing steps.

In a research context, physicians should comprehend machine learning terminology and try to understand the mechanics behind each computational method to provide suitable data and expertise.

Data cleansing should be driven by computer scientists, though they have less understanding of the medical problem itself, their knowledge of machine learning mechanics helps improve their decisions.

Acknowledgements. This work was supported by a grant of the Ministry of Research Innovation and Digitization, CNCS-UEFISCDI, project number PN-III-P4-PCE-2021–0057, within PNCDI III.

References

1. Shazly, S.A., Trabuco, E.C., Ngufor, C.G., Famuyide, A.O.: Introduction to machine learning in obstetrics and gynecology. Obstet. Gynecol. **139**, 669–679 (2022). https://doi.org/10.1097/AOG.0000000000004706
2. Wang, R., et al.: Artificial intelligence in reproductive medicine. Reproduction **158**, R139–R154 (2019). https://doi.org/10.1530/REP-18-0523
3. Pehrson, L.M., Lauridsen, C., Nielsen, M.B.: Machine learning and deep learning applied in ultrasound. Ultraschall Med. **39**, 379–381 (2018). https://doi.org/10.1055/A-0642-9545
4. Shen, Y.T., Chen, L., Yue, W.W., Xu, H.X.: Artificial intelligence in ultrasound. Eur. J. Radiol. **139** (2021). https://doi.org/10.1016/J.EJRAD.2021.109717
5. Fu, G.S., Levin-Schwartz, Y., Lin, Q.H., Zhang, D.: Machine learning for medical imaging. J. Healthc. Eng. **2019** (2019). https://doi.org/10.1155/2019/9874591
6. Madabhushi, A., Lee, G.: Image analysis and machine learning in digital pathology: challenges and opportunities. Med. Image Anal. **33**, 170–175 (2016). https://doi.org/10.1016/J.MEDIA.2016.06.037

7. Maletic, J.I., Marcus, A.: Data Cleansing. Data Mining and Knowledge Discovery Handbook, pp. 21–36 (2006). https://doi.org/10.1007/0-387-25465-X_2
8. Loshin, D.: Data Cleansing. Enterprise Knowledge Management, pp. 333–380 (2001). https://doi.org/10.1016/B978-012455840-3.50014-5
9. Kang, M., Tian, J.: Machine Learning: Data Pre-processing. Prognostics and Health Management of Electronics, pp. 111–130 (2018). https://doi.org/10.1002/9781119515326.CH5
10. Fayyad, U.M., Piatetsky-Shapiro, G., Uthurusamy, R.: Summary from the KDD-03 panel. ACM SIGKDD Explor. Newsl. **5**, 191–196 (2003). https://doi.org/10.1145/980972.981004
11. Pretrained Deep Neural Networks—MATLAB & Simulink. https://www.mathworks.com/help/deeplearning/ug/pretrained-convolutional-neural-networks.html
12. Bungărdean, R.M., Şerbănescu, M.-S., Streba, C.T., Crişan, M.: Deep learning with transfer learning in pathology. Case study: classification of basal cell carcinoma. Rom. J. Morphol. Embryol. **62**, 1017–1028 (2021). https://doi.org/10.47162/RJME.62.4.14
13. Nica, R.E., Şerbănescu, M.S., Florescu, L.M., Camen, G.C., Streba, C.T., Gheonea, I.A.: Deep learning: a promising method for histological class prediction of breast tumors in mammography. J. Digit. Imaging **34**, 1190–1198 (2021). https://doi.org/10.1007/S10278-021-00508-4
14. Şerbănescu, M.S., Oancea, C.N., Streba, C.T., Pleşea, I.E., Pirici, D., Streba, L., Pleşea, R.M.: Agreement of two pre-trained deep-learning neural networks built with transfer learning with six pathologists on 6000 patches of prostate cancer from gleason2019 challenge. Rom. J. Morphol. Embryol. **61** (2020). https://doi.org/10.47162/RJME.61.2.21
15. Şerbănescu, M.S., Manea, N.C., Streba, L., Belciug, S., Pleşea, I.E., Pirici, I., Bungărdean, R.M., Pleşea, R.M.: Automated gleason grading of prostate cancer using transfer learning from general-purpose deep-learning networks. Rom. J. Morphol. Embryol. **61** (2020). https://doi.org/10.47162/RJME.61.1.17
16. Şerbănescu, M.S., Bungărdean, R.M., Georgiu, C., Crişan, M.: Nodular and micronodular basal cell carcinoma subtypes are different tumors based on their morphological architecture and their interaction with the surrounding stroma. Diagnostics (Basel) **12** (2022). https://doi.org/10.3390/DIAGNOSTICS12071636
17. Florescu, L.M., Streba, C.T., Şerbănescu, M.S., Mămuleanu, M., Florescu, D.N., Teică, R.V., Nica, R.E., Gheonea, I.A.: Federated learning approach with pre-trained deep learning models for COVID-19 detection from unsegmented CT images. Life **12**, 958 (2022). https://doi.org/10.3390/LIFE12070958
18. Krizhevsky, A., Sutskever, I., Hinton, G.E.: ImageNet classification with deep convolutional neural networks
19. BVLC AlexNet Model. https://github.com/BVLC/caffe/tree/master/models/bvlc_alexnet
20. Szegedy, C., Liu, W., Jia, Y., Sermanet, P., Reed, S., Anguelov, D., Erhan, D., Vanhoucke, V., Rabinovich, A.: Going deeper with convolutions. In: Proceedings of the IEEE Computer Society Conference on Computer Vision and Pattern Recognition (2015)
21. BVLC GoogLeNet Model. https://github.com/BVLC/caffe/tree/master/models/bvlc_googlenet
22. He, K., Zhang, X., Ren, S., Sun, J.: Deep residual learning for image recognition. In: Proceedings of the IEEE Computer Society Conference on Computer Vision and Pattern Recognition, pp. 770–778 (2016). https://doi.org/10.1109/CVPR.2016.90
23. ImageNet. https://image-net.org/
24. Burt, A., Leong, B., Shirrell, S.: Beyond explainability: a practical guide to managing risk in machine learning models. Immuta Scholar; J.D. Candidate (2018)
25. Brusic, V., Brusic, V., Zeleznikow, J., Bono, E., Hammer, J., et al.: Data cleansing for computer models: a case study. In: 6TH International Conference on Neural Information Processing (ICONIP), pp. 2–603 (1999)

26. Barakat, N.H., Barakat, S.H., Ahmed, N.: Prediction and staging of hepatic fibrosis in children with hepatitis C virus: a machine learning approach. Healthc. Inform. Res. **25**, 173 (2019). https://doi.org/10.4258/HIR.2019.25.3.173
27. Rokham, H., Pearlson, G., Abrol, A., Falakshahi, H., Plis, S., Calhoun, V.D.: Addressing inaccurate nosology in mental health: a multi label data cleansing approach for detecting label noise from structural magnetic resonance imaging data in mood and psychosis disorders. bioRxiv. 2020.05.06.081521 (2020). https://doi.org/10.1101/2020.05.06.081521
28. Jauk, S., Kramer, D., Leodolter, W.: Cleansing and imputation of body mass index data and its impact on a machine learning based prediction model. Stud. Health Technol. Inform. **248**, 116–123 (2018). https://doi.org/10.3233/978-1-61499-858-7-116
29. Neira-Rodado, D., Nugent, C., Cleland, I., Velasquez, J., Viloria, A.: Evaluating the impact of a two-stage multivariate data cleansing approach to improve to the performance of machine learning classifiers: a case study in human activity recognition. Sensors **20**, 1858 (2020). https://doi.org/10.3390/S20071858
30. Lyan, G., Gross-Amblard, D., Jezequel, J.-M., Malinowski, S.: Impact of data cleansing for urban bus commercial speed prediction. SN Comput. Sci. **3**, 1–12 (2021). https://doi.org/10.1007/S42979-021-00966-1
31. Hara, S., Nitanda, A., Maehara, T.: Data cleansing for models trained with SGD. https://doi.org/10.5555/3454287
32. Ridzuan, F., Wan Zainon, W.M.N.: A review on data cleansing methods for big data. Procedia Comput. Sci. **161**, 731–738 (2019). https://doi.org/10.1016/J.PROCS.2019.11.177
33. Hosseinzadeh, M., et al.: Data cleansing mechanisms and approaches for big data analytics: a systematic study. J. Ambient. Intell. Humaniz. Comput. (2021). https://doi.org/10.1007/S12652-021-03590-2
34. Data quality and artificial intelligence—mitigating bias and error to protect fundamental rights|European Union Agency for Fundamental Rights. https://fra.europa.eu/en/publication/2019/data-quality-and-artificial-intelligence-mitigating-bias-and-error-protect
35. Stöger, K., Schneeberger, D., Kieseberg, P., Holzinger, A.: Legal aspects of data cleansing in medical AI. Comput. Law Secur. Rev. **42**, 105587 (2021). https://doi.org/10.1016/J.CLSR.2021.105587
36. Munappy, A.R., Bosch, J., Olsson, H.H., Arpteg, A., Brinne, B.: Data management for production quality deep learning models: challenges and solutions. J. Syst. Softw. **191**, 111359 (2022). https://doi.org/10.1016/J.JSS.2022.111359

Classification of Liver Abnormality in Ultrasonic Images Using Hilbert Transform Based Feature

Karthikamani R.[1(✉)] and Harikumar Rajaguru[2]

[1] Sri Ramakrishna Engineering College, Coimbatore, Tamil Nadu 641022, India
karthikamaniece@gmail.com

[2] Bannari Amman Institute of Technology, Sathyamangalam, Tamil Nadu 638 401, India

Abstract. The diagnosis of liver abnormalities from ultrasonic images is examined in this paper using transform Based features and classifiers. The liver ultrasonic images are acquired from cancer imaging archive database and Hilbert Transform based features are extracted from the liver ultrasonic images. The five classifiers Softmax Discriminant Classifier (SDC), Detrend Fluctuation Analysis, Naïve Bayesian Classifier (NBC), Harmonic search, Artificial Algae optimization (AAO) are utilized to identify abnormalities in liver ultrasound images. The classifiers performances are analyzed using standard parameters such as sensitivity, Specificity, Accuracy, Error Rate, Mathew Correlation Coefficient (MCC), and Jaccard Metric (JM). The Artificial Algae optimization (AAO) classifier outperforms with other classifiers with highest classification accuracy of 98.92% and an error rate of 1.08%.

Keywords: Hilbert transform · SDC · AAO · MCC · JM

1 Introduction

The liver is the major organ in the human body. It converts dietary nutrients into usable body substances, stores them, and supplies them to cells as needed. Also converts toxic substances into harmless ones [1]. The liver also produces bile, protein, glucose, hemoglobin, immune factors, and clears bilirubin. Thus, it is the most important organ, and maintaining its health is crucial for overall health [2]. With the increasing prevalence of unhealthy lifestyles and lack of physical activity, liver diseases are now a common thing. Most people worldwide suffer from acute to severe liver problems due to unhealthy lifestyles [3]. The Liver biopsy is the standard technique to detect liver diseases but it is an invasive method and it may result morbidity. The imaging technique, which is non-invasive, is an indirect means for diagnosing diseases. Computer Tomography (CT), MRI, X-Ray imaging, Ultrasonography, and Radiography are among the imaging techniques used. Ultrasonography is the most commonly used imaging technique due to its non-ionizing radiation, safety, non-invasiveness, and low cost [4].

S. Vlad and N. M. Roman (Eds.): MEDITECH 2022, IFMBE Proceedings 102, pp. 51–58, 2024.
https://doi.org/10.1007/978-3-031-51120-2_6

2 Materials and Methods

This work's overall process includes Acquisition of Image, Preprocessing, Feature Extraction, and Classification. Filters are used in preprocessing to remove noise. Hilbert transform features are extracted then Five Classifiers are employed to classify the liver abnormalities. The classifier's performance is assessed and compared using the benchmark parameters. Figure 1 shows the workflow of the liver cirrhosis detection.

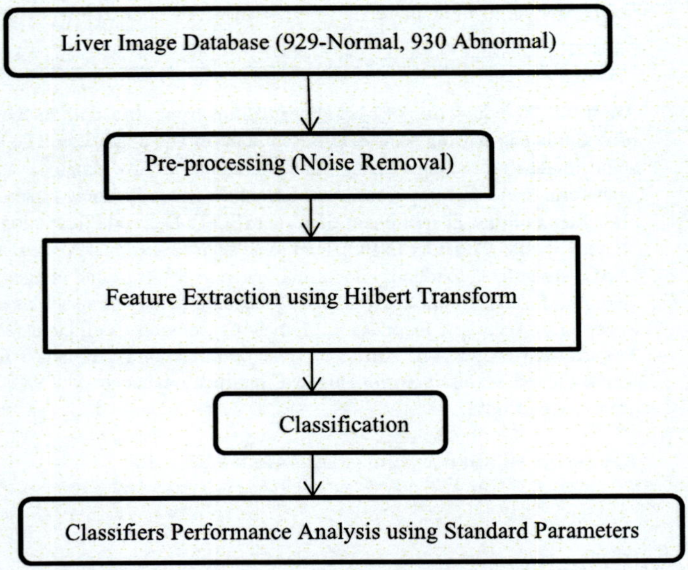

Fig. 1. Methodology of the proposed work.

2.1 Preprocessing

The database contains 1859 (B-mode) ultrasound images. The images captured are labeled "normal" and "cirrhosis liver." Ultrasound images are less effective due to the noise introduced during image acquisition. The speckle noise primarily affects ultrasonic images [5]. The following is a model for speckle noise

$$z(q, r) = x(q, r)y(q, r) \tag{1}$$

where $z(q, r)$ is observed signal, $x(q, r)$ is original signal and the noise component is $y(q, r)$. Generally the usefulness of computer aided diagnostic system can be improved by reducing this unwanted signal using suitable filtering techniques. The adaptive wiener filtering is used in this work to suppress speckle noise.

2.2 Feature Extraction Using Hilbert Transform

Feature extraction is a technique used for breaking down huge amounts of raw data into smaller chunks, more manageable groups for processing. The useful features of the ultrasonic images are extracted using Hilbert transform. The Hilbert Transform is a linear operator in mathematics and signal processing that gets a function Y(t) and produces a function, H(Y(t)), with the same domain. The Hilbert Transform is a fundamental tool in Fourier analysis that gives a tangible way to realize the harmonic conjugate of a given function or Fourier series [6].

$$Y_h(t) = H(Y(t)) = Y(t) * \frac{1}{\Pi t} = \frac{1}{\Pi}\int_{-\infty}^{\infty} \frac{y(\tau)}{t-\tau} d\tau == \frac{1}{\Pi}\int_{-\infty}^{\infty} \frac{y(t-\tau)}{\tau} d\tau \quad (2)$$

The convolution of Y(t) with(1/t) is the Hilbert transform of Y(t). It is the impulse response to Y(t) of a linear time-invariant filter also called a Hilbert transformer [7]. The impulse response is represented as $\frac{1}{\pi t}$.

Table 1. Extracted Features using Hilbert Transform.

Statistical parameters	Normal	Abnormal (Cirrhosis)
Mean	0.3183	0.3048
Variance	0.0382	0.0313
Skewness	0.5542	0.5907
Kurtosis	0.3491	−0.2859
Pearson correlation coefficient	0.5724	0.5091
CCA	**0.7607**	

The above Table 1 shows the result of statistical parameters obtained for the liver cirrhosis and normal data for Hilbert Transform feature extraction techniques. Skewness is based on the data distribution's symmetry. The Pearson Correlation coefficient describes the relationship between two continuous data sets. The two sets of data used in this work are normal liver case and abnormal liver (Cirrhosis) case. The association between the two sets of data is determined by Canonical Correlation Analysis (CCA).Here the CCA is 0.7607 indicates the features are correlated. Figure 2 shows the scatter plot of Hilbert transform based features. It indicates the features are overlapped. Therefore the classifiers are employed for classification of liver abnormality.

3 Liver Cirrhosis Detection Using Classifiers

The classifiers classify the data into classes or groups in order to predict or detect the desired output. Six classifiers are employed for this purpose.

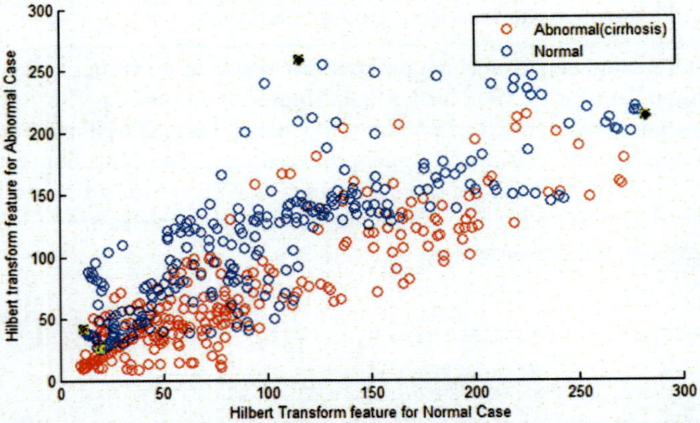

Fig. 2. Scatter plot hilbert transform for normal and abnormal liver ultrasonic images.

3.1 Softmax Discriminant Classifier (SDC)

The SDA classifier is more valuable and efficient. The SDA's goal is to detect a subclass where a specific test must be applied, which is accomplished through classification. It is accomplished especially by comparing and assessing the distance between the training and test samples [8]. The label information is assigned with the aid of a nonlinear transformation of the distance.

Consider the dataset from t distinct classes is represented by

$$Z = [Z_1, Z_2, Z_3, ... Z_t] \in R^{bc} \tag{3}$$

For tth class the sample Z_t is given as

$$Z_t = [Z_1^t, Z_2^t, Z_3^t, ..Z_c^t] \in R^{bc} \tag{4}$$

The SDA is represented as

$$h(x) = \arg \max_i e_z^i \tag{5}$$

3.2 Detrend Fluctuation Analysis (DFA)

The detrended fluctuation analysis technique has been effective in demonstrating the strength of long-range correlations in time-series data. It offers a simplified quantitative statistic called the scaled parameter α, which serves as a mark of the signal's correlation characteristics. A time series of length N termed y(k) is divided into N/n non-overlapping boxes using the DFA method A least-squares line is used to fit the data in each box of length n. (representing the trend in that box). y_n (k) stands for the straight line segments' y coordinate. Detrending is done by subtracting the local trend y_n (k) from each box from the integrated time series y(k) [9].

$$F_n = \sqrt{\frac{1}{N}\sum_{k=1}^{N}[y(k) - y_n(k)]^2} \tag{6}$$

3.3 Harmonic Search

The problem's description and parameter definition come first in the use of the Harmony Search Algorithm. This is a crucial stage since a practical approach to the optimization problem depends on the definition of the choice variables, their bounds, and their participation in the objective function [10].

The matrix containing the Harmony Memory is created following the declaration of the variables. The matrix has the dimensions m x n, where m is the size of the Harmony Memory and n is the total number of variables used in the objective function. The approach stipulates that the matrix must contain all starting values prior to the first execution. Typically, sets of random values for the decision variables are used to do this. The algorithm is now prepared to begin creating and evaluating new "Harmonies" by imitating the pursuit of musical harmony through the use of the following mechanisms in relation to the operations.

The idea is that the algorithm will pick a nearby value of the term x_i if it decides to slightly modify the term it chose from the harmonic memory, such as

$$x_i^{new} = x_i \pm Random(bw) \tag{7}$$

where Random (bw) represents the adjustment's bandwidth and is a random number between 0 and 1. This process is comparable to genetic algorithms' mutation. It is vital to remember that even while PAR can only accept very small numbers, it is thought to be crucial for the algorithm's convergence [11].

3.4 Artificial Algae Optimization (AAO)

The artificial algae algorithm (AAO), a recently developed bio-inspired optimization algorithm, was inspired by the living behaviors of microalgae. By idealizing the qualities of algae, artificial algae correspond to each solution in the problem space. Artificial algae may travel toward the light source to photosynthesize in a manner similar to actual algae. They can also adapt to their surroundings, alter the dominant species, and reproduce by mitotic division. The algorithm thus consisted of three fundamental components, referred to as "Evolutionary Process," "Adaptation," and "Helical Movement." Algae are the main genera in the algorithm. Algal colonies made up this population as a whole. Algal colonies are collections of live algae. One algal cell divides into two new algal cells, which live next to one another. When these two are divided again, another four cells live next to one another, and so on. Algal cells move collectively, behave like a single cell, and are susceptible to death in unfavourable environmental conditions. The colony may be divided into smaller parts by an external force like a shear strain or by unfavorable conditions, and as life continues, each divided component develops into a new colony. The colony of optimums, which is made up of the best-performing algae cells, is the one that currently exists at the optimum point [12].

$$\text{Population of Algal colony} = \begin{pmatrix} x_1^1 & \ldots & x_1^D \\ \vdots & \ddots & \vdots \\ x_N^1 & \ldots & x_N^D \end{pmatrix} \tag{8}$$

ith algal colony $= [x_i^1, x_i^2, \ldots x_i^D]$, where x_i^j is algal cell in jth dimension of ith algal colony.

3.5 Naïve Bayesian Classifier (NBC)

It is a feed forward neural network that is a member of the family of probability classifiers and it has the ability to solve classification and regression issues [13]. On the basis of its estimated probability, the Bayes rule is applied to new input data in order to assign it to a higher posterior probability class.

$$P(c/z) = \frac{P(z/c)P(c)}{P(z)} \tag{9}$$

4 Results and Discussion

The performance of the algorithm is analyzed using confusion matrix depicted in Table 2. The confusion matrix produces four types of results: TP (True Positive), TN (True Negative), FP (False Positive), and FN (False Negative) (False Negative). The classifiers analyze parameters such as Sensitivity, Specificity, Accuracy, Error rate, Mathew correlation coefficient (MCC), Jaccard Metric are examined.

Table 2. Confusion matrix - binary classification outcomes.

	Actual values	
Prediction	Positive	Negative
Positive	True Positive (#TP)	False Negative (#FN)
Negative	False Positive (#FP)	True Negative (#TN)

The Mean Squared Error is the ending criterion for all classifiers (MSE). MSE is defined as the average squared difference between obtained and actual values.

$$MSE = \frac{1}{M}\sum_{i=1}^{N}(T_i - O_j)^2 \tag{10}$$

Table 3. Confusion matrix and MSE of Hilbert transform.

S.No	Classifiers	TP	TN	FP	FN	MSE
1	Softmax Discriminant Classifier (SDC)	840	848	90	81	2.75E-05
2	Detrend fluctuation analysis	850	800	80	129	3.25E-05
3	Harmonic search	822	868	108	61	2.56E-05
4	Artificial Algae optimization (AAO)	919	920	11	9	1.85E-06
5	Naïve Bayesian Classifier (NBC)	898	888	32	41	3.61E-04

where M is Number of data points, Ti is observed values and Oj is the Predicted values.

The lower MSE value indicates the classifier is perfect and higher MSE indicates the model is least performing. From Table 3 it is observed that the classifier Artificial Algae optimization (AAO) obtained a lowest MSE of 1.85E-06 and the Naïve Bayesian Classifier (NBC) attained maximum MSE of 3.61E-04.

Table 4. Performance analysis of Hilbert transform in the detection of liver cirrhosis.

S.No	Classifiers	Sensitivity	Specificity	Accuracy	Error rate	Mathew correlation coefficient	Jaccard Metric (JM)
1	Softmax Discriminant Classifier (SDC)	91.21	90.41	90.80	9.20	0.8161	83.09
2	Detrend fluctuation analysis	86.82	90.91	88.76	11.24	0.7762	80.26
3	Harmonic search	93.09	88.93	90.91	9.09	0.8192	82.95
4	Artificial Algae optimization (AAO)	99.03	98.82	98.92	1.08	0.9785	97.87
5	Naïve Bayesian Classifier (NBC)	59.52	52.38	55.95	44.05	0.1194	40.32

The Sensitivity, Specificity, Accuracy, Error Rate, MCC, JM are the different parameters perceived when analyzing classifier performance. Because any medical diagnostic device is prone to error, performance analysis is an important consideration in any classification process. The percentage of accuracy of a classifier is determined by the number of occurrences of exact prediction of class, which is a primitive metric of measure of any classifier. As a result, after calculating the sum of the prediction of instances, the following formula 11 can be used to calculate the classifier's accuracy.

$$Accuracy = \frac{TP + TN}{TP + TN + FP + FN} * 100 \tag{11}$$

Table 4 shows the performance analysis of the classifier to detect liver cirrhosis from Hilbert transform based feature extraction. AAO classifiers outperforms with 98.92% accuracy compared with other classifiers with 1.08 of error rate.

5 Conclusion

The ultrasonic liver images are classified in this work using five classifiers. Because of the non-ionization radiation, ultrasonic images are widely used in medical imaging. Early diagnosis with an effective classification system is typically required in healthcare applications for appropriate treatment. The ultrasonic liver images are obtained from cancer image archive database. The features are extracted using hilbert transform. Out of five classifiers, Artificial Algae Optimization (AAO) algorithm has given more accurate result of 98.92% and with low error rate of 1.08% for hilbert transforms features, when compared to remaining classifiers. The Naïve Bayesian Classifier (NBC) classifier gives the lowest accuracy of 55.95% and highest error rate of 44.05%. Thus, the AAO classifier provides the more accurate results. In future the cluster based features along with hybrid classifiers will be used for classification of liver abnormality.

Conflict of Interest. The authors declare that they have no conflicts of interest.

References

1. Tanwar, N., Rahman, K.F.: Machine learning in liver disease diagnosis: current progress and future opportunities. IOP Conf. Ser.: Mater. Sci. Eng. **1022**, 012029 (2021)
2. Rabbi, M.F., Mahedy Hasan, S.M., Champa, A.I., Asif Zaman, M., Hasan, M.K.: Prediction of liver disorders using machine learning algorithms: a comparative study. In: 2020 2nd International Conference on Advanced Information and Communication Technology (ICAICT), pp. 111–116 (2020)
3. Alivar, A., Daniali, H., Helfroush, M.S.: Classification of liver diseases using ultrasound images based on feature combination. In: IEEE Proceedings 2014
4. Yeom, S.K., et al.: Prediction of liver cirrhosis, using diagnostic imaging tools. World J. Hepatol. **7**(17), 2069–2079 (2015)
5. Duarte-Salazar, C.A., Castro-Ospina, A.E., Becerra, M.A., Delgado-Trejos, E.: Speckle noise reduction in ultrasound images for improving the metrological evaluation of biomedical applications: an overview. IEEE Access **8**, 15983–15999 (2020)
6. Mukhopadhyay, S., Mitra, M., Mitra, S.: ECG feature extraction using differentiation, Hilbert transform, variable threshold and slope reversal approach. J. Med. Eng. Technol. **36**, 372–386 (2012). https://doi.org/10.3109/03091902.2012.713438

7. Stefan, Hilbert, L.: Transforms in Transforms and Applications Handbook. CRC Press Inc., Boca Raton, FL (1996)
8. Zang, Zhang, J.S.: Softmax discriminant classifier. In: 2011 Third International Conference on Multimedia Information Networking and Security, pp. 16–19, Shanghai, China (2011)
9. Rajaguru, Kumar Prabhakar S.: Bayesian linear discriminant analysis for breast cancer classification. In: 2017 2nd International Conference on Communication and Electronics Systems (ICCES), pp. 266–269, Coimbatore, India (2017)
10. Dubey, M.: A systematic review on harmony search algorithm: theory, literature, and applications. Math. Probl. Eng. **2021**, Article ID 5594267 (2021)
11. Kim, J.H.: Harmony search algorithm: a unique music-inspired algorithm. Procedia Eng. **154**, 1401–1405 (2016). ISSN 1877-7058
12. Korkmaz, S., Babalik, A., Kiran, M.S.: An artificial algae algorithm for solving binary optimization problems. Int. J. Mach. Learn. Cyber. **9**, 1233–1247 (2018)
13. Kaviani, P., Dhotre, S.: Short survey on naive Bayes algorithm. Int. J. Adv. Eng. Res. Dev. **4**(11) (2017)

Cataract Diagnosis Using Convolutional Neural Networks Classifiers. A Preliminary Study

Oana-Cristina Ciaca and Simona Vlad(✉)

Technical University of Cluj-Napoca, Cluj-Napoca, Romania
simona.vlad@ethm.utcluj.ro

Abstract. Cataract detection systems are meant to assist ophthalmologists in providing a more accurate diagnostic in a shorter period of time. In this paper, the functionality of four classifiers obtained with different pre-trained Convolutional Neural Networks (CNN) were tested and compared in order to determine a suitable way of achieving automated cataract classification. Thus, fundus images taken from two different datasets are to be classified in each of the two classes (normal eye and cataract) or three classes (normal eye, moderate cataract and severe cataract) by using four pre-trained CNNs (AlexNet, GoogleNet, InceptionV3 and Inception-ResNet-V2). Our paper also focuses on the challenges of obtaining a proper cataract detection system and proposes different approaches to improving its functionality.

Keywords: Cataract diagnosis · CNN · AlexNet · GoogleNet · InceptionV3 · Inception-ResNet-V2 · Fundus images

1 Introduction

Clear fundus images are of major importance when searching for different eye anomalies. Any image obturation may lead to a misinterpretation of the retinal structures, thereby causing problems in establishing a correct diagnosis. Apart from the conventional diagnosis methods, an automated cataract detection system could become useful tools in assisting ophthalmologists in both their work with patients and their research [1].

Detecting cataracts at an early stage is an important step in preventing the disease's natural evolution to blindness. According to the world health organization (WHO) 2021 report, one billion cases of vision impairments could have been prevented, out of which 94 million are undetected cataracts. When searching for a diagnosis, the medical history of each individual is to be considered, raising the chances of obtaining a subjective result and making it difficult for ophthalmologists to maintain constant control over a high number of patients [2]. Furthermore, underdeveloped countries lack both human resources and proper equipment for overcoming the increasing number of patients [1]. On this note, developing an automated system for cataract detection improves patients life quality by helping ophthalmologists focus more on the treatment and prevention of cataracts, rather than the diagnosis. Moreover, one such system not only could optimize

S. Vlad and N. M. Roman (Eds.): MEDITECH 2022, IFMBE Proceedings 102, pp. 60–68, 2024.
https://doi.org/10.1007/978-3-031-51120-2_7

the process of ophthalmologic screenings [1], but could also speed up the diagnosis of other eye diseases which are hidden by the cloudiness of the image.

The algorithm for automatic cataract detection uses CNN's to classify fundus images into several classes, thus being able to categorize any image into one of these classes. It is important that the algorithm is effective, has high sensitivity, and can provide accurate results promptly to detect not only the progression of the cataract but also possible changes that may appear during treatment. The retinal image can be taken either by an ophthalmologist or an optometrist and processed using a computer to detect the type of cataract. This alternative method can be used especially in the third world countries for reducing time, effort and costs.

In this paper, different classification methods were tested and compared in order to establish a suitable way of achieving automated cataract detection. Additionally, the paper aims to correctly identify the cataract cases especially, since cataract images classified as healthy eyes are more problematic than vice versa. Once classified as a cataract, the healthy eye will be retested and will eventually receive the correct diagnosis, while the misclassified cataract will progress.

2 Related Work

In 2017, Lingling Zhang et al. [3], proposed a model of cataract detection with deep CNN's, using a dataset comprised of 5620 images, out of which 1598 for mild cataract, 472 for moderate cataract and 281 for severe cataract. The results obtained for cataract detection (cataract, non-cataractous) had an accuracy of 93.52% and those obtained for cataract grading (normal eye and three types of cataract) had an accuracy of 86.69%.

A method using a pre-trained CNN for cataract diagnosis is proposed by Turimerla Pratap et al. [4]. The authors used both Support Vector Machine (SVM) classifier for feature extraction and the pre-trained CNN AlexNet for image classification. The green channel was extracted from the images and the results were obtained for both two-class classification (100% accuracy) and four-class classification (92.91% accuracy).

An interesting approach in terms of two-class cataract classification is proposed by Masum Shah Junayed et al. [5] with a novel pre-trained CNN, named CataractNet. The network has 16 layers, is optimized with the Adam optimizer and achieved accuracy of 99.13% for two-class classification (cataract and non-cataractous).

Testing the functionality of different pre-trained CNNs for cataract detection was studied by Md Kamrul Hasan et. al. [6] in 2021. The networks used were InceptionV3, InceptionResnetV2, Xception, and DenseNet121 for a two-class classification (cataract and normal eye) with a dataset consisting of 1088 fundus images. The best results were obtained with InceptionResNet-V2 model, which could classify cataract disease with a test accuracy of 98.17%, a sensitivity of 97%, and a specificity of 100%.

Apart from deep learning, other types of automatic systems were studied for cataract detection, either by using pattern recognition [7], principal component analysis [2], ensemble learning [1, 8], semi-supervised learning [9] or machine learning [10]. These methods have successfully achieved satisfactory results.

3 Methodology

3.1 Dataset

CNN training requires a high number of samples for the network to be able to properly learn the features. The retinal images used in this paper were taken from two open access datasets.

Cataract Dataset. [11] The first dataset consisted of 200 images, and was already classified in two classes: cataract (100 images) and normal eye (100 images). This dataset came in aid for obtaining both training and validation results.

Ocular Disease Intelligent Recognition. [12] The second dataset consisted of 1088 fundus images collected from various hospitals and medical institutions around China by Shanggong Medical Technology Co., Ltd. 5000 patients' ages, color fundus photographs of their right and left eyes, and diagnostic keywords provided by doctors are included in this database. Taking into account the fact that there were multiple eye diseases in this dataset, only normal eye images and cataract images were extracted for the purpose of this paper. Ocular Disease Intelligent Recognition dataset has been utilized for testing results only.

3.2 Image Classification

The classification was made manually, with the help of a medical professional with whom we collaborated, based on their personal experiences in the ophthalmological field. The classification criteria are as follows:

1. The visibility of the optic nerve's contour and details.
2. The visibility of the retinal structures, arteries and veins.
3. The visibility of the choroidal tissue.

Therefore, the cataract was divided into mild cataract, moderate cataract and severe cataract. As per the number of classes involved in the training, validation and testing processes, there were four: three types of cataracts and normal eye. Examples of images from each class can be seen in Fig. 1.

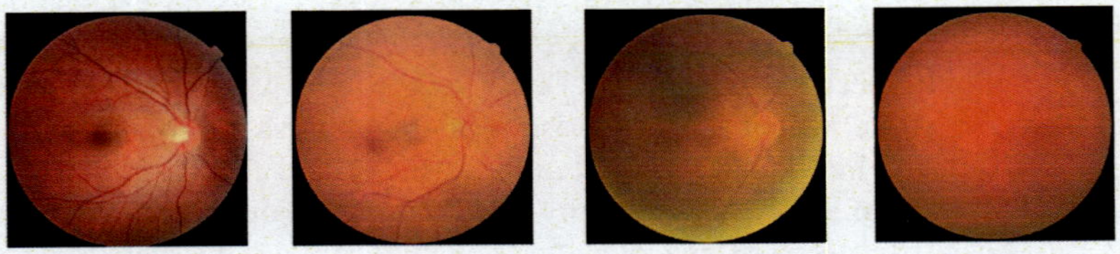

a) Normal eye b) Mild Cataract c) Moderate Cataract d) Severe cataract

Fig. 1. Examples of fundus images from each class

3.3 Pre-processing

All processes and procedures described in this paper were implemented by using deep learning toolbox and machine learning toolbox, available for Matlab. The networks were tested on both two-class classification and three-class classification, hence the images were pre-processed in order to improve the results.

The first step consisted on cropping the images from the first dataset to prioritize the useful information, minimize the black background, respectively, by using Matlab's Image Batch Processor application. At the end of this step, the images were both cropped and square (2400 × 2400). After analyzing the results obtained with 100 images in each class, in order to multiply the number of images, as the network needs a high number of samples, the images were augmented (roated in the possible directions) resulting in 400 images per class (normal eye and cataract).

Regarding the second dataset, the images were resized to correspond to the first dataset and they were manually selected as there were many flawed images (distorted, poorly illuminated, or presented various artifacts).

After a brief research on the current state-of-the-art, it was decided that the grayscale transformation, as well as the extraction of the green channel of the images were necessary. Improving luminance or contrast were also discussed and even implemented. Unfortunately, when re-examining the images, we observed some of the images changing their appearance, hence modifying their cataract type, and some others not. In order to avoid any confusion, these procedures were omitted.

Four datasets were obtained afterwards from both datasets (see Sect. 3.1): initial, cropped, gray scale and green channel dataset, all being involved in training, testing and comparison of the four networks. Images from each dataset can be seen in Fig. 2.

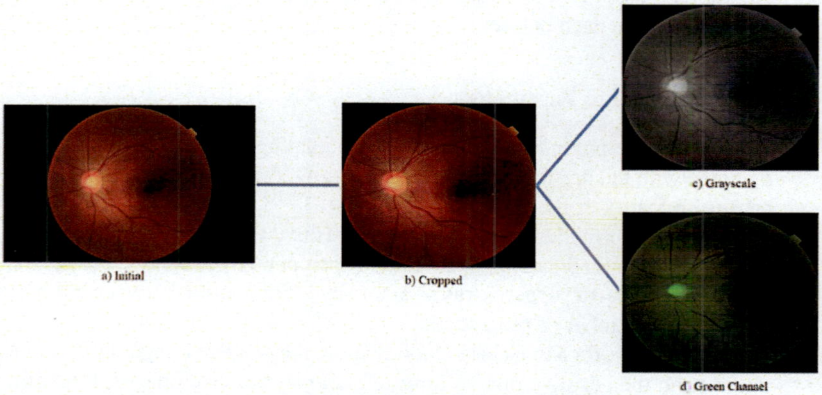

Fig. 2. Image examples from the four datasets, resulted after pre-processing (initial, cropped, grayscale, green channel extraction).

3.4 Proposed Models

As stated in the beginning of this paper, four pre-trained CNNs were tested and compared in terms of functionality according to their complexity, training time and classification accuracy. The models were implemented using Deep Network Designer application available on Matlab. In order to properly train, the input layers were modified to correspond to each individual network size requirements. Each network resizes the samples in the first layer according to their own input size for the images.

First CNN tested was the less complex one, AlexNet. This model is 8 layers deep, out of which 5 are convolutional layers and 3 are fully connected layers and require an input size for the images of 224 × 224 × 3 [13]. Compared to this model, GoogleNet is a more complex model, which includes an additional type of layer called inception layer. GoogleNet is 22 layers deep and can classify images into 1000 different object categories. The input size for this network is the same as the one AlexNet requires.

As one of the paper's main goal is to analyze CNNs for achieving automatic cataract classification, two additional networks were selected, with a more complex configuration (InceptionV3 and Inception-ResNet-V2).

InceptionV3 is 48 layers deep. This model combines many convolutional filters of various sizes to create a new filter, decreasing the number of parameters to be trained, respectively [14]. Inception V3 is most suitable when operating with large datasets but under limited conditions of computer memory, as well as under limited economic resources. The input size for InceptionV3 is 299 × 299 × 3.

Inception-ResNet-V2 merges the architecture of the Inception model with residual connections, mainly reducing training time. This model is 164 layers deep and the input size of the images is 299 × 299 × 3.

For all trainings, we used the ADAM optimizer, the initial learning rate was 0.001, the number of epoch was 15 and the Mini Batch Size varied depending on the number of samples from each dataset.

3.5 Performance Parameters

There are three parameters involved in calculating the performance of the classifiers obtained with the pre-trained models. Generally, the parameters are visible in either the confusion matrix or the ROC curve.

Sensitivity provides the percentage of positive images that were correctly classified (true positive rate). Specificity provides the percentage of negative images that were correctly classified (true negative rate). Accuracy is the fraction between correct predictions and the total number of predictions.

In this paper, for a two class-classification, the positive images term refers to cataract images and the negative images term refers to normal eye images. Regarding the three class classification, the positive images are the ones we are referring to during our discussion (e.g. if we are talking about moderate cataract, the positive images will only consist on those with moderate cataract), and the negative images term refers to the sum between the left aside classes (e.g. in this case, normal eye and severe cataract). The parameter of interest in this paper is the sensitivity, as the main goal is to properly identify cataracts.

4 Experimental Results

The classifiers were obtained using the four pre-trained CNNs above-mentioned. Table 1 presents the best results obtained by training the first dataset for two-class classification (cataract and normal eye), containing 100 images in each class. The dataset was divided in 70% images for training and 30% for validation and the classified images were those involved in the validation of the algorithm.

Table 1. Best results obtained for two-class classification, before augmentation.

First dataset	Pre-trained CNN	Performance		
		Sensitivity (%)	Specificity (%)	Accuracy (%)
Initial	GoogleNet	90	93.3	91.7
	Inception V3	96.7	73.3	85
	Inception-ResNet-V2	96.7	76.7	86.7
Cropped, color	Inception V3	90	83.3	86.7
	Inception-ResNet-V2	93.3	83.3	88.3
Cropped, grayscale	GoogleNet	86.7	96.7	91.7
	InceptionV3	93.3	90	91.7
	Inception-ResNet-V2	96.7	80	88.3

As seen in Table 1, regarding the initial dataset, both Inception V3 and Inception-ResNet-V2 obtained a sensitivity of 96.7%, meaning that only one cataract was classified as normal eye. Overall, the best classification was obtained with GoogleNet, with an accuracy of 91.7%. Regarding AlexNet, the classifier kept a low sensitivity and accuracy and was soon excluded from the trainings.

In order to improve the results, the images were cropped, but kept slightly similar results to the initial dataset, hence the decision to transform the images to grayscale. The sensitivity for Inception-ResNet-V2 increased, but it did not differ from the initial dataset, nor was far different from the sensitivity obtained with Inception V3. Moreover, Inception V3 had better results overall, with an accuracy of 91.7%, same as GoogleNet. Inception-ResNet-V2 was excluded as well from the trainings, as it also took a long training time (up to 8 h).

The comparison was made afterwards between GoogleNet and InceptionV3. The images from all datasets were augmented, the green channel was extracted and the trainings were resumed using the two CNNs. The results were obtained on the testing dataset (second dataset), as seen in Table 2.

Inception V3 could not recognize any of the cataracts, as its sensitivity was 0%, while GoogleNet improved significantly (96% sensitivity). As the results were better for GoogleNet and the training time for InceptionV3 (up to 6 h) was far longer compared to GoogleNet (up to 3 h), the latter one was the only one involved in the next trainings.

During all trainings, the misclassified images were re-analyzed and we have noticed the images from the mild cataract class being very similar to the ones from the normal

Table 2. Result obtained for the second dataset with cropped and green channel images.

Pre-trained CNN	Performance		
	Sensitivity (%)	Specificity (%)	Accuracy (%)
GoogleNet	96	98	97
Inception V3	0	100	50

eye class and thus creating confusions between the two classes. As a consequence, the mild cataract class was eliminated and set aside for further research. The results obtained for a three-class classification (normal eye, moderate cataract and severe cataract) with GoogleNet on both datasets, and for green-channel images are shown in Table 3.

Table 3. Results obtained for both validation and testing datasets, for green-channel images.

Dataset	Class	Performance	
		Sensitivity (%)	Accuracy (%)
Validation	Normal eye	82.2	88.1
	Moderate cataract	88.9	
	Severe cataract	93.3	
Testing	Normal eye	100	92.2
	Moderate cataract	90	
	Severe cataract	86.7	

Sensitivities for the three classes improved when using the testing datasets due to the manual selection of the images, those with mild cataract being avoided. The best accuracy obtained was with the green-channel dataset (92.2%). When classifying the validation dataset, there were mild cataracts which have been mixed with normal eyes, hence the 82.2% sensitivity for normal eye class. However, when eliminating the mild cataracts for the testing datasets, none of the normal eyes were misclassified.

5 Conclusion and Future Work

The paper has reached its purpose of testing and comparing four pre-trained CNNs for automatically detecting cataracts. The best model for this study was the CNN GoogleNet, which offered the best accuracies in both two-class classification (97%) and three-class classification (92.2%).

Fundus imaging is of high-maintenance when collecting patient images and can create ambiguities if the luminating technique or filter's colors are used improperly, for instance. Currently, the diagnosis of cataracts requires experienced ophthalmologists and advanced appliances for providing a high-quality fundus image. Consequently, for future work one could use a dataset received from the same ophthalmologists in order for the images to have the same appearances.

Furthermore, some segmentation procedures might be done to differentiate mild cataract from normal eye, regarding the exact dataset used in this paper. After segmentation, the number of objects could be counted and one classifier could be trained to classify images based on the number of elements.

For avoiding further confusions between the three types of cataracts, it is of major importance for the images to present no artefacts, nor to be shadowed by the pupil, as cataract diagnosis relies on the clearness degree of the image. One automatic system can be created in order to detect artefacts and indicate them to the ophthalmologists, so they can recollect the image.

Conflict of Interest. The Authors declare they have no conflict of interest.

References

1. Ji-Jiang, Y., et al.: Exploiting ensemble learning for automatic cataract detection and grading. Comput. Methods Programs Biomed. **124**, 45–57 (2016)
2. Fan, W., et al.: Principal component analysis based cataract grading and classification. In: 7th International Conference on E-health Networking, Application and Services (HealthCom) (2015)
3. Zhang, L., et al.: Automatic cataract detection and grading using deep convolutional neural network. In: 14th International Conference on Networking, Sensing and Control (ICNSC) (2017)
4. Pratap, T., et al.: Computer-aided diagnosis of cataract using deep transfer learning. Biomed. Signal Process. Control **53** (2019)
5. Junayed, M.S., et al.: CataractNet: an automated cataract detection system using deep learning for fundus images. IEEE Access **9**, 128799–128808 (2021)
6. Hasan, M.K., et al.: Cataract disease detection by using transfer learning-based intelligent methods. Comput. Math. Methods Med. **2021** (2021)
7. Yang, M., et al.: Classification of retinal image for automatic cataract detection. In: 15th International Conference on e-Health Networking, Applications and Services (Healthcom 2013) (2013)
8. Zheng, J., et al.: Fundus image based cataract classification. In: International Conference on Imaging Systems and Techniques (IST) Proceedings (2014)
9. Song, W., et al.: Semi-supervised learning based on cataract classification and grading. In: 40th Annual Computer Software and Applications Conference (COMPSAC) (2016)
10. Harini, V., et al.: Automatic cataract classification system. In: International Conference on Communication and Signal Processing (ICCSP) (2016)
11. Cataract dataset, [Online]. https://www.kaggle.com/datasets/jr2ngb/cataractdataset?select=README.md. Accessed 15 Apr 2022
12. Ocular Disease Recognition, [Online]. https://www.kaggle.com/datasets/andrewmvd/ocular-disease-recognition-odir5k. Accessed 20 May 2022

13. MathWorks, [Online]. https://www.mathworks.com/help/deeplearning/ref/alexnet.html. Accessed 02 Apr 2022
14. Nguyen, L.D., et al.: Deep CNNs for microscopic image classification by exploiting transfer learning and feature concatenation. In: IEEE International Symposium on Circuits and Systems (ISCAS) (2018)

Comparison Between Different Methods of Segmentation in Dental Image Processing

Cristina-Maria Stancioi(✉), Iulia Clitan, Marius Nicolae Roman, Mihail Abrudean, and Vlad Muresan

Technical University of Cluj-Napoca, Cluj-Napoca, Romania
stancioi_cristina@yahoo.com

Abstract. This paper presents three different methods of image segmentation and analysis of various panoramic dental radiographies. The images are analyzed from different perspectives depending on the dental condition of each patient's set of images, so the necessary information for establishing a correct diagnostic are extracted and analyzed. The algorithms are developed using Matlab work environment, so that if an image is hard to interpret, firstly is pre-processed using the Image Segmentation toolbox. Image segmentation methods are applied for analyzing the intra oral configuration of each patient based on the contour, size and intensity of specific surfaces identified by the dental specialist as being problematic. Each method will be detailed in this article and a comparison will be made between the three segmentation methods. Furthermore, another aim of this paper is find the best solution for processing this type of images, which are considered very hard to interpret using an automated tool and also to find even the hidden issues from a panoramic dental radiography. Some diagnostics can be identified from the first look of a specialist, but some images are very hard to interpret, so an automated tool is helpful in this cases. As a conclusion, the solution of processing such an image is developed, tested and finally, it will aid in the analysis of panoramic dental radiography.

Keywords: Image processing · Panoramic dental radiography · Segmentation

1 Introduction

Panoramic radiography is a method of investigation that uses a small amount of X-rays, through which one can visualize the dental ensemble in its entirety: dentition, maxillary bone, mandible, maxillary sinus and temporary-mandibular joints [1].

This type of radiography is a two-dimensional image-projection of the dental apparatus, which serves the dentist for diagnosis as a means of initial evaluation, but also in treatment, to establish the right work for each case.

Dental radiography allows the capture of black and white images, where white represents everything that is radio-opaque (X-rays cannot penetrate there), and black everything that is radio-transparent (X-rays can penetrate there). These images help the dentist to see exactly where the caries, infections, cysts, periodontal pockets or fractures are,

S. Vlad and N. M. Roman (Eds.): MEDITECH 2022, IFMBE Proceedings 102, pp. 69–74, 2024.
https://doi.org/10.1007/978-3-031-51120-2_8

these appearing as dark areas where they should not be. Very white areas, whiter than natural teeth, are represented by implants, fillings or prosthetic works [2].

The procedure of radiography has a number of clear advantages, which today makes it an indispensable procedure in dental treatment and extremely in demand. Among the advantages of panoramic radiography is the fact that this is a fast, non-invasive, comfortable and safe procedure for the patient [3].

Panoramic radiography is also useful in cases where it is aimed at mounting an implant or braces, in order to achieve prostheses perfectly appropriate to the patient's dentition [4].

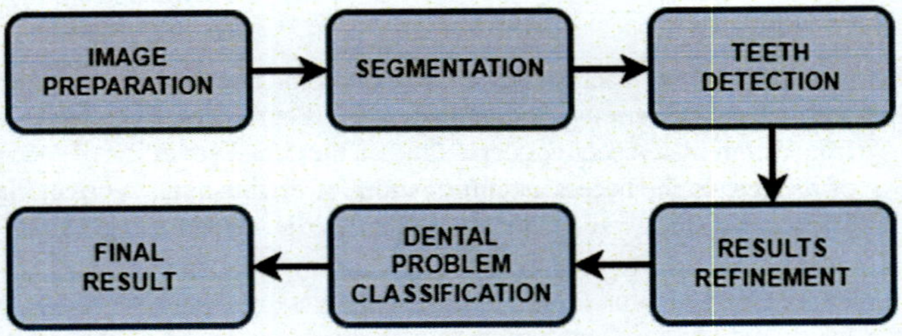

Fig. 1. The processing workflow

As it can be seen in Fig. 1, the interpretation of such an image has to be passed through some crucial steps in order to highlight all the information that is needed for establishing a proper and correct diagnostic. In the next sections are presented the steps in detail with the corresponding methods which will add to obtaining the best results for interpreting such an image.

2 Implementation

By following the schematic presented above, the first step in the process consists in preparing the original image which looks like in Fig. 2, for the segmentation. In this step, the noise is removed, the contour is defined and also the unnecessary information from the image is removed or not taken into consideration by selecting a region of interest which includes just the parts of interest from the panoramic dental radiography [5]. The image can be also split in different parts and each part to be considered in the process and after that to reconstruct the main image.

For removing the noise from the original image, Lee filter was applied and for each image, depending on the contrast and the visibility of the important parts, the Median filter was implemented to deal with such an image, in order not to remove important parts from the image which are crucial for determining the diagnostic.

The next step represents the segmentation of the image and it is done by implementing an algorithm which suits the best for this type of images. This algorithm is designed based on the Chan-Vese segmentation method, but with certain particularities that suit best for this images. The initial step of the segmentation was to use the Segmentation

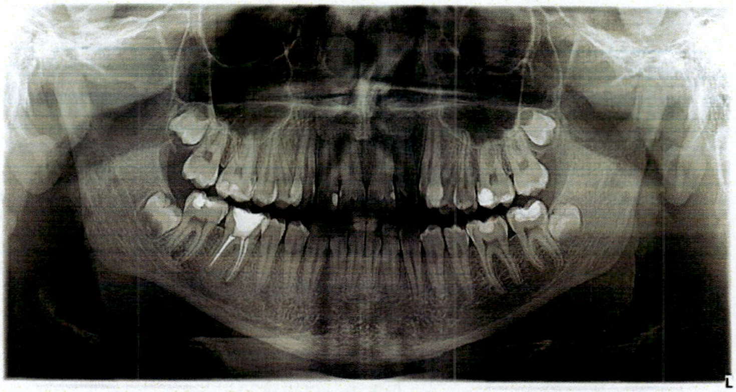

Fig. 2. The original image

Toolbox from Matlab, in order to compute and develop the segmentation algorithm. All the coefficients that have to be taken into consideration in the segmentation process were involved in order to obtain a very clear image after this step [6].

The well-known methods of segmentation also work, but there are images that need a better approach in order to obtain all the necessary information from the original image, so that with this algorithm all these aspects are met.

For the teeth detection (Fig. 3), after the segmentation process is performed and the image becomes easier to interpret, each tooth is detected and highlighted individually based on its position and size and this is helpful in terms of analyzing each part in particular, especially to determine if a cavity is present or the beginning of a cavity is present based on the contrast and on the color of the pixels from each part [7].

With this functionality, a dental specialist can easily analyze a patient's intraoral configuration by taking each component and deciding based on the computation of the color which is the stage of the cavity and how to proceed in this case.

The next step is the results refinement which is a procedure to eliminate the unnecessary information from the image and if some parts from the image are not problematic, it simply removes them from the final image. This is done by using mainly the Median filter combined with a zoom option which helps in deciding if a certain part of the image is problematic or not, as it can be seen in Fig. 4.

This can be done also without the zoom option, but for better results this option is considered [8–10].

After all these steps are performed, the dental specialist can establish a diagnostic and store it in the patient's database in order to have a clear overview.

3 Obtained Results

Dental panoramic radiography is an essential part of dentistry, one of the most common procedures used to examine teeth and gums. With this method and by following the workflow described above, it will help dentists to see the condition of the patient's teeth,

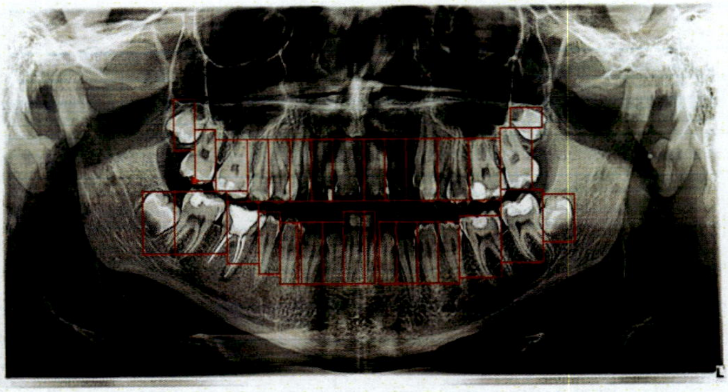

Fig. 3. Teeth detection

roots, jaw placement and composition of the facial bones. It also helps them to find dental problems that cannot be noticed on a simple physical examination and also to establish a treatment for them.

In the resulted image, after performing all the steps, the dental panoramic radiography shows different types of diagnostics like:

- Cavities (including if there are small damaged areas between the teeth);
- Damage to the tooth under the existing fillings;
- Bone loss in the jaw;
- Changes in the bone or root canal caused by infections;
- The condition and position of the teeth to help prepare dental implants, braces, dentures or other dental procedures;
- Abscesses (infections at the root of a tooth or between the gum and the tooth);
- Dental cysts and some types of tumors.

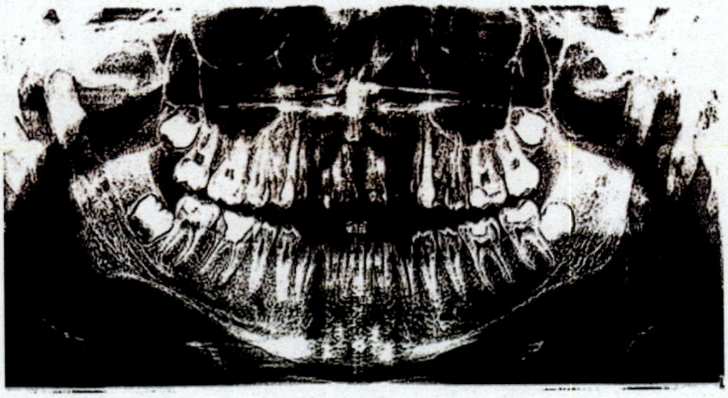

Fig. 4. Results refinement

The algorithm was tested on multiple images with different kind of possible diagnostics and the accuracy of detecting them was 92%. By processing the images, because some of them are very hard to interpret also because of the position of each tooth, the hidden problems can be discovered and solved in time.

Panoramic radiography is used when a full evaluation of the oral cavity is made, in order to establish a treatment plan, in the case of extractions, before mounting braces or in patients with periodontal treatments.

The time for analyzing such an image is also reduced, so the dental specialist can directly look on the specified areas and decide which is the problem and the cause for this.

Because most of the people are afraid in doing regularly this type of procedure, the previous images are stored for each patient and in some cases it is not necessary to do it again, depending on the issue which is addressed.

4 Conclusions

By taking into consideration the obtained results from above, we can say that image processing techniques play a major role in interpreting a panoramic dental radiography. This type of image is considered hard to interpret directly by a dental specialist and it can contain hidden dental issues that cannot be observed by the normal eye.

The developed algorithm incorporates different segmentation techniques, so that on the final resulted image can be easily observed all the details that help the dental specialist in determining in depth which is the problem for each patient.

In this case, after analyzing all the obtained results and different particularities depending on each image, for future work, an automatic tool will be helpful for interpreting this type of images and to establish the diagnostic automatically by considering all the necessary aspects that can be encountered depending on each patient intraoral configuration. In this way, infections, inflammations and cavities that require treatment can be observed and take action immediately.

References

1. White, S.C., Pharoa, M.J.: Oral Radiology: Principles and Interpretation, 5th edn. Mosby, Saint Louis (2007)
2. Kamburoglu, K., Kolsuz, E., Murat, S., Yüksel, S., Ozen, T.: Proximal caries detection accuracy using intraoral bitewing radiography, extraoral bitewing radiography and panoramic radiography. Dentomaxillofacial Radiol. Br. Inst. Radiol. **41**, 450–459 (2012)
3. Avendanio, B., Frederiksen, N.L., Benson, B.W., et al.: Estimate of radiation detriment: scanography and intraoral radiology. Oral Surg. Oral Med. Oral Pathol. Oral Radiol. Endod. **82**, 713–719 (1996)
4. Stella, J.P., Tharanon, W.: A precise radiographic method to determine the location of the inferior alveolar canal in the posterior edentulous mandible: implications for dental implants, II: clinical application. Int. J. Oral Maxillofac. Implants **5**, 23–29 (1990)
5. Jain, K.R., Chauhan, N.C.: Enhancement and segmentation of dental radiographs using morphological operations. In: Dental Image Analysis for Disease Diagnosis, pp. 39–58. Springer International Publishing, Berlin/Heidelberg, Germany (2019)

6. Valizadeh, S., Rahimian, S., Balali, M., Azizi, Z.: Effect of zooming, colorization, and contrast conversion on proximal caries detection. Avicenna J. Dent. Res. (2016) (in press)
7. Haiter-Neto, F., Casanova, M.S., Frydenberg, M., Wenzel, A.: Task-specific enhancement filters in storage phosphor images from the Vistascan system for detection of proximal caries lesions of known size. Oral Surg. Oral Med. Oral Pathol. Oral Radiol. Endod. (2009)
8. Mehr-Alizadeh, S., Sadri, D., Nemati, S., Sarikhani, S., Zafarfazeli, A.: Evaluation of the diagnostic efficacy of intra oral digital radiography with and without zoom option software in the detection of occlusal dentinal caries: an in vitro study. J. Islam. Dent. Assoc. Iran (2012)
9. Wang, Z., Zhang, D.: Progressive switching median filter for the removal of impulse noise from highly corrupted images. IEEE Trans. Circuits Syst. II **46**(1), 78–80 (1999)
10. Chen, T., Wu, H.R.: Adaptive impulsive detection using center weighted median filters. IEEE Signal Process. Lett. **8**(1), 1–3 (2001)

Health Technology Assessment

Assisted Assessment of Visual Stress – Method to Prevent and Reduce the Risk of Visual Function Loss

Barbu Braun(✉), Mitu Leonard, and Ional Serban

Transilvania University of Brasov, Brasov, Romania
{braun,leonard.mitu,ionel.serban}@unitbv.ro

Abstract. The paper deals with the problem of visual stress. In the first part, the concept of visual stress is explained, when it occurs and what risks it can involve. The second part presents a method by which the influence of visual stress can be effectively and objectively evaluated, in a form that occurs very frequently in everyday life. The method consists in evaluating 10 subjects, both in the absence and presence of visual stress, five of them being emmetropic, the others having different refractive errors. The assessment of people consisted of testing them in front of the Laptop screen, they had to identify and select from a list certain randomly generated words. In the first stage the subjects were tested under normal conditions, later they were tested under conditions where two large lights of different colors flickered randomly on the background of the screen. Assisted evaluation was possible thanks to a software interface that was designed, programmed and verified during this research. In one of the sections of the paper, the way in which the interface was created, as well as how to use it, is presented.

Keywords: Visual stress · Interface · Vision · Assessment

1 What Is Visual Stress

1.1 Visual Stress - Major Cause of Visual Function Deterioration

Visual stress could be defined as a factor that creates strong visual discomfort and can affect it in the short or long term. Generally, short-term exposure to visual stress can lead to vision impairment for a short period (a few minutes).

A long and repeated exposure, even in a low degree (when using the PC or smartphone) can lead to the visual function damage over time, including related effects (vertigo, nausea, dizziness, fatigue, lack of concentration, etc.). Another situation of this kind can be encountered in the case of working for long periods in artificially lit halls or rooms, with blue light bulbs, which can sometimes have fluctuations in intensity [1, 2].

S. Vlad and N. M. Roman (Eds.): MEDITECH 2022, IFMBE Proceedings 102, pp. 77–86, 2024.
https://doi.org/10.1007/978-3-031-51120-2_9

1.2 Visual Stress Assessment Methods

Currently, there are various methods of assessing visual stress, some of which involve sophisticated and very expensive equipment and devices. Others simply involve checking and recording how vision may be affected during and immediately after exposure to stress. All should have one main goal: to identify to what extent different situations involving a lower or higher dose of visual stress momentarily affect visual function [3, 4]. This aspect is extremely important, because in this way it is possible to extrapolate and draw up scenarios regarding the medium and long-term influence on vision for each of the stressors. Either this, once known, can be extremely useful to know which situations involve visual stress with major impact and, therefore, they should be avoided from the very beginning [5–7].

2 Proposed Method

2.1 Assisted Assessment of Visual Stress – Main Advantages

The assessment of visual stress in a computer-assisted form seems to be a practical option, while also being an efficient procedure, which allows an objective assessment of the results. On the other hand, this method helps the examiner, who, by means of a software application, can, based on the automatically generated results, quickly, but at the same time rigorously express certain conclusions regarding the testing done in the different situations.

Generally, the main aspect to be observed in terms of the presence or loss of visual stress seems to be the acuity, but it is not the only aspect targeted in the study of vision [8, 9].

2.2 Development and Use of a Specific Software Interface Within the Proposed Method

A simple method for an efficient investigation was the main concern of the research studies. For this reason, it was proceeded to program a software interface for visual function evaluation both in the absence or presence of visual stress. Moreover, it should, on the one hand, be able to induce visual stress and, on the other hand, to allow an objective visual acuity and reaction time assessment.

The environment in which the software interface was programmed is LabVIEW, developed by the National Instruments company. The reason for choosing this software environment was to be able to create a virtual instrument for simulations and measurements in conditions as close as possible to real ones. Another reason was that LabVIEW's graphical interface allows a very clear and quick visualization of all the parameters of interest. Specific to the LabVIEW graphical programming environment is the fact that, by means of two graphical windows, it is possible to view both the user interface and the programming algorithm diagram. Thus means a great advantage, as it is very easy to find and fix any syncope during the programming stage.

There are presented both situations during the software running: testing is done without visual stress, and when visual stress intervenes during testing.

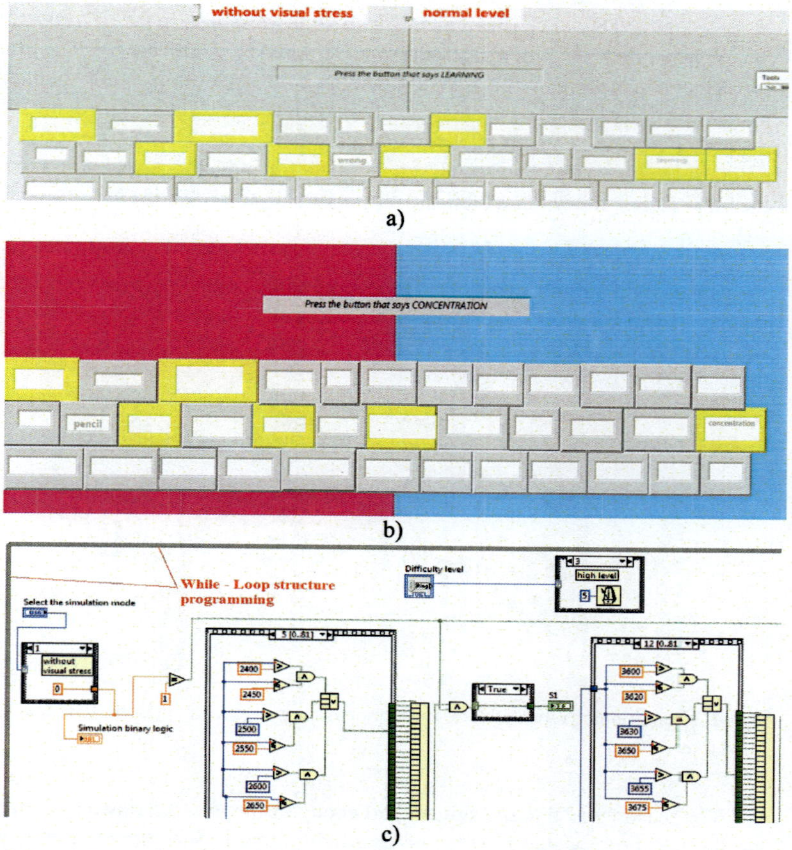

Fig. 1. Software interface during its using: a) Example of application running for testing without stress conditions; b) Example of application running for testing including visual stress; c) While – Loop structure for all logic events programming

The basis for programming was a repetitive While-Loop structure for conditioning all logical events during a test run cycle. An image meaning the use of the structure can be seen in Fig. 1 c).

In terms of the interface running, it means first of all the visual parameters testing.

For this, the logical events must refer to the visual stress inducing and also to the testing. It means that, while testing, different words, random apparition must take place, the concerned tested person must to recognize and to select the frame specific to the shown word. A particularly important aspect is that of the difference in the size of the characters, specific to testing the acuity, but also of the contrast difference compared to the background in which the words appear written in the border [12].

The first events involved the establishment of variable time intervals, with random occurrence, for the continuous on and off of two large rear buttons, throughout the period of the cycle. Both were defined as Boolean input variables, in the "0" logical state they are gray, and in the "1" logical state they are colored (Fig. 1a) and b)). The time intervals for successive turning on was related to the specific index of the While loop, imposing as many time constants as possible that define the intervals. The conditioning of switching on and off was done using two Boolean structures (True/False). The reason why the 2 colors (blue and purple) were chosen as lights for inducing visual stress are related to the fact that it is known that blue and purple radiation is the most harmful to the eye [10, 11].

The outputs of the two Boolean structures were connected to the two buttons with the role of light stimulus (Fig. 2). The conditioning of the logical events specific to the display of text-messages was made so that they start to be displayed only after a period of time after the start of the test cycle.

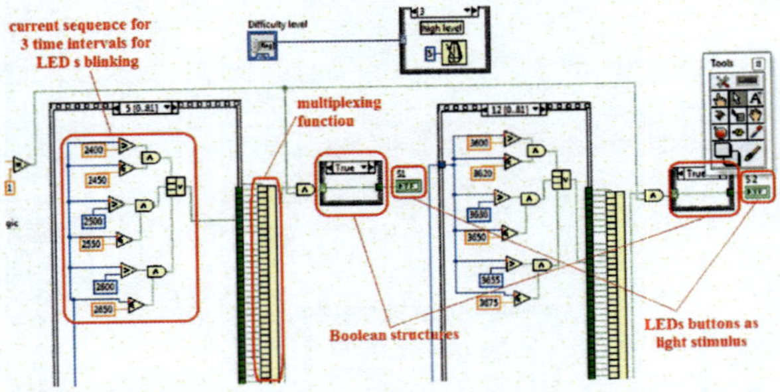

Fig. 2. Conditioning repeated for light stimuli turning on and off via Boolean structures and preset time intervals

The reason was that the subject had enough time to settle down and properly fixate on the text box located next to the two light stimuli. Specifically, the display of text messages was scheduled to begin about one-third of the way through the total test run.

Just as in the case of random flashes, time intervals have been predefined for which one word at a time will be displayed, in this case the time intervals are related by means of successive Boolean structures, as can be seen in Fig. 3. In Fig. 1b), an example can be seen in which, at a given moment, a text message is displayed, and the yellow boxes represent the answers of the subject by which he spotted the text messages that were displayed previously. For this, an appropriate number of virtual button-type Boolean input variables were used, which the test subject could switch to.

An important aspect referred to the possibility of establishing its degree of difficulty, using a selector Case function with three values, low level, medium level and high level of difficulty. It was related by a multi-case structure of Switch type, as can be seen in Fig. 4.

For each case, another specific time constant was established for the cycle timing, practically modifying the speed of the test. Besides, another almost equally important aspect in terms of programming referred to the possibility of establishing the regime for testing: with or without visual stress; for this, another selector function was used, this time with two cases.

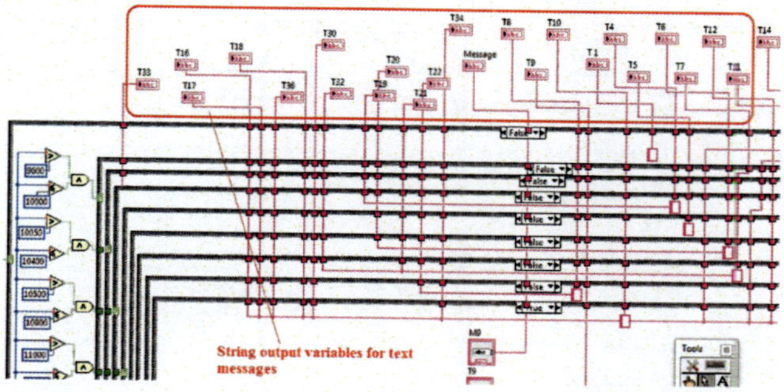

Fig. 3. Conditioning repeated for successively message text displaying during the test

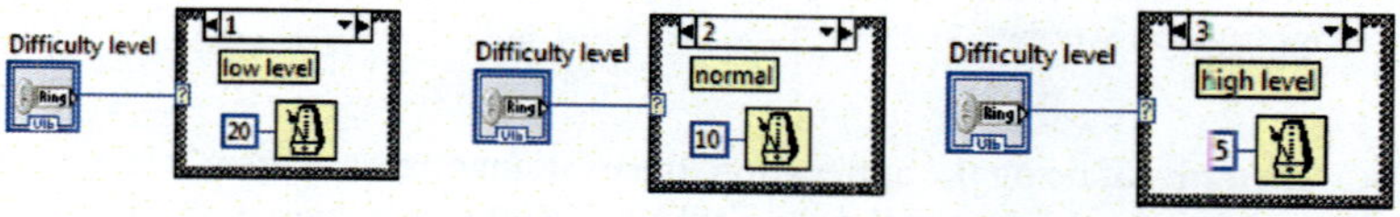

Fig. 4. Programming algorithm for degree of difficulty selection

The ability to automatically quantify subject responses during testing was another particularly important aspect of the application's programming. For this, an algorithm was created to add up all the positive and negative partial scores recorded for each answer. By partial positive scoring is meant the awarding of a score for the situation in which the subject correctly identified and spotted the current displayed word at a given time. By negative scoring is meant the penalty given for false-positive errors, more precisely for indicating a different word from the list than the one indicated during the test run. This meant that each string output variable must have a corresponding LED button, through which the subject can indicate the answer.

In the following, the specific program routine involving a specific partial score to an answer will be described, in total there are 30 possible answers, but only 18 of them being correct. If during the test run cycle the button associated with the word the subject believed to have identified was toggled at least once, then a partial positive or negative score will be given for that step, depending on the correctness of the response.

Otherwise, the partial score awarded will be 0. For this, an option to index Boolean values has been set on the output of the While loop, so that, through a vector of Boolean values, converted into binary code, it can be identified if in that vector there is at least one value equal to 1. If so, meaning that a partial score must be given, it will be equal to 10 or −10. Because this routine must be repeated 30 times, as many possible answers as can be given during the test, it was necessary to use a sequential structure with 30 sequences, each one containing a sequence.

Figure 5 shows an example showing two distinct sequences, one corresponding to the awarding of a positive score and another specific to a de-pointing for a wrong answer.

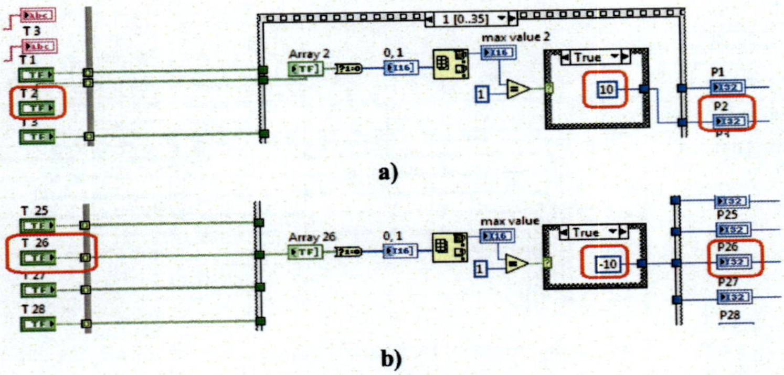

Fig. 5. Example of subroutines specific to the partial scoring approach: a) for positive scoring; b) for negative scoring

In terms of using the application, the examiner has a series of clear and simple steps to go through: the first of them would be to choose the degree of difficulty, through the dialog box on the interface - panel (Fig. 6).

The same procedure must to be applied by the examiner to select the how the test must be accomplished (with or without stress) (Fig. 7).

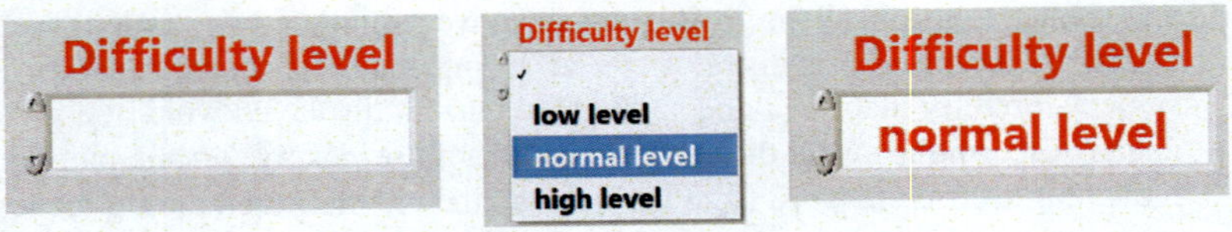

Fig. 6. Selecting the degree of difficulty

In general, the application serving for a comparative, it is recommended that, for the same subject, first the test is carried out under normal conditions and, after a period of time, but under the same physiological and environmental conditions to repeat the test in the presence of visual stress. Ideally, the test should be repeated on the next day at a time close to the time when the stress-free test was taken.

The next stage means the test running, after all settings for testing have been made previously. An example of this stage can be seen in Fig. 1b).

The last stage, and the most important one, is the visualization of the results after the test, an example is illustrated in Fig. 8.

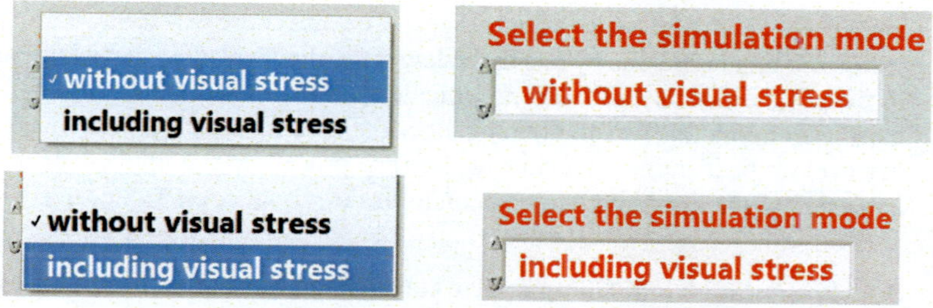

Fig. 7. Selecting the way to proceed for testing

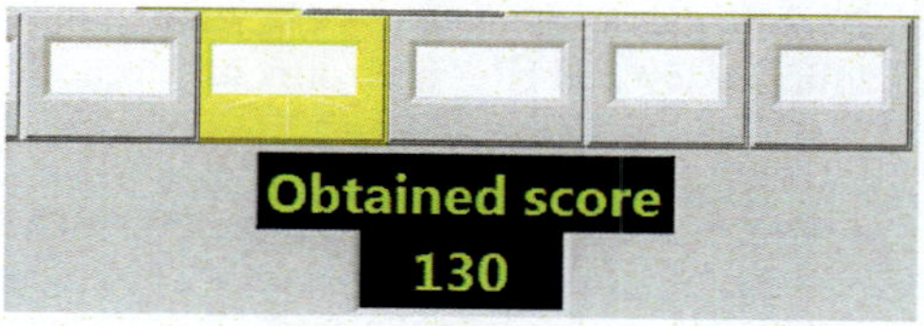

Fig. 8. Example of final score displaying

3 Results and Discussion

3.1 Selection and Preparation of Subjects for Testing

Once the software has been completed, 10 people were identified who gave their consent to be tested both under normal conditions and under visual stress conditions. These were identified in the 40–50 age group, all of whom were male. 5 of these were identified as emmetropic, while another 5 were found to have myopia ranging from −0.75DS to −1.5DS.

To complete the tests, the subjects were clearly explained what they would consist of and what they had to do during the test. More specifically, they were told that they would first go through the test without any kind of visual stress, all subjects being evaluated, one by one, then they, in the same order, would be retested, but this time under conditions of visual stress [9].

3.2 Assessment Procedure

All tests, both in normal mode and in visual stress mode, were supervised by an examiner, as a graduate of the Optometry specialization, so that there is no risk that, at some point, any of the people would no longer know what to he had to do. In addition, supervision was also useful to avoid certain fraud attempts (i.e. not keeping the distance from the laptop screen). In this idea, the distance imposed from the screen during testing was set at 0.8 m, considered an intermediate viewing distance, and the screen was tilted at an angle of 10°–15° so that the visual axis of the subjects came perpendicular to screen.

The two stages, each, in turn, involved three sub-stages of evaluation, namely: reduced degree of difficulty, medium degree of difficulty and high difficulty (with the highest speed of displaying text messages). The procedure was followed, so that all subjects to be first tested one by one in the low difficulty level, then the testing was repeated in the same order for the medium difficulty and then for the high difficulty level. The reason for doing this was to not remember the order in which the text messages appear in a cycle to be identified. Obviously, the same procedure was applied identically for the 2nd stage of the assessment, under conditions of visual stress [9].

3.3 Presentation and Comparative Interpretation of the Obtained Results

Tables 1 and 2 show the results obtained after testing the 10 subjects in the 2 postures. It should be noted that the score awarded was considered between 0 and 180. For the tests the following abbreviations were made: LL - testing in the reduced level of difficulty; NL - medium difficulty test and HL - high difficulty test.

Table 1. Testing the first 5 subjects, considered emmetropic

1st Subject			2nd Subject			3rd Subject			4th Subject			5th Subject		
Without visual stress														
LL	NL	HL	LL	NL	HL	LL	NL	HL	LL	NL	HL	LL	NL	HL
180	180	170	150	130	130	180	160	160	170	170	160	180	180	160
Including visual stress														
170	150	130	130	120	120	150	140	120	150	130	110	150	140	130

Table 2 displays the results for the other tested persons (having myopia).

Table 2. Testing the last 5 subjects, having myopia

6th Subject			7th Subject			8th Subject			9th Subject			10th Subject		
Without visual stress														
LL	NL	HL	LL	NL	HL	LL	NL	HL	LL	NL	HL	LL	NL	HL
130	110	70	100	70	50	100	90	70	90	80	60	100	90	70
Including visual stress														
120	70	50	90	60	40	70	70	50	80	70	50	90	80	60

It should be specified that the subjects with myopia were evaluated without any correction of refractive errors (no glasses or contact lenses). The reason was to observe to what extent visual stress can affect more a subject with uncorrected or poorly corrected vision problems. This is because it is known that very often even if a person wears corrective glasses, they may no longer correspond to current needs [9].

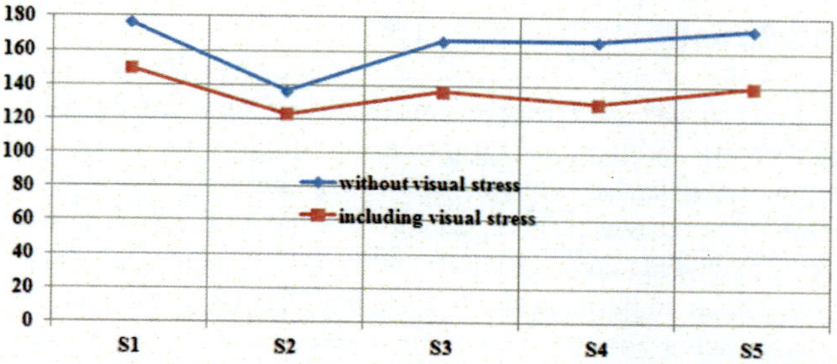

Fig. 9. Distribution of the values of the average scores of the first 5 men (emmetropics)

Figure 9 shows the distribution plots of the mean score values of the first 5 emmetropic subjects. Average scores mean the arithmetic mean of the scores obtained by a subject for all difficulty levels.

Figure 10 shows another distribution plot of the mean score values of the other 5 subjects (having myopia).

From this finding one could, by extrapolation, draw a conclusion, namely that a person with low vision could be more affected in the case of visual stress, but to a small extent, compared to a person without vision problems.

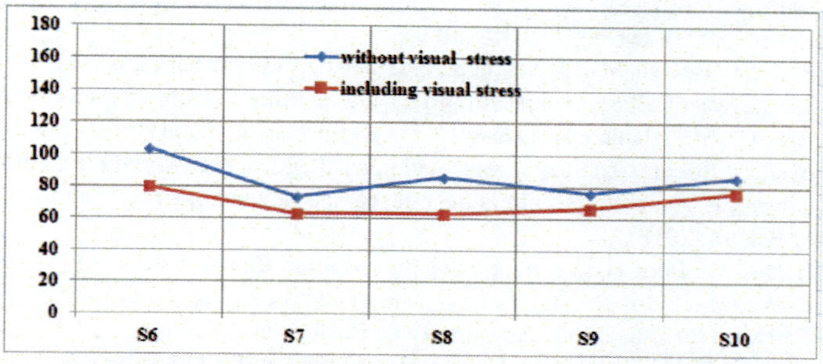

Fig. 10. Distribution of the values of the average scores of the last 5 persons (with myopia)

Obviously, a decrease in performance under conditions of visual stress could be observed, for both categories of people investigated. One of the aspects targeted was to observe which of the two categories would be more affected by the induction of visual stress. For this, starting from the data, as average values of the scores, for each category, the following could be found: For the first the decrease in performance as a result of the presence of visual stress it was about 17% compared to the case of no stress. For the second category the decrease in performance as a result of the presence of visual stress was approximately 18% compared to the case of the absence of stress.

4 Conclusion

The method proved to be effective and conclusive regarding the influence of visual stress on visual acuity and work performance. Although it was based only on the study of a single type of visual stress, it can be considered as a basis for further research, the expansion of assisted assessment methods of the influence of visual stress, the research can also be extended to prevent short- and long-term exposure to blue light and ultraviolet radiation. The main purpose was to raise concerns, through practical, objective and fast methods, in being able to prevent, as much as possible, the exposure of the eyes to as many forms of stress as possible. The main areas targeted would be occupational medicine optometry, military, occupational optometry and even sports optometry.

Acknowledgment. The research described in the paper was largely due to the contribution of Optometry graduate students, 2021–2022 promotion, within the Diploma Project, the practical activity being carried out in the laboratories of Transilvania University, as well as in medical clinics Specialized.

References

1. Jackson, A., Bailey, I.: Visual acuity. Optom. Pract. **5**, 53–70 (2004)
2. Barbu, D.: Analysis and modeling of the visual function. Transilvania University Publishing House (2003). ISBN:973-635-130-0
3. Paton, J., Belova, M., Morrison, S., Salzman, D.: The primate amygdala represents the positive and negative value of visual stimuli during learning. Nature **439**, 865–870 (2006)
4. Alanazi, M., Alanazi, S., Osuagwu, L.: Evaluation of visual stress symptoms in age-matched dyslexic, Meares-Irlen syndrome and normal adults. Int J Ophthalmol **9**(4), 617–624 (2016)
5. Cowan, P.: Do coloured filters benefit reading beyond placebo? Doctoral Thesis, University of Bristol (2018)
6. Baritz, M.: Poor vision and glasses prescription. Course notes (2017)
7. Baritz, M.: "Serious games" for serious vision problems of children. In: 12th e-Learning and Software for Education Conference eLSE, Bucharest, Romania (2018)
8. Baritz, M.: Using "Serious Game" for Children and Youth Education in Sustainable Energy Field and Environment Protection. SpringerLink (2017)
9. Donici, M.: Determination of visual acuity according to eye fatigue. Diploma Project, Coordinator: Lecturer Dr. Eng. Braun, B. (2021)
10. Tosini, G., Ferguson, I., Tsunota, K.: Effects of blue light on the circadian system and eye physiology. Mol. Vis. **22** (2016)
11. Ernst, C.: A thesis presented for the Master of Science Degree, The University of Tennessee, Knoxville (1996)
12. Wilkinson, M.: Contrast sensitivity testing: when visual acuity testing alone is not enough. J. Am. Soc. Ophthalmic Regist. Nurses **35**(4) (2010)

Influence of the Conventional and Planar Yagi Uda Antenna on Human Tissues

Claudia Constantinescu(✉), Claudia Pacurar, Adina Giurgiuman, and Calin Munteanu

Technical University of Cluj-Napoca, Cluj-Napoca, Romania
Claudia.Constantinescu@ethm.utcluj.ro

Abstract. In an era in which all devices tend to be smaller, the conventional and planar devices are functioning together. The present study aims at determining the influence of a conventional and a planar Yagi-Uda antennas, each functioning at the same frequency of approximately 2.6 GHz, on three types of human tissue present in their vicinity, namely skin, fat and muscle. For this, the Specific Absorption Rate (SAR), electric field and magnetic field are determined and compared in order to reach some conclusions. Also, the distance of the tissues from the antenna was varied and it was determined if the antennas can be placed near tissue layers without producing damages to them. The values obtained are analyzed and compared with the ones suggested by ICNIRP (International Commission on Non-Ionizing Radiation Protection) in order to determine if the limits are according to the standard.

Keywords: Yagi Uda antenna · Classical construction · Planar construction · Tissue influence · ICNIRP limits

1 Introduction

Conventional Yagi-Uda antennas were first constructed in Japan by Shintaro Uda and Yagi, and the first study about them was published in 1928. The Yagi Uda antennas were used even in the Second World War for radar systems, and after that their mainly use was for TV transmission. Considering the directivity, this type of antenna is unidirectional and allows the minimization of interference level for emission and reception. They have a gain which allows the reception of low intensity signals and in comparison with other antennas they are easy to manufacture due to their simple construction from robust and resistant metallic rods [1, 2].

Among their disadvantage is the limited gain value because for a higher gain the dimensions of the antenna are too big.

Once the technology progressed and considering the breakthroughs in the material study and the printed circuit, the planar antennas became more spread in a lot of domains, among them being also the Yagi-Uda antenna. This type of antenna was proposed for the first time in 1998, and has as advantages reduced weight, compactness, low manufacturing costs. Another big advantage is their easy integration together with other electronic components in different circuits. They are highly used in wireless communication systems, radar systems, direction detection portable systems, medical devices and devices from the military domain [3–7].

S. Vlad and N. M. Roman (Eds.): MEDITECH 2022, IFMBE Proceedings 102, pp. 87–98, 2024.
https://doi.org/10.1007/978-3-031-51120-2_10

2 Modeling and Comparison Between Conventional and Planar Yagi Uda Antenna

The main elements of a Yagi Uda antenna are the reflector, the dipole and the directors. The two antennas were modeled to function at approximately the same frequency for a better comparison between their specific parameters and after that to better evaluate their influence on the human tissues present in their vicinity.

2.1 Construction and S Parameters of the Conventional and Planar Yagi Uda Antenna

In Fig. 1 the conventional Yagi Uda antenna modeled with the help of HFSS program can be seen. The antenna is constructed with 3 directors, while the dipole feeding the antenna is presented with a different shade of green. The total length of the antenna is 102.7 mm, and the width is 63.4 mm, while the rods are considered to be constructed from aluminum. The radius of the rods is considered to be 2 mm. Even though the dimensions are smaller than most of the Yagi Uda conventional antennas present on the market, it is normal because of the higher frequency for which the antenna was constructed.

The planar antenna was constructed on a flexible dielectric material called polyimide, with a relative permittivity of $\varepsilon r = 3.5$. The constitutive elements are the same, the reflector being placed on a side of the dielectric, while the directors and dipole are on the other side, the number of directors being increased at 5. In Fig. 2 the structure is represented. The directors have different lengths and a width of 1.5 mm. The total length of the structure is 65 mm, while the width is 56 mm, the thickness being 0.71 mm. Considering the conventional structure, it can be stated that the dimensions are reduced. Also, because of the dielectric substrate keeping the conductors in place the second structure is more robust and trustworthy, while the first one is more fragile.

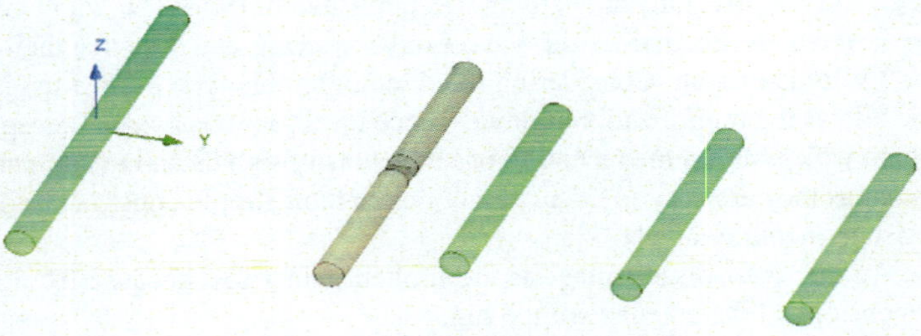

Fig. 1. The modeled conventional Yagi Uda antenna.

2.2 Comparison of the Characteristic Parameters of the Conventional and Planar Yagi Uda Antenna

Among the parameters of interest for Yagi Uda antenna are the gain, bandwidth, and front to back ratio. In this study we also determined the electric and magnetic distribution

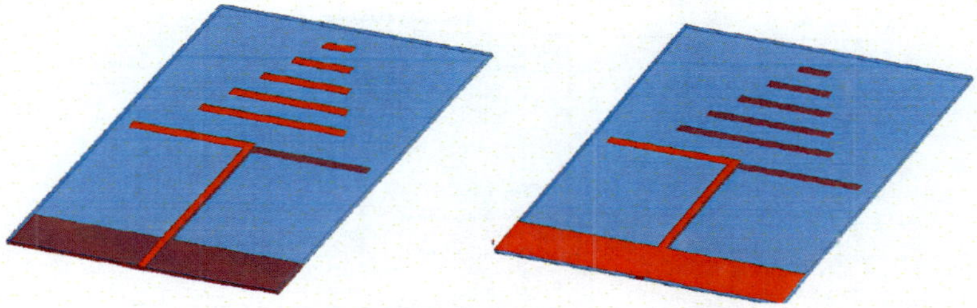

Fig. 2. The modeled planar Yagi Uda antenna.

around the antenna and SAR when the tissues are considered in order to better understand their functionality and also where would the antenna impact more a tissue present in its vicinity.

After modeling the conventional antenna from Fig. 1 it was discovered that it is functioning in the frequency range between 2.04–2.75 GHz as it can be observed from the S parameter representation from Fig. 3. The S parameters for the planar antenna were also obtained and presented in Fig. 4 and the bandwidth, which for this case is between 2.36–2.99 GHz, is approximately with the same width for both antennas.

The second parameter considered was the gain of the antennas. The representations can be seen in Figs. 5 and 6. The maximum values, as expected for a Yagi Uda antenna, are low namely the conventional antenna has a maximum gain of 6.4, while the planar antenna has an even lower value for the gain, 4.1. The direction of the gain is, as expected, along the directors due to the fact that the reflector does not let the antenna to emit in the other direction, but there is a surprise with the planar antenna constructed where the gain is higher in one corner and not along the dipole which is fed.

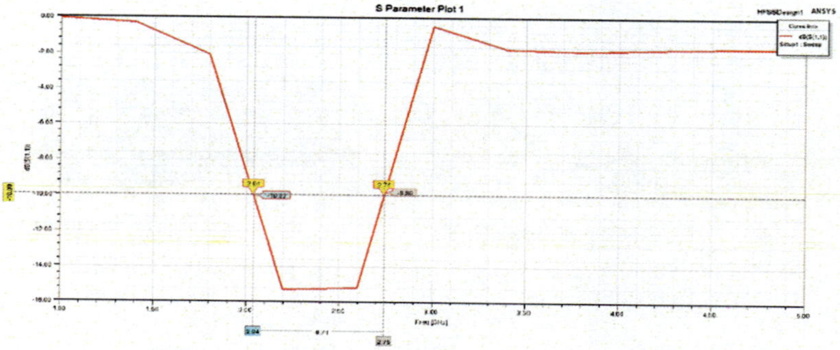

Fig. 3. The S parameters representation for the conventional antenna.

The human exposure to electric and magnetic fields are limited by standards in force. Considering the guidelines for limiting radiofrequency EMF exposure given by ICNIRP in 2020 [8], the frequency of 2.6 GHz is not considered, but in the case of the frequency of 2 GHz for general public for an exposure over 30 min the incident E field strength

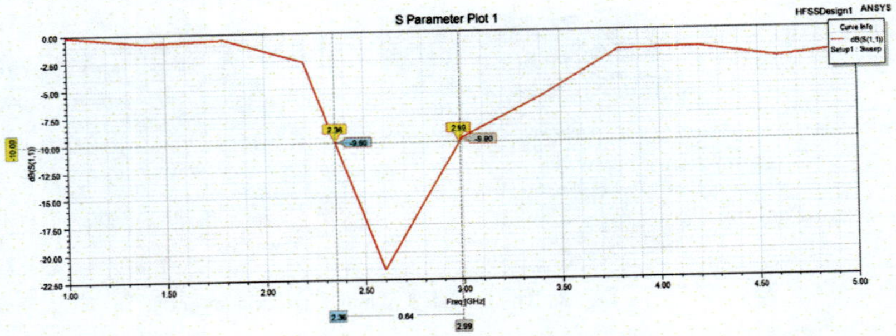

Fig. 4. The S parameters representation for the planar antenna.

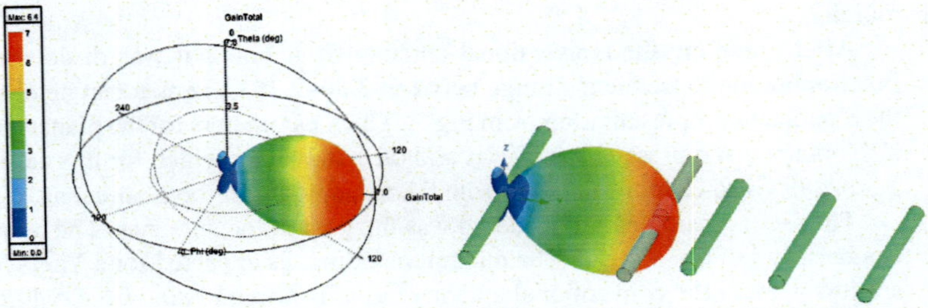

a)3D polar representation b) Representation on the antenna geometry

Fig. 5. The gain representation for the conventional antenna.

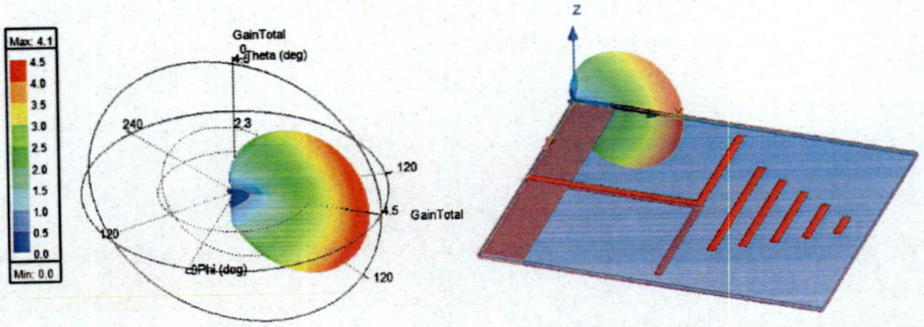

a)3D polar representation b) Representation on the antenna geometry

Fig. 6. The gain representation for the planar antenna.

reference level can be calculated with formula (1). The magnetic field for general public for an exposure over 30 min is calculated with formula (2). The resultant values are not that far from values that should be considered as a threshold for the 2.6 GHz frequency.

$$E = 1.375 f_M^{0.5} \tag{1}$$

$$H = 0.0037 f_M^{0.5} \tag{2}$$

where f_M is the frequency in MHz.

Thus, for the electric field after calculating we obtain a value of 67.36 V/m, while for the magnetic field we obtain a value of 0.1812 A/m.

For an exposure between 6 and 30 min the exposure limits are higher than the previous ones, being calculated with formulas (3) and (4), for electric field 134,101 V/m and magnetic field 0.3494 A/m but still they are exceeded by the ones obtained near the studied structures.

$$E = 4.72 f_M^{0.43} \tag{3}$$

$$H = 0.0123 f_M^{0.43} \tag{4}$$

After analyzing the results obtained for the antennas, we can say that the limits are exceeded thus a human is not safe in the proximity of such an antenna and should not stay close to them. The higher values are, as expected, near the feeding point and along the directors and conductor parts for the electric field as seen in Figs. 7 and 8 and magnetic field as it can be observed in Figs. 9 and 10.

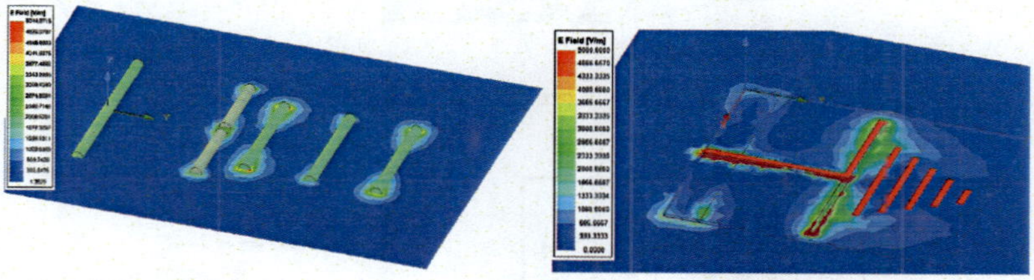

a)conventional b) planar

Fig. 7. Electric field representation for the antennas in the XY plane.

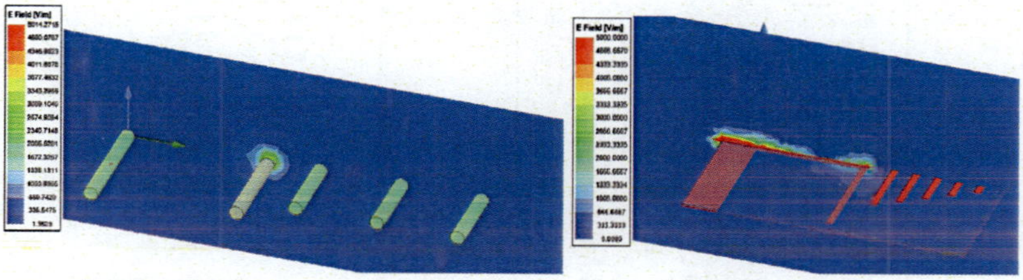

a) conventional b) planar

Fig. 8. Electric field representation for the antennas in the YZ plane.

The characteristic parameters can be also obtained as a table for each antenna. These specific tables can be seen in Fig. 11.

After analyzing the results, it can be concluded that even though the conventional antenna has a higher peak gain value, the front to back ratio has the lowest value for the smaller and more robust planar antenna, making it the better choice from more points of view.

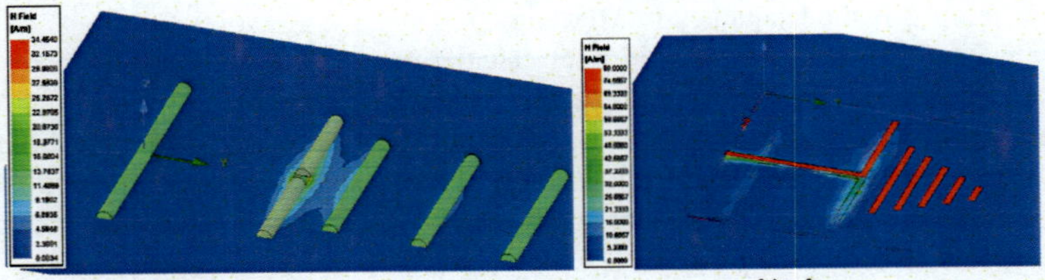

a) conventional b) planar

Fig. 9. Magnetic field representation for the antennas in the XY plane.

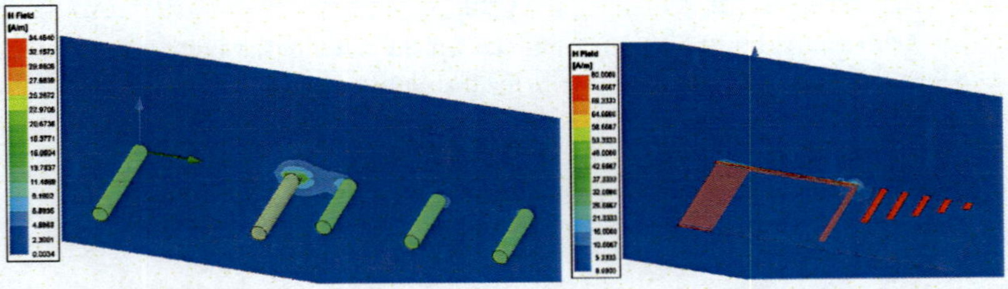

a) conventional b) planar

Fig. 10. Magnetic field representation for the antennas in the YZ plane.

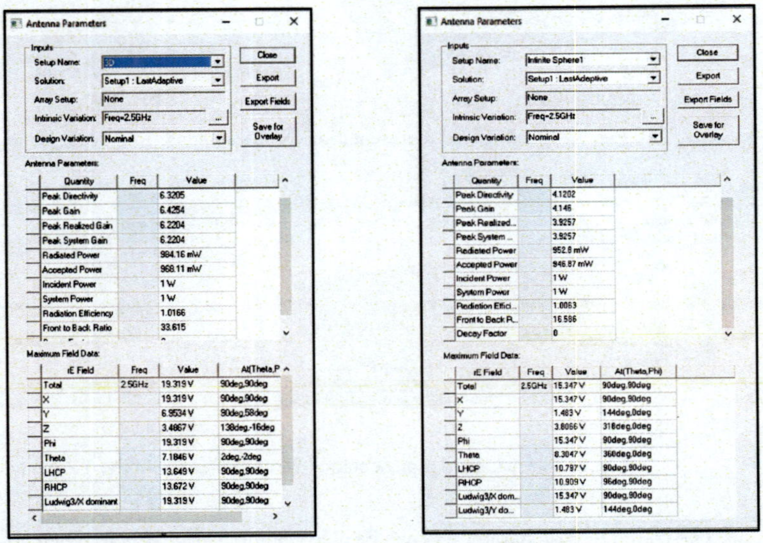

a) conventional b) planar

Fig. 11. Characteristic parameters of the modeled antennas.

3 Comparison of the Influence of the Antennas on Different Types of Human Tissues

The two analyzed antennas were considered to be placed near three layers of human tissue. The characteristics of the tissues are presented in Table 1 and have the following thicknesses: skin 4 mm, fat 4 mm and muscle 30 mm [8–13]. The tissues are considered to cover all the antenna surface, thus for the conventional antenna the tissues are wider. In Fig. 12 an exploded view of the tissues is presented for the 2 cases. The first studied case was when the antenna is placed directly on the skin tissue and after that the tissues are moved further from the antenna to see the effect of distance on the parameters that could negatively influence the human body according to ICNIRP exposure levels limits.

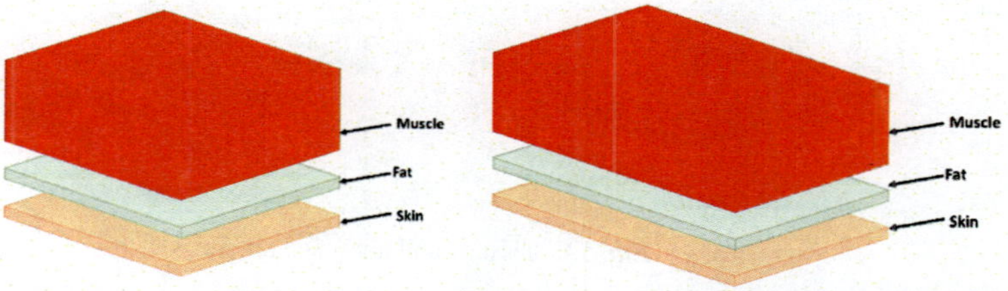

a) tissues above the planar antenna b) tissues above the conventional antenna

Fig. 12. Tissue considered in the vicinity of the antennas – exploded view.

Table 1. Characteristics of the tissues considered.

Type of tissue	Relative permittivity	Conductivity	Loss tangent
Skin	38	1.46	0.283
Fat	5.28	0.1	0.145
Muscle	52.7	1.74	0.242

3.1 Tissues Placed Directly on the Antennas

The first considered case to be studied was the one where the antennas are on the skin tissue, as it can be seen in Fig. 13. For this scenario, the average SAR (Specific Absorption Rate) and electric and magnetic fields values were obtained inside the three types of tissues.

According to ICNIRP the values for SAR for the general public exposure scenario [8], for intervals higher than 6 min in the frequency range 100 kHz–300GHz is 2 for the local Head/torso and 4 for the local limb, values which are highly exceeded in the 3 types of tissue in this study as it can be observed in Fig. 14 for the planar antenna, the highest value present being approximately 190 W/kg. For the conventional structure the conclusions remain the same (Fig. 15), the limits are highly exceeded in the proximity of the antenna, the highest value obtained being of 294 W/kg. The maximum values are encountered in the skin layer, the values decreasing as the distance from the antenna increases. Also, the highest values are present near the feeding point.

A transversal section on YZ axis was made in the middle of each of the antennas and the SAR values were represented there because the highest values are present near the feeding point. As expected, the higher values are in the skin and fat layer, while in the muscle layer the values exceed the limits on a small surface.

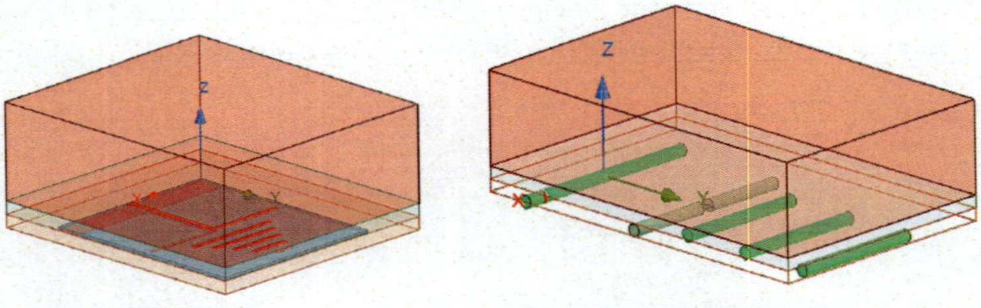

a) planar antenna b) conventional antenna

Fig. 13. Tissues and analyzed antennas.

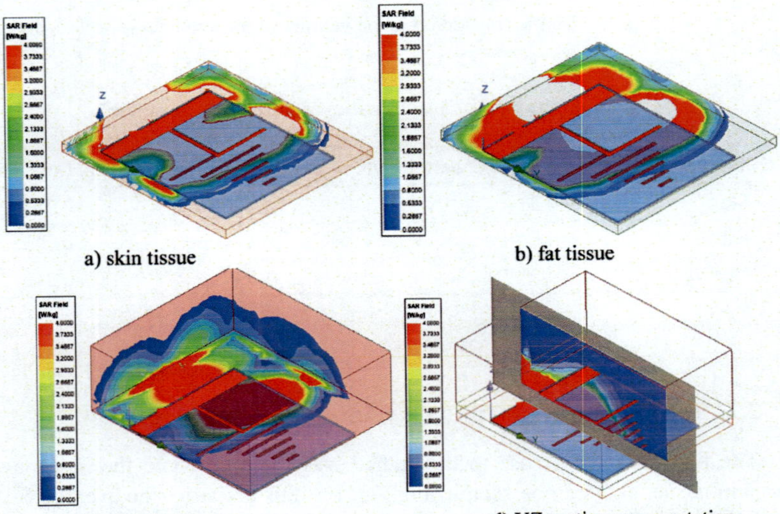

a) skin tissue b) fat tissue

c) muscle tissue d) YZ section representation

Fig. 14. SAR values in the tissues present above the analyzed planar antenna.

In Fig. 16 the electric field in the YZ section for the two types of antennas is presented. Given the limits calculated according to ICNIRP, it can be seen that the values are exceeded in the tissue layers for both antennas and also it can be seen that the distribution

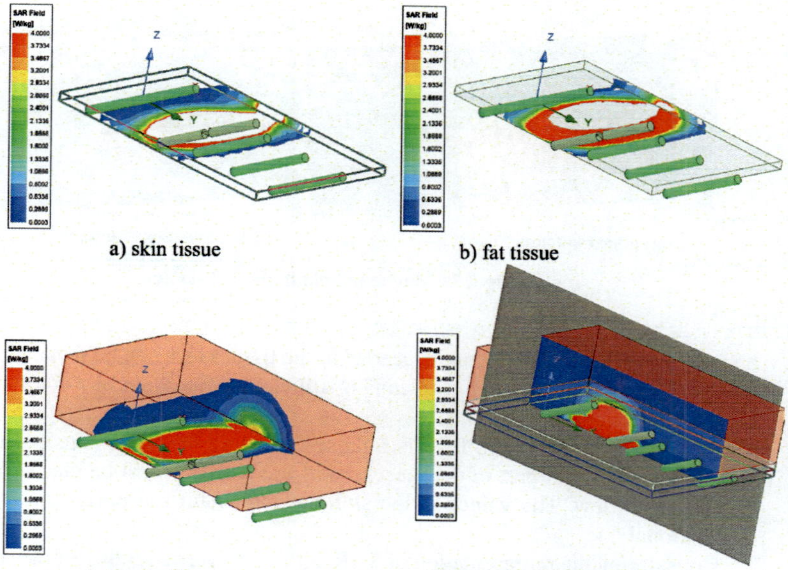

a) skin tissue b) fat tissue

c) muscle tissue d) YZ section representation

Fig. 15. SAR values in the tissues present above the analyzed conventional antenna.

is affected by the transition between different types of tissue. The values are better in the muscle tissue for both cases. Also, the higher values are more concentrated for the conventional antenna, while for the planar antenna they are more evenly distributed along the antenna conductor elements.

The magnetic field values also exceed the imposed values by the standard, but in this case the exceeding values are found in all 3 tissue layers, as can be seen in Fig. 17.

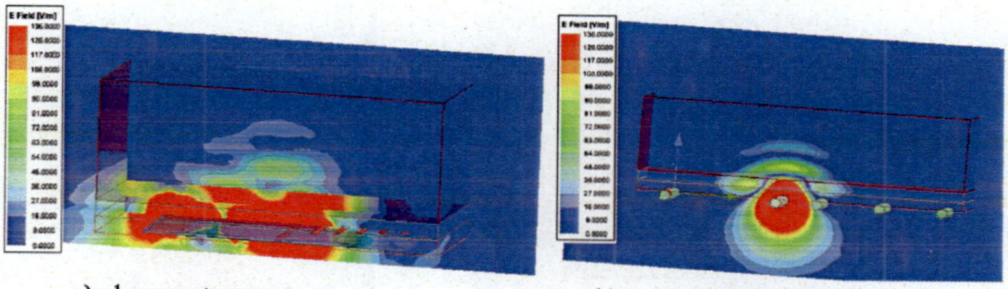

a) planar antenna b) conventional antenna

Fig. 16. Electric field in the YZ section.

3.2 Tissues Placed at 10 mm from the Antennas

When considering the increase of the distance between the tissues and the antenna, the highest values are present near the antenna and the values of the electric field imposed

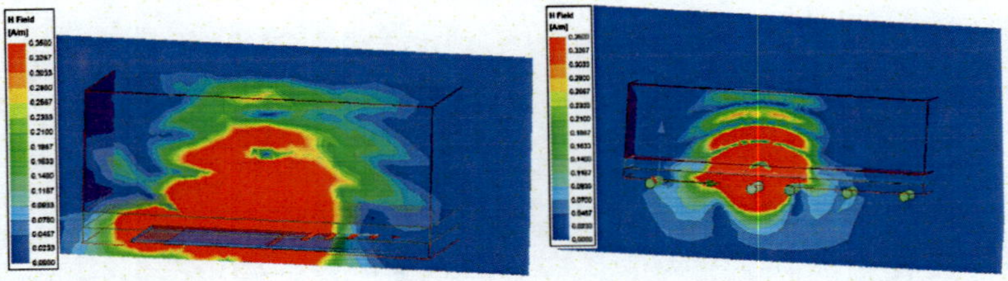

a) planar antenna b) conventional antenna

Fig. 17. Magnetic field in the YZ section.

by the standards in force are not exceeded in the tissues as it can be seen in Fig. 18, thus the distance of 10 mm from the antenna is sufficient to be safe near it for a time interval higher than 6 min.

In Fig. 19 the magnetic field is represented. Here the values are exceeded in the skin and also a small part of the muscle, thus the antenna must be placed farther from this point of view. The values in the skin are higher for the planar antenna than the conventional one.

Considering the representation of SAR in the transversal section of the tissue layers, it can be stated that the limit values are not exceeded, thus being safe to be near the antennas from this point of view.

Considering all 3 parameters analyzed, the main conclusion is that the increase of the distance between the tissue layers and antennas is efficient, and the distance must be more than 10 mm (Fig. 20).

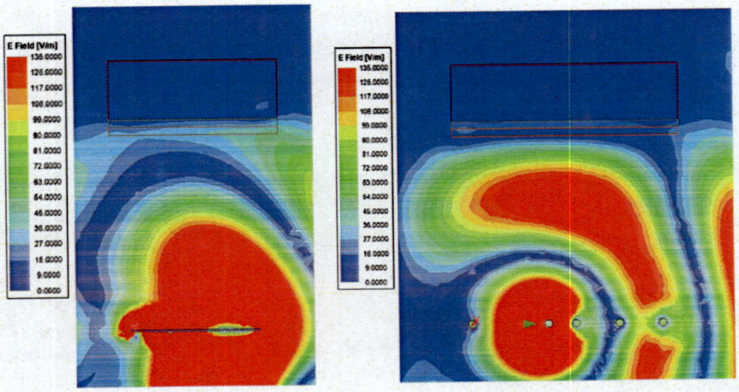

a) planar antenna b) conventional antenna

Fig. 18. Electric field in the YZ section.

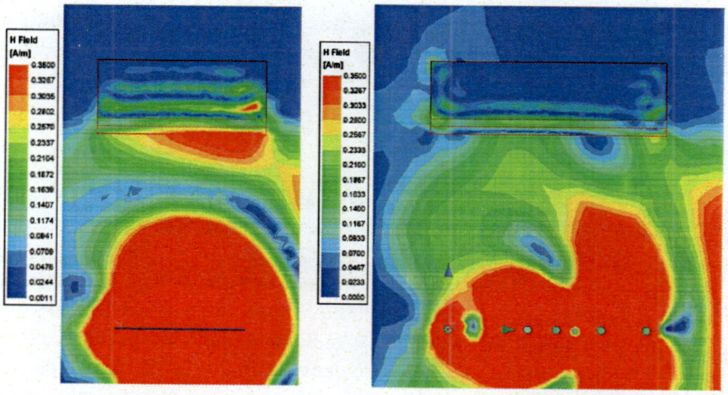

a) planar antenna b) conventional antenna

Fig. 19. Magnetic field in the YZ section.

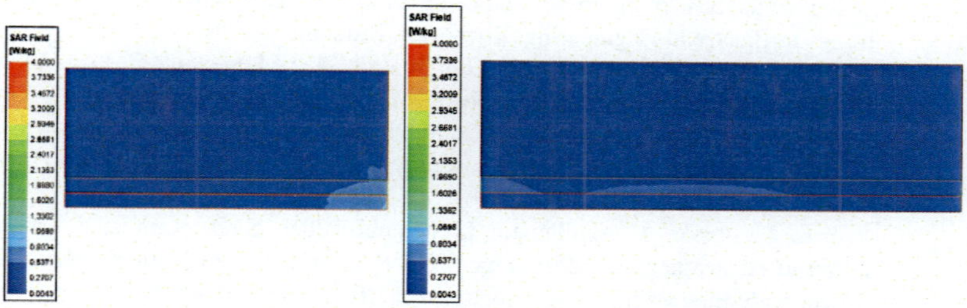

Fig. 20. SAR values in the tissues present above the analyzed conventional antenna.

4 Conclusion

The present study aims at comparing the influence of a conventional and a planar Yagi Uda antenna on tissue layers present in their vicinity. After determining their dimensions considering the operating frequency at approximately 2.6 GHz, the antennas were first compared from the dimension point of view and it was determined that for the same frequency, the planar antenna is smaller and more reliable from the mechanical point of view. Even though the conventional antenna has a higher peak gain value, the front to back ratio has the lowest value for the planar antenna.

The higher values of the electric and magnetic fields are, as expected, near the feeding point and along the directors and conductor parts. Thus, after considering the tissue layers in the vicinity of the antenna it was concluded that according to ICNIRP, the limits for both electric and magnetic field are exceeded near the feeding and along the directors. The SAR values are also exceeded in all three types of the tissue; thus a human would be seriously affected if the antenna would be placed on him for longer periods of time.

The authors considered placing the antenna at 10 mm from the human skin layer and major improvements were seen. Even though the values are still high, in the tissues only the magnetic field exceeds the limits, thus showing that even a small distance from the tissues diminishes the exposure a lot.

References

1. Balanis, C.A.: Antenna Theory Analysis and Design, 4th edn. Wiley (2016)
2. Kraus, J.D., Marhefka, R.J., Khan, A.S.: Antennas and Wave Propagation, 4th edn. Tata McGraw Hill Education Private Limited (2010)
3. Ramos, A., Varum, T., Matos, J.N.: Compact multilayer Yagi-Uda based antenna for IoT/5G sensors. Sensors **18**(9), 2914 (2018). https://doi.org/10.3390/s18092914
4. Fan, Y., Liu, X., Li, J., Chang, T.: A miniaturized circularly polarized antenna for in-body wireless communications. Micromachines **10**(1), 70 (2019). https://doi.org/10.3390/mi10010070
5. Xianming, Q., Chen, Z.N., See, T., Goh, C., Chiam, T.M.: Characterization of RF transmission in human body, pp. 1–4 (2010). https://doi.org/10.1109/APS.2010.5561841
6. Constantinescu, C., Munteanu, C., Pacurar, C., Racasan, A., Gliga, M., Andreica, S.: High frequency analysis of bowtie antennas. In: 2019 11th International Symposium on Advanced Topics in Electrical Engineering, Bucharest, Romania (2019)
7. Constantinescu, C., Pacurar, C., Giurgiuman, A., Munteanu, C., Andreica, S., Gliga, M.: Numerical modelling and analysis of circular patch antenna array for further use determination. In: 9th International Conference on Modern Power Systems (MPS) (2021)
8. ICNIRP guidelines for limiting exposure to electromagnetic fields (100 kHz to 300 GHz). Health Phys. **118**(5), 483–524 (2020)
9. Aguirre, E., Arpon, J., Azpilicueta, L., Miguel Bilbao, S. D., Ramos, V., Falcone, F.: Evaluation of electromagnetic dosimetry of wireless systems in complex indoor scenarios with human body interaction. Prog. Electromagn. Res. B **43**, 189–209 (2012). https://doi.org/10.2528/PIERB12070904
10. Ibraheem, A., Manteghi, M.: Performance of an implanted electrically coupled loop antenna inside human body. Prog. Electromagn. Res. **145**, 195–202 (2014). https://doi.org/10.2528/PIER14022005
11. Bottiglieri, A., Ruvio, G., O'Halloran, M., Farina, L.: Exploiting tissue dielectric properties to shape microwave thermal ablation zones. Sensors **20** (2020)
12. Pacurar, C., et al.: High frequency analysis of the influence of Yagi-Uda antenna on the human head. In: 11th International Conference and Exposition on Electrical and Power Engineering—EPE 2020, Iași, Romania (2020)
13. Constantinescu, C., Pacurar, C., Giurgiuman, A., Munteanu, C., Andreica, S., Gliga, R.: The Influence of Electromagnetic Waves Emitted by PIFA Antennas on the Human Head. Springer Nature (2022)
14. Khraisat, Y.S.H., Al-Zoubi, A.S., Al-Ahmadi, A., Mbaideen, O.A.: Design implantable antennas with human body effect. Int. J. Innov. Technol. Explor. Eng. (IJITEE) **9** (2020)
15. Ali, U., et al.: Design and SAR analysis of wearable antenna on various parts. J. Electr. Eng. Technol. **12** (2017)

Air Quality Monitoring in a Home Using a Low-Cost Device Built Around the Arduino Mega 2560 Platform

C. Drugă(✉), Ional Serban, A. Tulică, and Barbu Braun

Faculty of Product Design and Environment/Product Design, Mechatronics and Environment Department, Transilvania University, Braşov, Romania
druga@unitbv.ro

Abstract. The article is aimed to present the construction and test of a low-cost prototype device for monitoring indoor air quality to enhance human comfort, health, and safety. The device was built around the Arduino Mega 2560 platform to which several sensors are connected, such as DHT11, MQ-2, MQ-3, MQ-4, MQ-7, MQ-9, and MQ-135. The main objective was to incorporate in a single device as many sensors as possible, each detecting a certain type of gas (methane, ethanol, LPG, liquefied methane, hydrogen) or dangerous substances (carbon monoxide, alcohol vapors, smoke) to respond to the widest possible range of factors that can affect people's health and safety. Neither the temperature nor the humidity has been forgotten, which can contribute to the discomfort of the inhabitants. For each of the risk factors, a certain level can be set, which if exceeded will cause the device to warn (sound and through messages displayed on an LCD display or transmitted via Bluetooth to a smartphone) the residents. The device was built and tested at the Transilvania University of Brasov in the Medical Engineering Laboratory.

Keywords: DHT11 · MQ-2 · MQ-3 · Arduino mega 2560 · Air quality

1 Introduction

Air quality depends on atmospheric emissions from ambient sources, mainly in large cities, and long-range transport of pollutants. Poor indoor air quality is particularly harmful to children, the elderly, and vulnerable groups of people suffering from cardiovascular and respiratory diseases. Major indoor air pollutants include cigarette smoke, gases or particles from burning fuel, chemicals, and allergens [1]. The presence of toxic gases, in high concentrations, harms people's health, as well as the environment [1]. So, using the device of monitoring significantly improves process control and helps prevent incidents [2]. Gas sensors are used in many industrial applications, and home protection is cheap compared to other technologies. They have a long life, are relatively cheap, and have high sensitivity and fast response time [2]. Home security consists of using devices to monitor the causes of risk to detect gases and toxic substances, caused by wood or coal stoves, thermal plants, fires, etc. [2, 3].

S. Vlad and N. M. Roman (Eds.): MEDITECH 2022, IFMBE Proceedings 102, pp. 99–104, 2024.
https://doi.org/10.1007/978-3-031-51120-2_11

2 Materials and Methods

2.1 The Perspectives of Low-Cost Sensors

Although low-cost sensors cannot provide the same precision, stability, sensitivity, and accuracy as traditional routine monitoring stations, they can potentially be a valuable supplement in the monitoring programs, and perhaps partly replace traditional reference stations [4]. Employing low-cost sensors can give a better temporal and spatial resolution of pollution on maps, improve the knowledge about pollution dynamics, identify hot spots, and validate or reconsider the location of routine monitoring stations [4, 5]. Furthermore, the sensors can be used as a monitoring tool by municipalities, consultants, or researchers, as personal exposure monitors, for emergency response and hazard-warning systems, and as monitoring and controlling emissions at the source [6, 7].

2.2 MQ-2 Gas Sensor

The module MQ-2 can be used to detect gas leaks and is a precautionary method for poisoning and fires. The sensor has high sensitivity and it is used to detect: LPG, isobutane, propane, methane, alcohol, hydrogen, and smoke [8].

The sensor consists of a comparator, so you can read analog data in real time or identify if gas concentrations have exceeded a certain limit. In this experiment, the buzzer will beep to warn if harmful gases reach a certain concentration.

2.3 MQ-3 Semiconductor Sensor for Alcohol

The module MQ-3 is a sensor with high sensitivity but also a fast response time. The sensor returns a value directly proportional to the concentration of alcohol in the exhaled air. The sensor is stable and can be used for a long time. The analog output voltage can be found between 0–5 V. In this interval, the output voltage increases relatively with the concentration of alcohol vapors coming in contact with the sensor [9]. If the concentration of alcohol vapors is greater than the threshold value set, the digital output will display LOW. This will be easily monitored when the DOUT LED lights up. Additionally, rotating the potentiometer clockwise can result in higher sensitivity [9].

2.4 MQ-4 Semiconductor Sensor for Monitoring Natural Gas

The MQ-4 Gas Sensor Module detects the presence of methane (CH_4) at a concentration between 300 to 10,000 ppm. The sensor needs only one analog input from the microprocessor [10]. The MQ-4 sensor is a sensor with a high sensitivity in methane detection. It can also detect propane or butane very well. The MQ-4 is a low-cost sensor that can detect a variety of gases, especially natural gases.

2.5 MQ-7 Semiconductor Sensor for Carbon Monoxide

The MQ-7 module is a highly sensitive gas sensor and can detect carbon monoxide concentrations, between 10 to 10,000 ppm, in the air. MQ7 sensor consists of a small heater inside with an electrochemical sensor that is able to measure different kinds of gas combinations. The gas sensor module can be used at room temperature [11].

2.6 MQ-9 Sensor for Measuring CO/Combustible Gas

The MQ9, low-cost, sensor is sensitive/able to detect Carbon Monoxide, Methane, and LPG. It can detect carbon monoxide density between 10 to 1000 ppm and flammable gases density between 100 to 10000 ppm. MQ9 consists of an internal heater that starts warming up if a 5V voltage is applied. The sensor is sensitive and can be adjusted by using the potentiometer [12]. It can be used in areas as: Domestic gas leakage detectors, Industrial gas detectors, and Portable gas detectors [12].

2.7 MQ-135 Sensor for CO/Combustible Gas

The MQ-135 sensor belongs to the MQ series that detect different gasses in the air. The MQ-135 module is used to detect gases: NH_3, NO_x, alcohol, benzene, smoke, CO_2, etc. The conductivity of the MQ-135 is low in clean air. The conductivity of the sensor increases directly proportional to the increasing gas concentration. The supply voltage is 5 VDC, and the output voltage has an increment of 0.1 V for every 20 ppm [13].

2.8 DHT11 Digital Relative Humidity and Temperature Sensor

The DHT11 sensor monitors, with good accuracy, temperature, and humidity. The sensor has outstanding long-term stability, a good transmission distance of up to 100 m, and low power consumption.

A negative temperature coefficient thermistor (NTC) is used to measure temperature and a capacitive sensor for the relative humidity. These sensing elements are pre-calibrated and the output is provided as a digital signal. The DHT11 sensor is compatible with most of microcontroller development boards, like Arduino Uno. Arduino Mega 2560, etc.

3 Design of the Electrical Circuit and Implementation of the Device Programming

The creation and simulation of the electric circuit were done with the help of the circuito.io website (Fig. 1). The electrical circuit of the device consists of the Arduino Mega 2560 platform, the 7 sensors for the detection of flammable and dangerous gases for human health, a Bluetooth module, a buzzer, LEDs, LCD 4 × 20 display and 9 V battery.

The first step is to install the Arduino IDE, and afterward to identify and install all the libraries needed for the: LCD, Bluetooth module, and gas and temperature sensors. In the next step, each sensor was tested, and then proceed to integrate the 7 source codes into one, and repeat the measurements. The device's practical realization consists of an expansion shield for the Arduino Mega 2560 board, a buzzer, a 9VDC battery, a Bluetooth module, two LEDs of different colors, and a housing (3D printed)- Fig. 2.

If the maximum allowable concentrations for carbon monoxide, carbon dioxide or other gases are exceeded, the human personnel are notified by lighting the red LED or by a message sent to a smartphone via Bluetooth device. By attaching a Bluetooth module

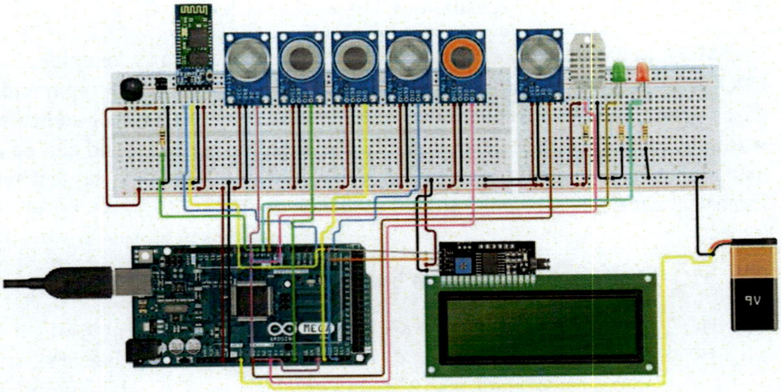

Fig. 1. Electrical circuit of the device

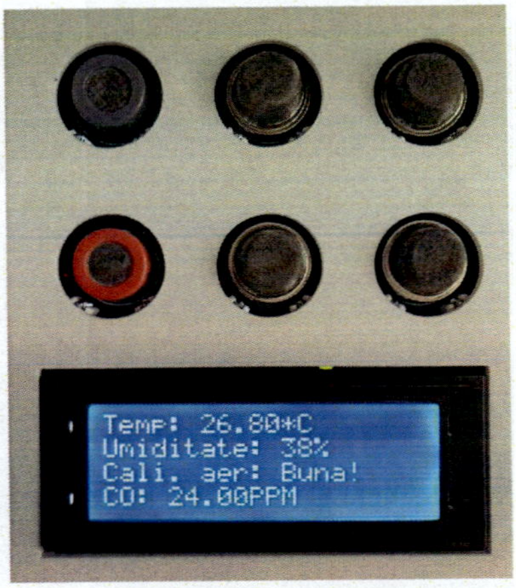

Fig. 2. The front panel of the device

to the device and installing the Arduino Bluetooth Terminal application, which can be purchased from Google Play, the device user can see the values recorded by the system directly from the mobile, in real-time (Fig. 3).

4 Conclusions

This device for monitoring the causes of risk in a home is a prototype created to record values of gas concentrations to warn individuals in the room if the limit is exceeded normal and to avoid possible dangers and incidents that affect the human body. The device was created to be a simplified, portable, reliable, and economical system. Applications are exclusively for people's comfort, health and safety, quality of life, and technology

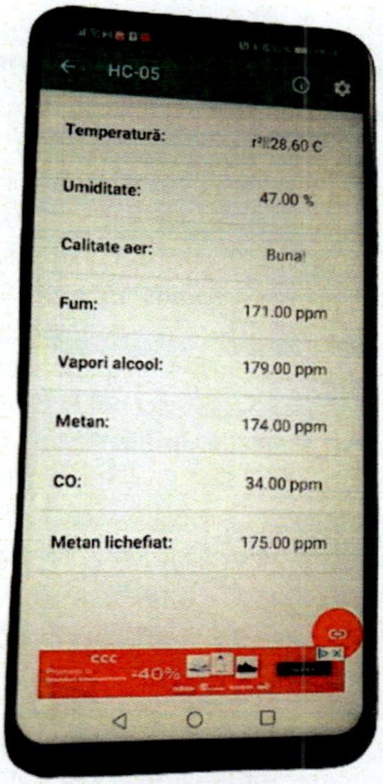

Fig. 3. View the sensors' values using the Arduino Bluetooth Terminal application on a mobile phone

development. In the case of this system, no specialized training is needed to use it, and not require special storage conditions. The gas monitor provides data security for a customized level of exposure and manages at a low cost to display the measurements in a relatively short time. By making the system we can thus gradually advance through simple changes and fewer investment expenses in terms of energy consumption. The device for monitoring the causes of risk in a home proves its usefulness and qualitative functionality through the prism of the measurements performed. Thanks to the mobile app, the device is very useful for monitoring parameters in real time from sensors. Wireless communication allows users to use the device from a relatively long distance.

Acknowledgment. Considering their involvement in the development of this paper, we would like to thank students Vrînceanu Claudia and Budău Larisa, and also to the team from the County Center for Medical Equipment of Brasov (CJAM-Bv).

References

1. Roberts, W.E.: Air pollution and skin disorders. Int. J. Women's Dermatol. Rancho Mirage, CA 6 USA 92270. https://doi.org/10.1016/j.ijwd.2020.11.001 (2020)
2. Korotcenkov, G.: Senzorii de gaz şi rolul lor în industrie, agricultura, medicina şi monitorizarea mediului. Akademos- Ştiințe Inginereşti și Tehnologice **4**(6), 20–28 (2019)
3. Yamazoe, N.: Toward innovations of gas sensor technology. Sens. Actuators B **8** (1–2), 2–14 (2005). https://doi.org/10.1016/j.snb.2004.12.075

4. Castell, N., et al.: Can commercial low-cost sensor platforms contribute to air quality monitoring and exposure estimates? Environ. Int. **99**, 293–302 (2017)
5. Aleixandre, M., Gerboles, M.: Review of small commercial sensors for indicative monitoring of ambient gas. Chem. Eng. Trans. CET **30** (2012). https://doi.org/10.3303/CET1230029
6. Gerboles, M., Buzica, D.: Evaluation of micro-sensors to monitor ozone in ambient air. Joint Res. Center Environ. Sustain. EUR 23676 EN (2009). https://doi.org/10.2788/5978
7. Mead, M.I., et al.: The use of electrochemical sensors for monitoring urban air quality in low-cost, high-density networks. Atmos. Environ. **70**(5), 186–203 (2013)
8. Sun Funder, Lesson 22 Gas Sensor. https://docs.sunfounder.com/projects/sensorkit-v2-pi/en/latest/lesson_22.html. Last accessed 15 September 2022
9. Microcontrollerslab, Interface MQ3 Alcohol Sensor Module with Arduino. https://microcontrollerslab.com/mq3-alcohol-sensor-arduino-tutorial/. Last accessed 14 September 2022
10. Utmel Electronic, How to Use MQ4 Gas Sensor? https://www.utmel.com/components/how-to-use-mq4-gas-sensor?id=821. Last accessed 14 September 2022
11. Circuits Diy, MQ7 Carbon Monoxide (CO) Gas Sensor Module. https://www.circuits-diy.com/mq7-carbon-monoxide-co-gas-sensor-module/. Last accessed 15 September 2022
12. Optimus Digital, MQ-9 Gas Sensor Module. https://www.optimusdigital.ro/en/gas-sensors/1129-modul-senzor-de-gaz-mq-9.html. Last accessed 10 September 2022
13. Druga, C.N., Braun, B., Serban, I., Tulica, A.: Device for Measurement Concentration of Toxic Gas in an Enclosure, Macromolecular Symposia, vol. 404, issue 1, Special Issue: Conference on Design and Technologies for Polymeric and Composites Products—POLCOM 2021, Issue Edited by: Giuseppe Lamanna, Constantin G. Opran, Wiley Online Library (2022)

BE-AI: A Beaconized Platform with Machine Learning Capabilities

Tatar Simion-Daniel(✉) and Gheorghe Sebestyen

Technical University of Cluj-Napoca, Cluj-Napoca, Romania
{Simion.Tatar,Gheorghe.Sebestyen}@cs.utcluj.ro

Abstract. The genomic and metagenomic data sources currently available offer many possibilities to access and analyze them. Machine learning provides a suite of well-known intelligent algorithmic tools for interpreting genomic and metagenomic data. These data can come in different formats and serve different purposes. Integrating these heterogenous data sources is a necessary task in order to use different pipelines to obtain the actionable information. Once the data is processed it can be made available for querying in the beacon network for others for different purposes, among which are alleles of interest. To address machine learning necessities and the sharing of data through a beacon, BE-AI was developed.

Keywords: Machine learning · Genomic Python platform · Beacon

Abbreviations and Acronyms

A	Adenine
API	Application Programming Interface
AST	Antimicrobial Susceptibility Testing
C	Cytosine
CARD	Comprehensive Antibiotic Resistance Database
CNN	Convolutional Neural Networks
DNA	Deoxyribonucleic Acid
DT	Decision Trees
G	Guanine
GCP	Google Cloud Platform
GPU	Graphical Processing Units
HMM	Hidden Markov Models
HTTP	Hypertext Transfer Protocol
ICGC	International Cancer Genome Consortium
IDE	Integrated Development Environment
INSDC	International Nucleotide Sequence Database Collaboration
JSON	Javascript Object Notation
KNN	K Nearest Neighbors
PATRIC	Pathosystems Resource Integration Center
RPC	Remote Procedure Call

S. Vlad and N. M. Roman (Eds.): MEDITECH 2022, IFMBE Proceedings 102, pp. 105–114, 2024.
https://doi.org/10.1007/978-3-031-51120-2_12

REST	Representational State Transfer
RNA	Ribonucleic Acid
SVM	Support Vector Machines
T	Thymine
TCGA	The Cancer Genome Atlas

1 Introduction

1.1 Introduction to Genomics

The genome comprises all the genes necessary to the functioning of an organism and its cell reproduction. Besides active genes, there are other portions of genomic sequences that are non-coding genes, signals and repeated sequences.

The coding sequences are named codons and the non-coding ones are called introns. This gives a greater complexity in analyzing the genome structure in search for the protein coding sequences. The genes are built from basic blocks of bases: adenine (A), cytosine (C), guanine (G) and thymine (T). They are used in building the whole DNA (deoxyribonucleic acid). The RNA (ribonucleic acid) has uracil (U) instead of thymine. These determine the amino acid sequences in proteins.

The genomics field studies the genome's structure, the phenotype and its relation to the genome, the evolutionary aspects of related genomes, its editing, etc.

The most interesting genome is of course the human one [1–4].

There are also other Eukaryote genomes and genomic data in different databases like Genbank [5, 6], ENCODE [7], Ensembl [8–14] etc. These data can be accessed in various ways, ranging from FTP (File Transfer Protocol) or web interface. Ensembl offers the possibility of access via REST (Representational State Transfer) API (Application Programming[1] Interface).

1.2 Introduction to Metagenomics

The metagenomics is the field that studies organisms in the Prokariota empire, comprising Bacteria and Archaea. These are organisms that lack a nucleus and organelles with membrane.

Their genome has a circular or linear structure, lacking the division between introns and codons and therefore easier to analyze.

The metagenomics field explores environments like soil, wastewater, human body, lakes, thermal vents, the oceans, rivers, biomass, etc.

An interesting aspect of the metagenome is that not all of it is culturable, but it can be sequenced. If data from laboratory cultures is unavailable, then a promising route is that of genomic sequencing.

Public databases exist with metagenomic datasets available via various means of access.

1 *Tatar Simion-Daniel, Simion.Tatar@cs.utcluj.ro, Cluj-Napoca, Romania.

Important projects referring to metagenomes are the "Human Microbiome Project" [15–17] and MetaHIT (Metagenomics of the Human Intestinal Tract). It is estimated that the human metagenome is tenfold the number of human cells and encode 100-fold more unique genes [187].

Another data sources are EMBL-EBI (European Molecular Biology Laboratory - European Bioinformatics Institute) [18] and DDBJ [20] which provide also RESTful APIs. They are part of INSDC (International Nucleotide Sequence Database Collaboration) [21].

1.3 Antimicrobial Resistance

The antimicrobial resistance is recognized as a global crisis [22]. The infectious agents obtain resistance to diverse classes of drugs through survival of the fittest by gene mutations or acquiring resistance genes through horizontal gene transfer. There are not only bacteria involved, but also fungi, viruses and parasites. Their genomes are known as the resistome.

Some agents are resistant to a specific class of drugs, other have resistance to whole classes of drugs. Another factor is decreasing the manufacturing of novel drugs to combat the agents [23].

These problems are known for years and are documented in the literature. Initiatives to address these issues resulted in collecting samples and performing laboratory analyses and genomes sequencing. These data were aggregated in databases like PATRIC (now BV-BRC) [24–30], CARD [31–37] and ARDB [38].

The analysis on PATRIC allowed RPC (Remote Procedure Call) to manipulate the data and the new BV-BRC site allows FTP (File Transfer Protocol) access [39] and the web interface.

These databases are interesting from the point of view of interpreting the phenotype – antimicrobial resistance – based on whole-genome sequences. Therefore, they provide data related to AST (antimicrobial susceptibility testing) linked to curated genomes.

1.4 Cancer Data

The cancer is a major disease and a subject of a major research effort. The databases contain plenty of genomic and phenotypic data: TCGA (The Cancer Genome Atlas) [40], ICGC (International Cancer Genome Consortium) [41], etc.

There is an interest in machine and deep learning applications on cancer data: assessment of cancer based on microscopy, molecular subtyping, prognosis prediction, precision oncology, tumor microenvironment, etc. [42].

1.5 RESTful APIs

REST stands for Representational State Transfer.

It is an architectural mode to describe in the uniform way the communication between different components. It can be used in the Internet and is useful in a client – server architecture. For web applications it is often based on the HTTP (Hypertext Transfer

Protocol) and it uses standards as JSON (Javascript Object Notation) or XML (Extended Markup Language), and the ubiquitous HTML (Hypertext Markup Language).

The HTTP methods are used to identify resources, manipulate resources and pass descriptive messages using: GET (for retrieving data), POST (creating data on the server), PUT (modifying existing data on the server), DELETE (for removing data on the server) and some more as exemplified in Fig. 1.

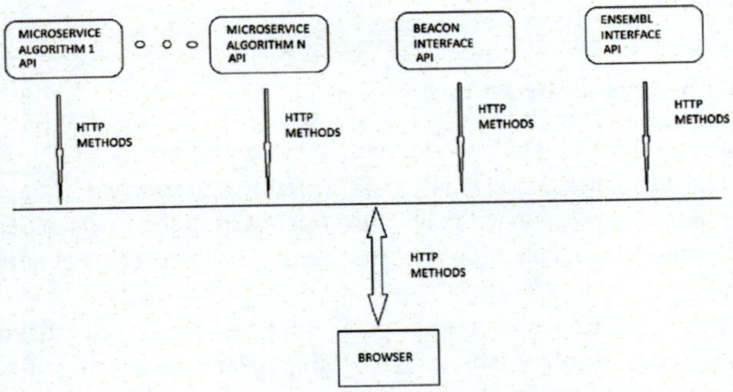

Fig. 1. REST communication over HTTP

These methods are standardized and can be used in building RESTful conformant APIs. They allow not only communication between a client and a server, but also between servers, creating a mesh of interconnected web servers that obey this specification.

APIs can be developed in different programming languages (Java, Python, C#), using different paradigms and even more they can be used because of the communication standards.

1.6 Machine Learning

There are many applications of machine learning in the field of biomedicine: gene identification, disease and patient categorization, treatments of patients, imaging applications, text applications, electronic health results, gene expression, splicing, transcription factors, microRNA, protein structure, protein-protein interactions, single-cell data, metagenomics, sequencing and variant calling, drug development, etc. [43].

The field of machine and deep learning is a part of artificial intelligence that uses algorithms able to learn from data and make predictions on unknown and new data. They can be applied in unsupervised learning, supervised learning and semi-supervised learning.

Their performances are affected by the quantity of data and the availability of earlier models for that data.

The machine learning applied to biomedicine is a hot topic with promises regarding personalized medicine.

Two well-known platforms that provide machine learning capabilities for biomedical computing are KBase [44] and Galaxy [45]. KBase does not currently support machine learning applications. Galaxy offers some machine learning algorithms but there are still many to implement; it does have a REST API, but misses the beaconized human data part.

1.7 Microservices

Microservices provide an architecture where the domain functionality is grouped and communicate through means of lightweight protocols, such as HTTP for web. A combination of these two concepts: REST und microservices is a successful solution for biomedical problems.

1.8 The Beacon Network

The Beacon for genomics is a discoverability and data sharing protocol [46, 47]. It enables queries of the human genome regarding the presence or absence of a specific allele at a position within the genome. It can have a great impact on clinical data and ensures security and privacy of genomic data. The beacon can be used for metagenomics datasets like SARS-Cov-2 [48].

2 Method

The three main concepts that the current platform implements are: REST calls to acquire and distribute data using a microservices architecture that offers the possibility of scaling and the cloud deployment, the machine learning component and the use of the Beacon protocol to make the data discoverable and accessible.

2.1 Datasets

The datasets were provided by the Python libraries, and they are publicly available. They were used as a proof of concept to show the platform functionality. The possibility for new datasets is open.

2.2 Framework and Tools

The framework used for this application was Django (version 3.2.7) and was chosen because of flexibility, robustness, easy and fast development and deployment.

The Python programming language was 3.10 using a PyCharm IDE (Integrated Development Environment). The Python library used was scikit-learn version 1.1.2 [49].

ReactJS was used for the frontend as it is widely used and with accessible documentation.

2.3 The Machine Learning Algorithms

The choice of programming language implementation had to do with available libraries that provide the needed functionality. Java, C# and Python were evaluated. Python was the winner because of machine learning existing algorithms that could be easily integrated in the program's logic.

The scikit-learn library offers a plethora of computational solutions. As such, SVM (Support Vector Machines), knn (K Nearest Neighbors) and DT (Decision Trees) were chosen as first algorithms to deal with biomedical data. They are used very often for biomedical machine learning experiments, and they show good results in practice as algorithms of choice.

The mentioned algorithms offer interpretable and explainable models in healthcare. They are simpler than deep learning algorithms and are successful applied to a variety of biomedical problems. They compete in terms of performance metrics and interpretability with deep learning algorithms.

These algorithms integrated in the platform are the first steps for a multi-omics solution. Multi-omics is a newly developing branch in machine learning that accounts for different aspects of the biomedical domain.

2.4 Microservices Implemented

A REST based microservices architecture allows different implementations to communicate using a standardized way through HTTP means. From the software engineering point of view, it makes sense to choose such an implementation for interoperability and integration of heterogenous resources. The microservices-based architecture is depicted in Fig. 2.

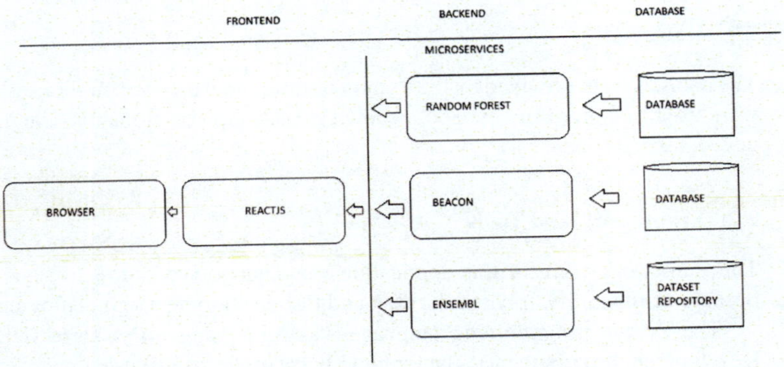

Fig. 2. The microservices-based architecture

The algorithms were allocated in the same microservice, as they provide the computational functionality of the application.

Another microservice was dedicated to Ensembl over RESTful API calls to get the data from the available metagenomic or genomic datasets. This way the data necessary for genomic analysis pipelines can be easily accessed. The other RESTful calls allow to transfer data from and to the Ensembl database.

The other microservice implemented access to the Beacon network over REST calls. For human genomes and SARS-Cov-2 the Beacon version 1 provided query results to answer the question: was there a nucleotide observed at a specific location in the genome? The Beacon version 2 provides richer phenotype informations and clinical data thorough the same federated model. It also has uses for rare diseases and cancer. The data in the Beacon network is secured with different access levels.

3 Results and Discussion

The microservices architecture allows a clean separation of concerns and domain functionality, and for this case it is achieved. The algorithms are separated from retrieved datasets and the datasets can be easily put into the beaconized network.

From the software engineering point of view, they can be developed and deployed separately, independent of each other, hiding the implementation details at microservice's boundaries. Using a public interface allows decoupling of microservices.

Deploy auf cloud has the advantage of scaling as number of processors, memory and storage. This means that higher data quantities could be used. A laboratory instance of the platform enables a researcher to tweak it and save money working on own data. The proposed pipeline concept follows the information flow as in Fig. 3.

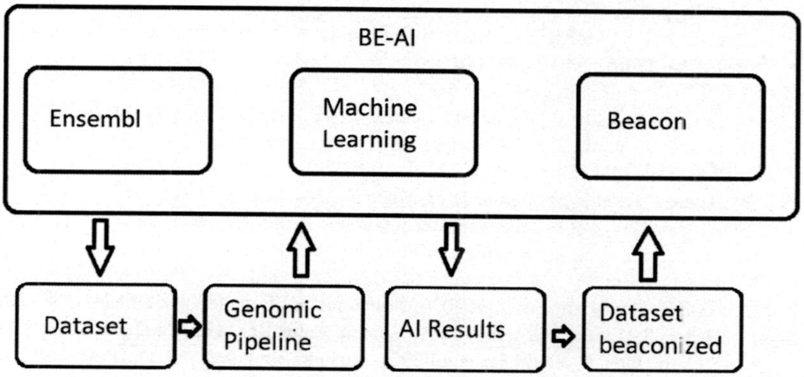

Fig. 3. The information pipeline

4 Conclusion

The use of a platform with machine learning algorithms provides insights for various problems in the genomics and metagenomics fields. The integration and interoperability of different heterogenous data sources enables diverse research analyses. The different technologies like REST APIs, microservices and Beacon networks are put together in a platform that provides also machine learning capabilities.

5 Future Research

As next steps it is possible to use this machine learning platform to connect with various other databases that hold data or web servers that provide access to data through REST APIs or RPC technologies. Another step could be deployment of the microservices solution into the cloud (for example in GCP - Google Cloud Platform) to benefit from dynamic scalability under increased data load.

Other directions would be an increase in the number of artificial intelligence algorithms provided by the platform (for example deep learning architectures CNN – convolutional neural networks) and other basic genomic pipelines based on Biopython. The number of machine learning algorithms provided by the current platform would be increased.

Conflicts of Interest. The authors declare no conflicts of interest.

References

1. Dulbecco, R.: A turning point in cancer research: sequencing the human genome **231**(4742), 1055–1056 (1986)
2. Collins, F., Galas, D.: A new five-year plan for the U.S. human genome project. Science **262**(5130), 43–46 (1993)
3. Collins, F.S., Fink, L.: The human genome project. Alcohol Health Res. World **19**(3), 190–195 (1995)
4. Collins, F.S., McKusick, V.A.: Implications of the human genome project for medical science. JAMA **285**(5), 540–544 (2001)
5. www.ncbi.nlm.nih.gov/genbank/
6. Benson, D.A., et al.: GenBank. Nucleic Acids Res. **45**(D1), D37–D42 (2017)
7. Lee, B.T., et al.: The UCSC Genome Browser database: 2022 update. Nucleic Acids Res. **7;50**(D1), D1115–D1122 (2022)
8. Aken, B.L., et al.: Ensembl 2017. Nucleic Acids Res. **4**;45(D1): D635–D642 (2017)
9. Zerbino, D.R., et al.: Ensembl 2018. Nucleic Acids Res. **46**(D1), D754–D761 (2018)
10. Hunt, S.E., et al.: Ensembl variation resources. Database (Oxford) bay119 (2018)
11. Cunningham, F., et al.: Ensembl 2019. Nucleic Acids Res. **47**(D1), D745–D751 (2019)
12. Yates, A.D., et al.: Ensembl 2020. Nucleic Acids Res. **48**(D1), D682–D688 (2020)
13. Howe, K.L., et al.: Ensembl 2021. Nucleic Acids Res. **49**(D1), D884–D891 (2021)
14. Cunningham, F., et al.: Ensembl 2022. Nucleic Acids Res. **50**(1), D988–D995 (2022)
15. Kaminski, J., Gibson, M.K., Franzosa, E.A., Segata, N., Dantas, G., Huttenhower, C.: High-specificity targeted functional profiling in microbial communities with shortBRED. PLoS Comput. Biol. **11**(12), e1004557 (2015)
16. Sinha, R., Abnet, C.C., White, O., Knight, R., Huttenhower, C.: The microbiome quality control project: baseline study design and future directions. Genome Biol. **16**, 276 (2015)
17. Human Microbiome Project Consortium: Structure, function and diversity of the healthy human microbiome. Nature **486**(7402), 207–214 (2012)
18. Qin, J., et al.: A human gut microbial gene catalogue established by metagenomic sequencing. Nature **464**(7285), 59–65 (2010)
19. Kanz, C., et al.: The EMBL nucleotide sequence database. Nucleic Acids Res. **33**, D29–D33 (2005)

20. Fukuda, A., Kodama, Y., Mashima, J., Fujisawa, T., Ogasawara, O.: DDBJ update: streamlining submission and access of human data. Nucleic Acids Res. **49**(D1), D71–D75. European Mo- lecular Biology Laboratory (2021)
21. Cochrane, G., Karsch-Mizrachi, I., Takagi, T., et al.: The international nucleotide sequence database collaboration. Nucleic Acids Res. **44**, D48–50 http://www.insdc.org/ (2016)
22. McEwen, S.A., Collignon, P.J.: Antimicrobial resistance: a one health perspective. Microbiol. Spectr. **6**(2) (2018)
23. Brinkac, L., Voorhies, A., Gomez, A., Nelson, K.E.: The threat of antimicrobial resistance on the human microbiome. Microb. Ecol. **74**(4), 1001–1008 (2017)
24. Antonopoulos, D.A., et al.: PATRIC as a unique resource for studying antimicrobial resistance. Brief. Bioinform. **20**(4), 1094–1102 (2019)
25. Davis, J.J., et al.: The PATRIC bioinformatics resource center: expanding data and analysis capabilities. Nucleic Acids Res. **48**(D1), D606–D612 (2020)
26. Gillespie, J.J., et al.: PATRIC: the comprehensive bacterial bioinformatics resource with a focus on human pathogenic species. Infect. Immun. **79**(11), 4286–4298 (2011)
27. Parrello, B., Butler, R., Chlenski, P., Pusch, G.D., Overbeek, R.: Supervised extraction of near-complete genomes from metagenomic samples: a new service in PATRIC. PLoS One **16**(4), e0250092 (2021)
28. Wattam, A.R., et al.: PATRIC, the bacterial bioinformatics database and analysis resource. Nucleic Acids Res. **42**(Database issue), D581–91 (2014)
29. Wattam, A.R., et al.: Improvements to PATRIC, the all-bacterial bioinformatics database and analysis resource center. Nucleic Acids Res. **45**(D1), D535–D542 (2017)
30. Snyder, E.E., et al.: PATRIC: the VBI Pathosystems resource integration center. Nucleic Acids Res. **35**(Database issue), D401–6 (Jan)
31. McArthur, et al.: The comprehensive antibiotic resistance database. Antimicrob. Agents Chemother. **57**, 3348–3357 (2013)
32. Jia, et al.: CARD 2017: expansion and model-centric curation of the comprehensive antibiotic resistance database. Nucleic Acids Res. **45**, D566-573 (2017)
33. Tsang et al.: Pathogen taxonomy updates at the comprehensive antibiotic resistance database: implications for molecular epidemiology. Preprints 2019070222 (2019)
34. Faltyn et al.: Evolution and nomenclature of the trimethoprim resistant dihydrofolate (dfr) reductases. Preprints 2019050137 (2019)
35. Guitor, et al.: Capturing the Resistome: a robust and reliable targeted capture method for detecting antibiotic resistance determinants. Antimicrob. Agents Chemother. **64**, e01324-e1419 (2019)
36. Chen, et al.: Detection of antimicrobial resistance using proteomics and the comprehensive antibiotic resistance database: a case study. Proteomics Clin. Appl. **14**, e1800182 (2019)
37. Alcock, et al.: CARD 2020: antibiotic resistome surveillance with the comprehensive antibiotic resistance database. Nucleic Acids Res. **48**, D517–D525 (2020)
38. Liu, B., Pop, M.: ARDB—antibiotic resistance genes database. Nucleic Acids Res. **37**(Issue suppl_1), D443–D447 (2009)
39. VanOeffelen, M., et al.: A genomic data resource for predicting antimicrobial resistance from laboratory-derived antimicrobial susceptibility phenotypes. Brief Bioinform. **22**(6), bbab313 (2021)
40. https://www.cancer.gov/tcga
41. Zhang, J., Bajari, R., Andric, D., et al.: The international cancer genome consortium data portal. Nat. Biotechnol. **37**(4), 367–369 (2019). doi:https://doi.org/10.1038/s41587-019-0055-9
42. Tran, K.A., Kondrashova, O., Bradley, A., Williams, E.D., Pearson, J.V., Waddell, N.: Deep learning in cancer diagnosis, prognosis and treatment selection. Genome Med. **13**(1), 152 (2021)

43. Ching, T., et al.: Opportunities and obstacles for deep learning in biology and medicine. J. R. Soc. Interface. **15**(141), 20170387 (2018)
44. Arkin, A.P., Cottingham, R.W., Henry, C.S., Harris, N.L., Stevens, R.L., Maslov, S., et al.: KBase: the United States department of energy systems biology knowledgebase. Nat. Biotechnol. **36**, 566 (2018)
45. Afgan, E., et al.: The Galaxy platform for accessible, reproducible and collaborative biomedical analyses: 2018 update. Nucleic Acids Res. **46**(W1), W537–W544 (2018)
46. Fiume, M., et al.: Federated discovery and sharing of genomic data using Beacons. Nat. Biotechnol. **37**(3), 220–224 (2019)
47. Rambla, J., et al.: Beacon v2 and Beacon networks: a "lingua franca" for federated data discovery in biomedical genomics, and beyond. Hum. Mutat. **43**(6), 791–799 (2022)
48. https://covid19beacon.crg.eu/
49. Pedregosa et al.: Scikit-learn: machine learning in Python. JMLR 12, pp. 2825–2830 (2011)

eHealth Mobile Application Using Fitbit Smartwatch

Adela Pop[1], Alexandra Fanca[1](✉), Honoriu Valean[1], Dan-Ioan Gota[1], Ovidiu Stan[1], Marius Nicolae Roman[2], Iulia Clitan[1], and Vlad Muresan[1]

[1] Faculty of Automation and Computer Science, Department of Automation, Technical University of Cluj Napoca, Cluj Napoca, Romania
alexandra.fanca@aut.utcluj.ro

[2] Faculty of Electrical Engineering, Electrical Engineering and Measurements Department, Technical University of Cluj Napoca, Cluj Napoca, Romania

Abstract. Health is one of the most precious aspects of every person's life. Whether we're talking about a well-functioning heart, nervous system, respiratory system, or simply body weight, each of these branches contributes to a person's overall health. It is important to monitor certain body functions and characteristics as often as possible so that we can prevent or, in unfortunate situations, treat health problems early. The developed mobile application facilitates the monitoring of heart rate, ideal weight, basal metabolic rate, and body mass index. The data used by the mobile app is collected by the FITBIT smartwatch. Based on the data, heart rate statistics and nutritional calculation results (body mass index, basal metabolic rate, and ideal body weight) are generated according to the user's gender, age, weight, and height.

Keywords: Heart rate · Body mass index · Basal metabolic rate · Ideal weight

1 Introduction

Heart rate tells us how many times a person's heart beats in a minute. It is important to know your heart rate and normal heart rate values so that you can make a comparison and know where you stand [1]. Certain conditions have a direct impact on heart rate: arrhythmia (causes an irregular heartbeat, making it beat either too fast or too slow), tachycardia (this condition occurs when the heartbeat exceeds 80–110 beats/minute) [2], or bradycardia (with a heart rate ranging from 40 to 50 beats/min and hypotension with systolic blood pressure (SBP) in the 80 mm Hg and mean arterial pressure (MAP) in the 50 mm Hg) [3]. Also, complications of SARS-CoV-2 infection can include cardiac effects [4–6].

Unfortunately, we can suffer from these problems without having any symptoms, so heart rate monitoring [7] can help us discover whether we are suffering from one of these disorders or whether we are healthy, and whether our heart rate is within normal parameters.

Users of Fitbit smartwatches, which have heart rate measurement as their main functionality [8], can generate an Excel file containing the number of heartbeats per

S. Vlad and N. M. Roman (Eds.): MEDITECH 2022, IFMBE Proceedings 102, pp. 115–125, 2024.
https://doi.org/10.1007/978-3-031-51120-2_13

minute in a given day. Based on this file, the app will generate a graph of the heart rate over a time interval chosen by the user. In this way, the user can track certain disorders they might be suffering from or present this result to their doctor for more information and expert details. Another functionality that the application has achieved is the possibility of nutritional calculations body mass index, basal metabolic rate and ideal weight based on the user's personal information (gender, age, weight, height).

The Body Mass Index indicates the weight group to which each person belongs (degree of obesity). Identifying this value is also identifying the number of kilos a person needs to lose or gain to reach the ideal weight for user height [9].

The basal metabolic rate is the daily energy requirement of a resting body. Nowadays, most people, especially women, are in a constant battle with calories, trying as much as possible to burn as many and perhaps often they even end up burning some of the calories the body needs every day to function properly. Thus, knowing your basal metabolic rate can be of great help in maintaining the health of your body [10].

Body weight is a factor that greatly influences the proper functioning of the whole body and all vital functions. Comparing personal weight with calculated based on a formula that considers height, age, and gender can help a person in becoming aware of certain problems related to this aspect if they exist [11].

2 State of the Art

Below are the four aspects that the app includes heart rate, body mass index, basal metabolic rate and ideal body weight.

2.1 Heart Rate

In addition to indicating the heartbeat, the heart rhythm is a source of information about the condition of the blood vessels and can sometimes also indicate that the cardiovascular system is not functioning within normal parameters. Knowing your heart rhythm and trying to its normal values when necessary is very important for the health of every human.

In an adult, the normal heart rate varies between and beats per minute. Thus, the most common heart rhythm disorders are:

1. *Tachycardia* over beats per minute: this condition may be accompanied by: palpitations, sweating, dizziness, fatigue, or even fainting.
2. *Bradycardia* below beats/minute): this condition may be accompanied by: shortness of breath, fatigue and trouble concentrating.

2.2 Body Mass Index (BMI)

Body mass index is a value that primarily helps to classify you into a certain weight group (degree of obesity) [12]:

$<$18.5 Underweight

$>$18.5 Normal weight

>25 Overweight

>30 Obese

>40 Morbidly obese

As the body mass index increases, so does the risk of acquiring diabetes or other metabolic diseases. The Body Mass Index is based on a very simple formula, the ratio of a person's weight to their height.

2.3 Basal Metabolic Rate (BMR)

The basal metabolic rate is the amount of energy a person's body needs to function properly when at complete rest. The energy consumed by the body at rest is transferred to blood circulation, and respiration and helps maintain body temperature. The formula used to calculate the basal metabolic rate is as follows:

$$\boldsymbol{Women} : [655 + (9.5 * \text{weight}) + (1.8 * \text{height}) - (4.7 * \text{age}) \tag{1}$$

$$\boldsymbol{Men} : [655 + (9.5 * \text{weight}) + (1.8 * \text{height}) - (4.7 * \text{age}) \tag{2}$$

2.4 Ideal Body Weight (IBW)

The ideal body weight is represented by a value calculated according to several criteria for each person. The implemented application calculates this using a formula that considers age, height and weight, the calculations being different from woman to man. The ideal weight is calculated according to a person's gender:

$$\boldsymbol{Women} : [50 + 0.75 * (\text{height} - 150) + (\text{age} - 20)/4] * 0.9 \tag{3}$$

$$\boldsymbol{Men} : [50 + 0.75 * (\text{height} - 150) + (\text{age} - 20)/4] * 0.9 \tag{4}$$

3 Core Concept

The system allows the user to acquire and monitor the data collected from the smartwatch and view the heart rate in a graphic form and calculates body mass index, basal metabolic rate and ideal weight. In Fig. 1 it is presented the global system architecture.

The global system architecture presents the module composed of the Fitbit smartwatch, which is connected via Bluetooth to a Smartphone, this module sends data to the database threw a web service. Firebase represents the database, in which the values of the parameters measured by the smartwatch are stored.

Figure 2 represents the use-case diagram and shows all the actions that the user can do within the application.

A user of the application can create a new account based on email and password and can log into the application using email and password. If they wish to change their

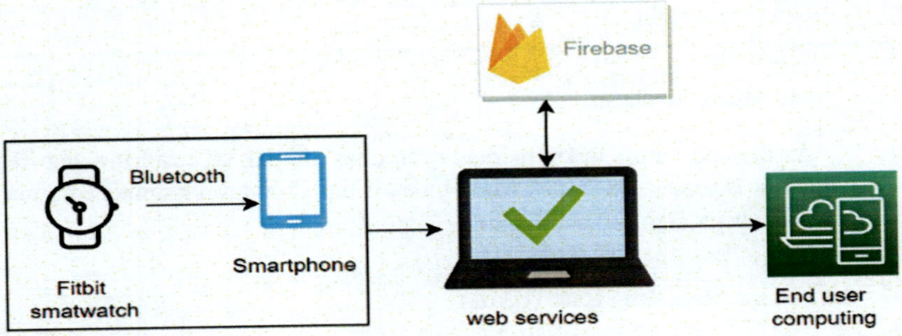

Fig. 1. The global system architecture

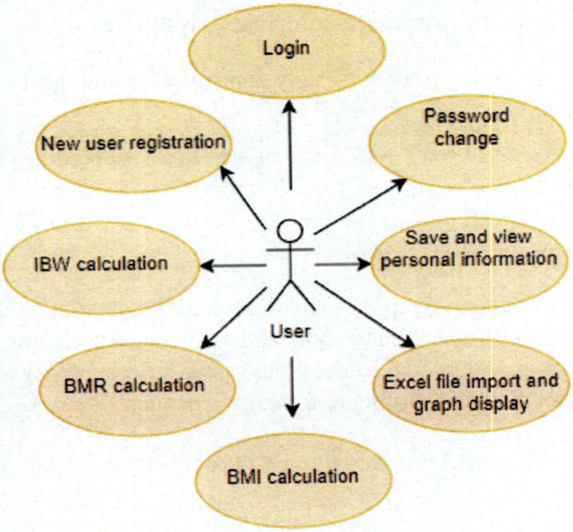

Fig. 2. Use-case diagram

password, they can do so using a link received in their email. Once the account is created, the user has the following functionalities in the application: calculation of basal metabolic rate, calculation of body mass index, calculation of ideal weight and importing a file containing the number of heartbeats per minute. Once the file is loaded into the application, an hourly interval can be selected from which a graph will be generated. In addition to these options, the user can view the data entered after registering in the application and updating it.

3.1 Software Design

When the application opens, the first activity is displayed, the one in which the user creates a new account Fig. 3. After entering the email, and password and clicking on the *Register* button, the application will display the activity that asks for personal data

(Fig. 4). If the user already has an account created in the application, he/she can switch from the registration activity to the login activity by clicking on *Already registered? Login here*, which will open the login activity (Fig. 5).

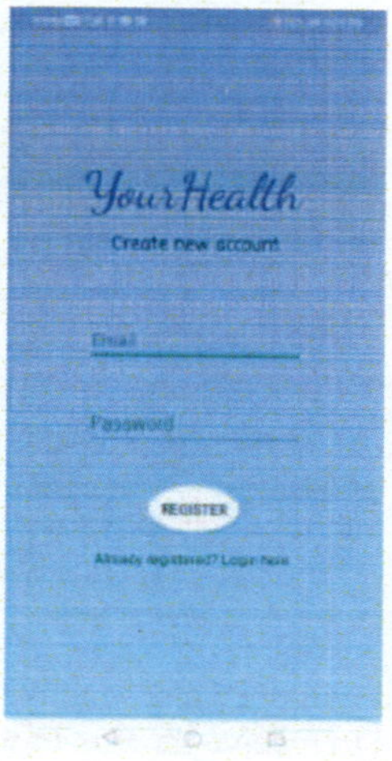

Fig. 3. Registration account

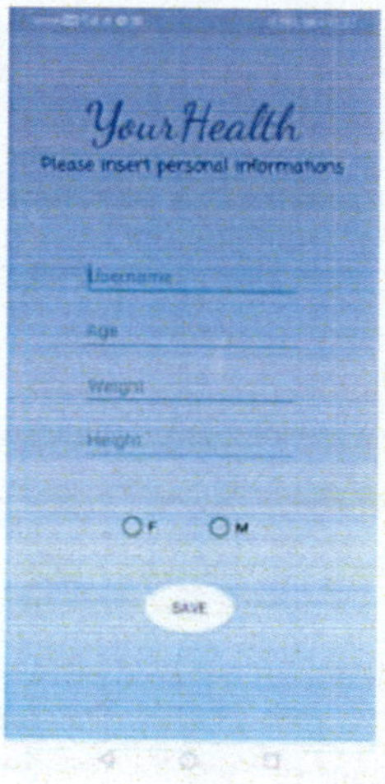

Fig. 4. New user registration

Similarly, the user can go from the login activity to the registration activity by clicking on *New here. Create account*. Another functionality available to the user is to change the password in case it is forgotten. In the login activity, there is also a *Forgot the password*

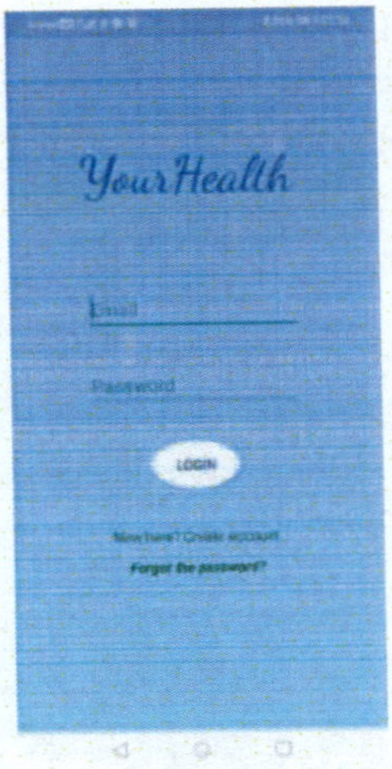

Fig. 5. Login

button that once accessed will open a new activity where the user has to enter the email address that he/she wants to receive the link to reset the password (Fig. 6).

Once successfully logged in, the application displays a fragment called *Home*, which contains a minimum of information related to the application and its functions (Fig. 7). In the upper left corner, there is a button in the form of horizontal lines, which when accessed brings the navigation menu in front of the user, from where he/she can select which functionality of the application he/she wants to use (Fig. 8). The navigation menu contains:

- 5 fragments: Home fragment, IBW where the ideal weight is calculated, BMI where the body mass index is calculated and BMR where the basal metabolic rate is calculated and the fragment for Logout the user logs out from the current account, the application goes to the registration page;
- 2 activities: Upload Fitbit Data this is where the Excel file is uploaded and the User account (here the user can see the personal data entered when creating the account).

4 Results

The ideal weight is calculated in the Body Mass Index (BMI). The method used for this calculation is the ratio of a person's weight to their height. To obtain a result, we read from the database the values of these two parameters. The reading was implemented in such a way that the data obtained belonged to the current user and not to others in the database. Based on this value, a person can fit into a certain standard of obesity.

In the method implemented to calculate the body mass index value, we also added an alert message to let the user know which obesity standard they fall into. To do this, we compared the result with the limits of each obesity category a person can fall into, as can be seen in Fig. 9.

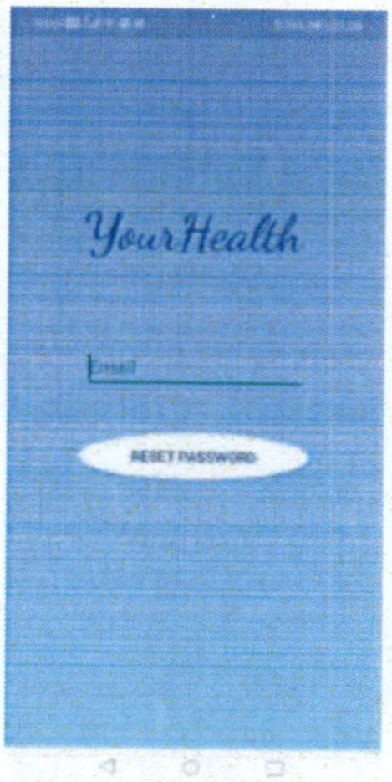

Fig. 6. Password change

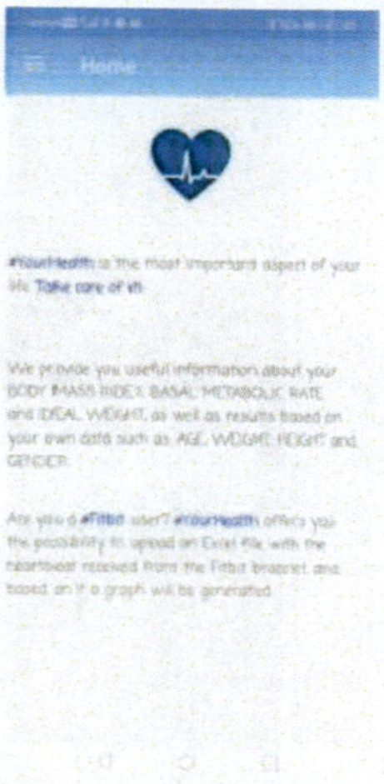

Fig. 7. Home page

After choosing a time for the start of the interval (Fig. 10) and one for the end the OK button is pressed which will open the activity in which the graph will be displayed.

The graph in Fig. 11 is for the time interval 11:00:00–12:00:00. Because the more data the larger the interval, we have enabled the option that allows the user to zoom in on the graph so that they can see the exact value at a particular time without the problem of overlap.

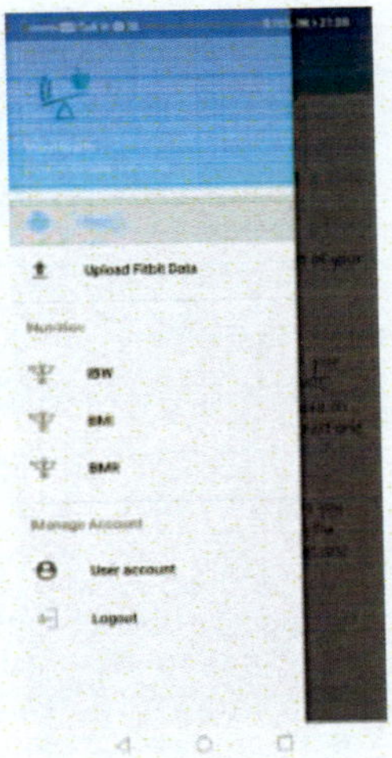

Fig. 8. Menu

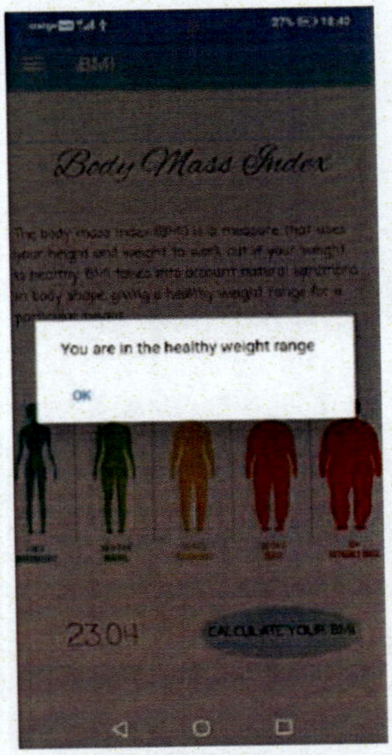

Fig. 9. Body mass index

This app is especially for people with heart conditions, but also for people who want to change their body weight. The major advantage of this app is that it facilitates the monitoring of 4 very important aspects of maintaining a healthy body. At the same time, it is much more practical to have all these functionalities in a single application on your

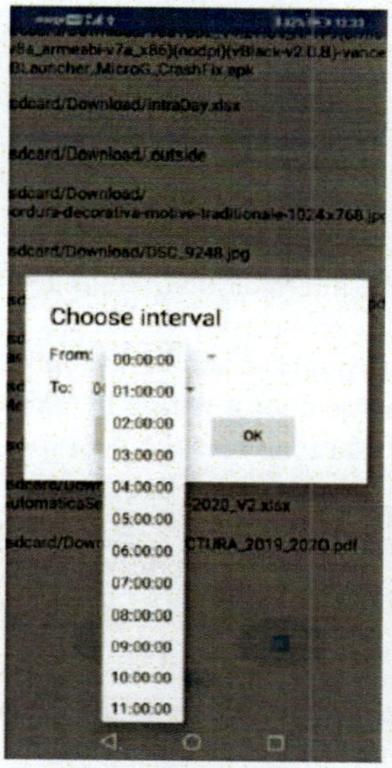

Fig. 10. Choose interval

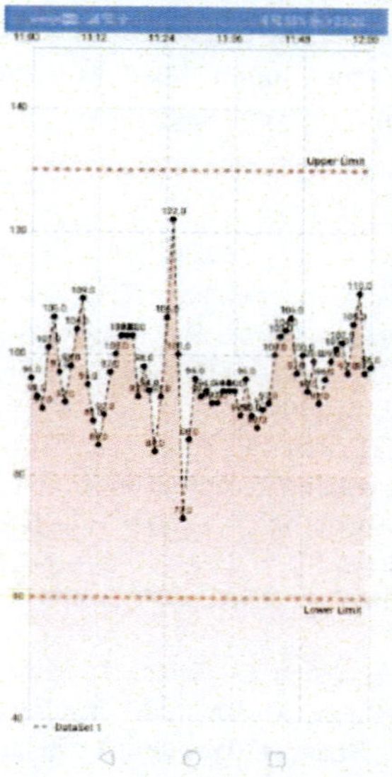

Fig. 11. Heart rate evolution

mobile phone making everything much easier, not having to access different web links to calculate certain indices or to obtain statistics based on heart rate values.

4.1 Discussions

The objectives we had in mind for the realization of this project were to build a mobile application, using the Java programming language, in the environment of Android Studio development environment, using the Firebase database.

The app has the following functionalities:

1. Implementation of an interface that facilitates user interaction with the application and the functionalities provided.
2. Implementation of the register and login function.
3. Saving the user's personal information in the database.
4. Possibility to modify in real time the data that the user has specified at the time of registration.
5. Implementation of Excel file upload functionality.
6. Graphing of the file within a time interval set by the user.
7. Perform nutritional calculations based on personal user information.

The specifications of the application correspond to the proposed objectives. The user can create an account, with an email and password, and then fill in some fields with his/her data: name, height, weight, gender, and age. All this data will be stored in real-time in the Firebase database. If the user forgets the password, they can set a new password using a link sent to their email address. The application provides the possibility to modify the personal data filled in at the time of registration. All these changes are made in the database in real-time. The rest of the specifications correspond exactly to the objectives mentioned above. The interface facilitates user interaction with the application, everything is very suggestive and easy to use.

References

1. Mayo Clinic staff. Know your numbers: Heart rate. https://www.mayoclinichealthsystem.org/hometown-health/speaking-of-health/know-your-numbers-heart-rate, 2021/02/16
2. Simpson, J., Yates, R., Sharland, G.: Irregular heart rate in the fetus—not always benign. Cardiol. Young **6**, 28–31 (1996)
3. Gearges, C., Haider, H., Rana, V., Asghar, Z., Kewalramani, A., Kuschner, Z.: Bebtelovimab-induced bradycardia leading to cardiac arrest. Crit. Care Explor. **4**, e0747 (2022)
4. Sinclair, J., Zhu, Y., Xu, G., Ma, W., Shi, H., Ma, K., Cao, C., Kong, L., Wan, K., Liao, J., Wang, H.Q., Arentz, M., Redd, M., Gallo, L., Short, K.: The role of pre-existing chronic disease in cardiac complications from SARS-CoV-2 infection: a systematic review and meta-analysis (2020)
5. Weber, B., Siddiqi, H., Zhou, G., Vieira, J., Kim, A., Rutherford, H., Mitre, X., Feeley, M., Oganezova, K., Varshney, A., Bhatt, A., Nauffal, V., Atri, D., Blankstein, R., Karlson, E., Carli, M., Baden, L., Bhatt, D., Woolley, A.: Relationship between myocardial injury during index hospitalization for SARS-CoV-2 infection and longer-term outcomes. J. Am. Heart Assoc. **11**(22010) (2021)
6. Almamlouk, R., Kashour, T., Obeidat, S., Bois, M., Maleszewski, J., Omrani, O., Tleyjeh, R., Berbari, E., Chakhachiro, Z., Zein-Sabatto, B., Gerberi, D., Tleyjeh, I., Mondolfi, A., Finn, A., Duarte-Neto, A., Rapkiewicz, A., Frustaci, A., Keresztesi, A.A., Hanley, B., Grime, Z.: COVID-19-associated cardiac pathology at post-mortem evaluation: a Collaborative systematic review. Clin. Microbiol. Infect. **28** (2022)

7. Netalkar, D., Gowrika, H.: Review on IoT based heart rate monitoring system. Int. J. Adv. Res. Sci. Commun. Technol. 354–356 (2022)
8. Hajj Boutros, G., Landry-Duval, M.A., Comtois, A.S., Gouspillou, G., Karelis, A.: Wrist-worn devices for the measurement of heart rate and energy expenditure: a validation study for the apple watch 6, Polar Vantage V and Fitbit sense. Eur. J. Sport Sci. (2021)
9. Van de Moortel, K.: The body mass index recalculated (2022). https://doi.org/10.13140/RG.2.2.24205.00481
10. Leiner, G.C., Abramowitz, S.: Basal Metabolic Rate. Can. Med. Assoc. J. **7611**, 977 (1957)
11. Kuzmenko, N., Tsyrlin, V., Pliss, M., Galagudza, M.: Seasonal body weight dynamics in healthy people: a meta-analysis. Hum. Physiol. **47**, 676–689 (2021)
12. https://pilates1901.com/wp-content/uploads/2015/01/body-mass-index.gif

Experimental Research upon Neutralisation with Ozone of Chemical and Microbiological Pollutants from Sewage Wastewater

Budu Sorin Radu(✉)

Technical University of Cluj-Napoca, Memorandumului 28, 400114 Cluj-Napoca, Romania
Sorin.BUDU@ethm.utcluj.ro

Abstract. The main purpose of the work is to provide practical information regarding the sterilization and reuse of sewagewaters and domestic wastewater, infested with biological and chemical compounds that endanger human health. The research carried out is based on a long experience in the field of sterilization of water infested with pathogenic germs. Water samples were taken from the sewagewater in Cluj-Napoca, containing massive loads of biological micro-pollutants various species of Coliforms, bacilli, bacteria, viruses), specific residues (fats, detergents, cyanides, nitrites, nitrates, sulfur compounds, etc.) that pose severe risks to human health and the environment. To carry out the experiments, the author created an original, versatile experimental stand, which provides a variable voltage source (U = 230V-22 kV), with variable frequency between 1Hz-1 MHz, fed with various waveforms: sine, step, train of pulses, sawtooth, with smooth or fast attack and/or rest ramp. The tests were carried out using two types of electrodes: brush type and with needle discharge tips, for two ozone concentrations: $3g/m^3$ and $5g/m^3$. Sample exposure times were 3, 5 and 7 min. The results indicate a total annihilation of microbiological compounds, total reduction of detergents and nitrites and a partial reduction of cyanides. The microbiological and physico-chemical tests were carried out in accredited specialized laboratories.

Keywords: Ozone · Sewagewater · Sterilization

1 Introduction

Due to the phenomenon of global warming which implicitly determines the decrease of water reserves, the reuse of waste water becomes a priority nowadays.

The purpose of this work is to highlight the effects of ozone on the chemical and microbiological pollutants present in wastewater, including those originating from urban collecting channels, which are usually later discharged into watercourses.

The results obtained from the tests are very promising and this method, used on an industrial scale, can become a standard in the field.

Due the cooperation between LCEI (HIEF—High Intense Electric Field Laboratory) with the Water Company "Someşul" S.A., the Water-Sewerage Autonomous Administrations in Cluj-Napoca (RAJAC) and its branch in Gilău City, allowed to perform

S. Vlad and N. M. Roman (Eds.): MEDITECH 2022, IFMBE Proceedings 102, pp. 126–134, 2024.
https://doi.org/10.1007/978-3-031-51120-2_14

preliminary tests [1] in order to study the possibility of ozone treatment of municipal sewage wastewater and their chemical and microbiological load sterilization [2–4].

Several experiments were performed by the author on the treatment plant. Chemical and microbiological tests were performed in the specialized laboratories of the Water Company "Someşul" S.A. in Cluj-Napoca.

Water samples were taken from the sewagewater in Cluj-Napoca, containing massive loads of biological micro-pollutants (various species of Bacteria and excremental Coliforms, bacillus, Streptococcus, viruses as Esterichia Coli, detergents, cyanides, nitrites, etc. [4–6] with a severe degree of risk for the population's health.

The massive chemical, organic and microbiological load of sewagewaters require fast and efficient measures in order to ensure the sterilisation of these waters. Consequently, due to the climate heating, the sterilised wastewaters can be reused, including as drinking water.

Currently, industrial sterilizers show low yields, high energy costs and low efficiency for large volumes of processed waste water. One of the causes is the use of voltage sources that operate at low voltages (from hundreds of volts to about 3–4 kV) and mainly at industrial frequencies (50Hz or 60Hz).

However, from a microbiological and chemical point of view, the microbiological pathogenic compounds are irreversibly affected at high frequencies and voltages.

For these reasons, the author had built a variable high voltage source up to 22 kV and frequencies between 1 Hz and 1 MHz. The present tests were carried out at 22 kV and 15.625 Hz.

The testing of the samples, after taking the water from the areas infested with chemical and microbiological pollutants (sewage wastewater collected from emisary) and the subsequent treatment of this kind of used wastewater were carried out in specialized laboratories accredited according to international standards.

2 Preliminary Sampling of Chemical and Bacteriological Load of Sewagewater

In Table 1 the chemical and bacteriological load of sewagewater taken from the urban sewage waters in Cluj-Napoca is presented. Also the preliminary experimental results obtained by ozone treatment in thin layer of wastewater with the author method are presented in the same table.

2.1 Experimental Stand

The author had developed an original experimental stand (Fig. 1), which operates at frequencies between 1 Hz ÷ 1MHz, at maximum 22 kVvoltage average, in order to ensure the treatment for sterilisation of wastewater and sewagewater. Tests upon sewagewaters were carried upon the experimental high frequency (15,625 Hz) ozonifier stand.

Sterilization stand can provide variable amplitudes of the applied voltage (from 230V up to 22kV) and different shapes of voltage (sine, step, rectangular, triangular, sawtooth, with smooth or fast ramp of rise/decrease shape, pulse train) can be applied to the discharging electrodes and water sterilizers devices [8].

Table 1. Chemical and bacteriological load of sewagewater befre and after treatment

Sample	NF	U = 22 kV Sine f = 15 kHz	Treatment results (in mg/l, pathogens in no. of germs/100 ml)							
Type of germs		Time	Total Coli	Excremental Coliforms	E-coli	Strept	CCO-Mn	Det	CN^-	NO^-
M1	3gr.O^3		> 18x10^5	> 17,5x10^5	> 17,5x10^5	> 8,4x10^5	192	1	0.019	0.850
P1.1	NF 1 pass	1.5min 3 min 7 min	< 14x10^5 < 1.9x10^3 < 1.4x103	< 1.8x10^3 < 1.2x10^3 < 0.5 x10^3	< 0.8 x10^3 < 0.8 x10^3 < 0.4 x10^3	1.2 0 0	11087 65	0.43 0.37 0.23	0.016 0.014 0.012	0.018 0.014 0.01
M2	5gr. O^3		> 18x10^5	> 17,5x10^5	> 17,5x10^5	> 8,4x10^5	192	1	00.19	0.850
P2.1	NF 1 pass	1.5min 3 min 7 min	< 1.7 x10^3 < 1.5 x10^3 < 1.4 x10^3	0.3 x10^3 0 0	> 0.2 x10^3 0 0	0 0 0	42 38 48	0.302 0.289 0.263	0.005 0.003 0.001	1 0.102 0.088

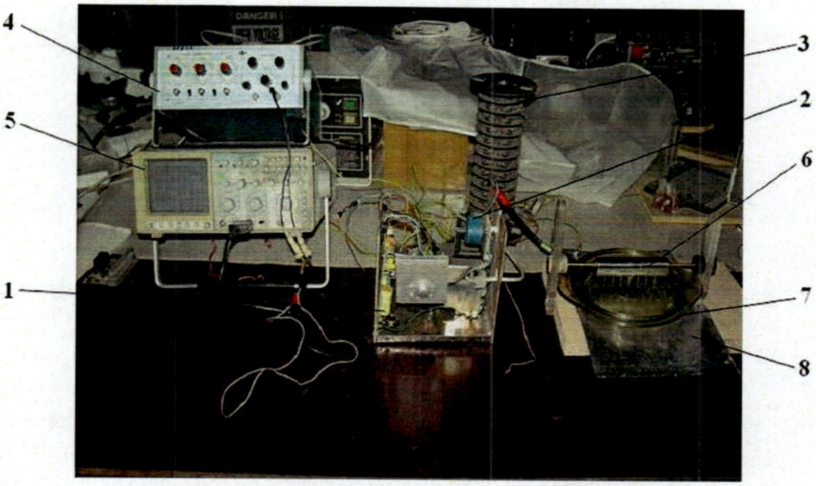

Fig. 1. Original experimental stand for high frequency ozone generation, used in sewage and wastewater direct treatment cells; 1—control block and sync processor with TBA 950 integrated circuit; 2—high voltage transformer (22 kV); 3—ohmic divider (475 Mohm); 4—variable frequency from 1 Hz ÷ 1MHz function generator; 5—TR 4653 oscilloscope; 6, 7—wastewater direct treatment cell, equipped with electrode with point-shaped or brush type discharge electrodes placed upon a Petri dish (Jena glass); 8—grounded electrode.

The power supply of the high voltage transformer works with the help of a TBA 950 syncronised processor [8], modified by the author in order to can adjust the frequency (otherwise constant) and shape of the signal generated by the sync processor in the range 1 Hz ÷ 1MHz.

Experimental stand mainly consist of an high voltage step up transformer (toroidal transformer on ferrite core with 150 W maximum power). The voltage apllied to the corona discharge electrodes (U = 22 kV) act by Corona discharges upon the wastewater direct treatment cells, in order to produce ozone [7, 9].

The kit is provided with protection devices to overvoltage or overcurrent that occur during arc or spark discharges in case of accidental breakdown of the discharge gap (protection by reversing the characteristic of the electronic control unit and mechanical spark gaps). Two types of electric discharging electrodes were used in order to perform the carried tests: brush type electrodes (Fig. 2,a) and three needle point electrodes (Fig. 2,b) [5, 9–11].

2.2 Experimental Method

From the study of the control samples taken at the points of sewagewater discharge in the emissary, result that the classical water treatment by method of clorination does not completely eliminate the pathogen microbiological compounds. Also, chlorine is carcinogen on long term.

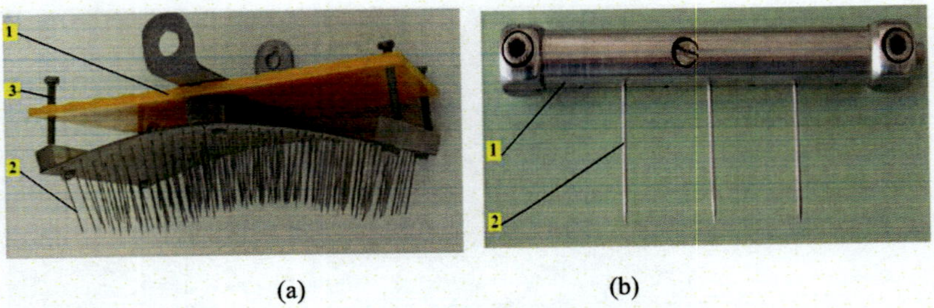

Fig. 2. Corona discharge electrodes: (a)—brush-type; 1—electrode holder support; 2—needle-type point-shaped tips; 3—brush-type electrode curvature adjustment system; (b)—1—electrode holder support; 2-multiple needles type electrode.

Moreover, there are a relatively large number of micro-polluting compounds, both chemical (nitrites, nitrates, sulphates) and microbiological pathogens with high risk for human life (Esterichia Coli, various Streptococcus, excremental Coliforms and multiple types of other kind of Coliforms, various species of bacteria, such as Coliform bacteria). Their presence in the waste waters are very dangerous for the human health [7, 10, 11].

The samples of sewagewater were treated on two sets of tests each, related to the use of two values of ozone concentration: 3g O_3/m^3 and 5g O_3/m^3. Samples were processed for 3 times each, at 1.5 min, 3 min. And 7 min.

Control samples were chemical and microbiologically assessed too, according to the European quality standards, in specialized laboratory of Water Company "Someşul" S.A. in Cluj-Napoca. Results of treated water were assessed by means of four groups of specific tests, using treated water, both on culture media (in samples of 0.01 ml, 0.1 ml, 1 ml and 10 ml), as well as by direct quantitative assessment (no. of pathogens / 100 ml).

The results of the experiments regarding the chemical and microbiological load present in the sewagewaters and the neutralization of the living and chemichal micro-pollutants (additional to Table 1), were performed at high frequency (15,625 Hz) and are presented in **Fig. 3** and **Fig. 4**.

The mainly experimental conditions under which the tests were performed are: AC voltage supply U = 22 kV, frequency f = 15,625 Hz [9]. Successive passages (exposures) of the sewage wastewater samples were performed (3 passages), at an average velocity of sewagwater of 0.3 m/s.

2.3 Experimental Results

Synthesis of the obtained results, related to two values of the amount of ozone generated (3gO3/100 ml and 5gO3/100ml), related to the volumes of the treated wastewater samples are presented in Fig. 3 and Fig. 4:

The results of the global experiments regarding the microbiological and chemichal load neutralization of the micro-pollutants are presented in Fig. 5.

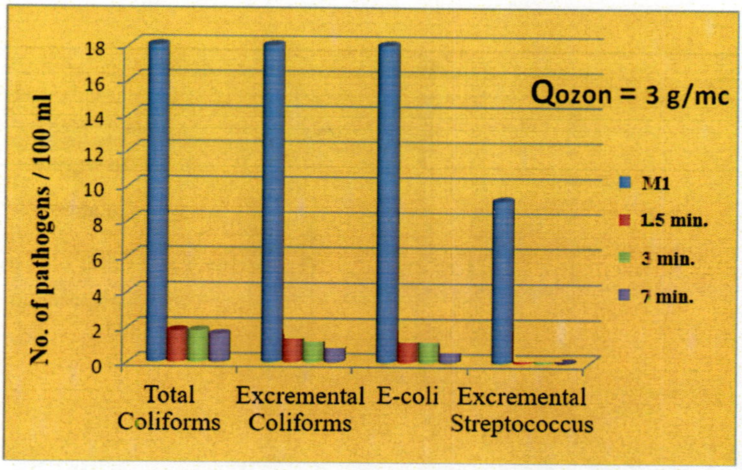

Fig. 3. Efficiency of neutralization of pathogens found in treated waters, at the discharge into the emissary (from the Wastewater Treatment Plant in Gilău); Experimental conditions: no. of germs / 100 ml (ratio 1 ‰); $Q_{ozone} = 3g\ O_3/m^3$, $t_{exposure} = 1.5—3—7$ min., U = 22 kV, f = 15,625 Hz.

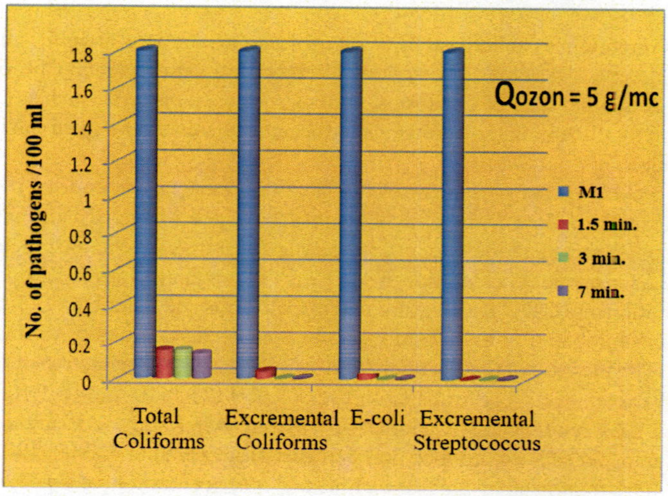

Fig. 4. Efficiency of neutralization of pathogens found in treated waters, at the discharge into the emissary (from the Wastewater Treatment Plant in Gilău); Experimental conditions: no. of germs / 100 ml (ratio 1 ‰); $Q_{ozone} = 5g\ O_3/m^3$, $t_{exposure} = 1.5—3—7$ min., U = 22 kV, f = 15,625 Hz.

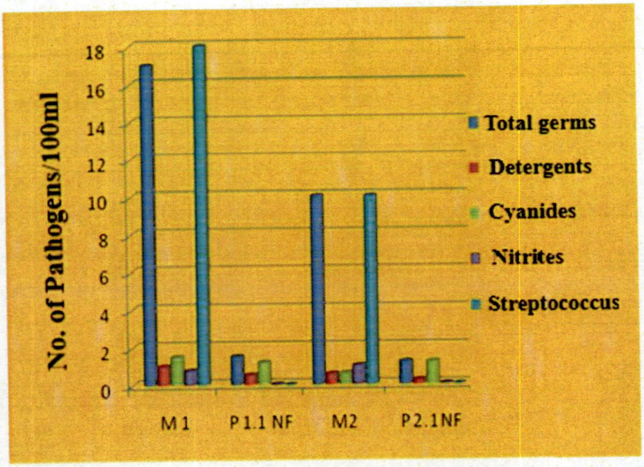

Fig. 5. Results of municipal wastewater treatment in ozone generation by corona discharge field, samples not further filtered through a bed of sand. NF—"not filtered samples".

3 Analysis of the Results

It is important to notice that by using ozone concentrations of 5g/m^3 all the microbiological load ((Esterichia Coli, various Streptococcus, excremental Coliforms and multiple types of other kind of Coliforms, various species of bacteria, such as Coliform bacteria) were totally anihilated and the water became absolute pure from microbiological point of view.

Beside of the presented results, also the odour and colour of the water have significantly improved, the effects being determined olfactorily and visually. The water becomes clear and the odour of the sewage becomes pleasant, ozonated.

At an ozone concentration of 3g O_3/m^3, at treatment times of 1.5 min, the total number of coliforms (CT/100 ml), excremental Coliforms and Esterichia Coli decreased 8 times, as the number of units /100 ml. Also Streptococcus decreased 7.5 times.

The increase of the treatment time to 3 min leads to a reduction of Coliform Bacteria, and excremental Coliforms from over 18,000 units /100 ml to 1,100 units, Esterichia Coli has been reduced by another 50% (from over 1,800 to 830 units); and excremental Streptococcus have dropped dramatically (from 1,600 to 7 units /100 ml).

The treatment of control samples at a concentration of 5g O_3/m^3 and exposure times of 1.5 min of each sample (in a single passage through of samples) resulted in an extremely severe reduction of total Coliforms (from over 18,000 units to 5 units /100 ml), and of the excremental Coliforms and Esterichia Coli from over 18,000 at 3 units. Streptococcus were totally annihilated.

At exposure times of 5 min and 7 min, all microorganisms present in the water samples were completely annihilated, the water becoming 100% microbiologically pure.

4 Conclusions

The results highlight the special effectiveness of ozone treatment of treated seawagewater, in order to neutralize biological and chemical micropollutants, so that these waters can be reintroduced after treatment in the industrial circuit and even for usual domestic use.

Sterilization of sewagewater and domestic water against chemical and microbiological pollutants, as well as its reuse, can be achieved by treating water with ozone in an intense electric field, at relatively high voltages (15–22 kV), frequencies of the order of kilohertz and average ozone concentrations generated between 3–5 gO_3/m^3.

The duration required for the total sterilization of sewagewater or householdwater, respecting the data above, is approx. 3–5 min.

Experimental results allow us to conclude that the treatment of wastewater before discharge into the emissary waters and before distribution to secondary consumers must be subjected to ozone treatment for the total elimination of pathogens, which cannot be completely annihilated by classical methods.

The method of sewage waters treatment is about five times faster and much more effective as the classic methods, i.e. clorination or sand bed filtering.

References

1. Biluca, Ş., Budu, S., Suărăşan I.: An Electronic High Voltage and Frequency Supply Used for Corona Discharging Field. In: Proceedings of International Conference Quality, Automation and Robotics. Q&A-R 2000. May 19th–20th, 2000. I.P.A. & U.T.C.N., Casa Cărţii de Ştiinţă Publishing, Cluj-Napoca, p. 343–348, ISBN 973–686–058–2, (2000)
2. L.Onga, I. Kornev, S Preis: Oxidation of reactive azo-dyes with pulsed Corona discharge: Surface reaction enhancement, Journal of Electrostatics, Elsevier (2020)
3. Zhu, Y., Chen, C., Shi, J., Shangguan, W.: A novel simulation method for predicting ozone generation in Corona discharge region. Chem. Eng. Sci. Elsevier (2020)
4. Morar, R., Suărăşan, I., Budu, S., Bologa, M., Dăscălescu, L.: Einfluss Des Korona-Entladungsfeldes Auf Einige Physikalisch—Chemische Parameter Des Wassers", International Meeting on Chemistry Engineering, Environmental Protection and Biotechnology ACHEMA'2000, Frankfurt, pp. 376–382, (2000)
5. Morar,R., Suărăşan,I., Mudura, M., Neamtu,V., Budu, S., Petru,C., Munteanu, I., Ghizdavu, L., Munceleanu,I., Ceclan, C., Botezan, M.A., Popa, V.C., Oros, O., Chira, R., Mic, L., Ciortea, V.: Experimental research on the implementation of complex technologies for treatment in intense electric fields, with controlled generation of ozone and ozonators in the process of rehabilitation of wastewater from public sewage. Scientific research grant no. 33532/2003, Theme A 31, CNCSIS Code 720. Benef.: Minist. Educ. Res.
6. Muncelean, I., Suărăşan, I., Budu, S., Muntean, I., Morar, R.: The influence of the corona discharging field upon some physical and chemical parameters of the polluted waters. In: 3th International Conference on Renewable Sources and Environmental Electro-Technologies, RSEEE'2000, University of Oradea, In: Annals of the University of Oradea, ISSN 1223–2106, pp. 103–108, May, (2000)
7. Rasberger, H., Hulsheger, H., Niemann, E.G.: – "Lethal Effect of High Voltage Pulse on E-Coli K12." Radiat. Environ. Biophys.. Environ. Biophys. **18**, 281–288 (1980)
8. Sincroprocesorul TBA 950 [TBA 950 Sync Processor]—IEI Electronica Bucharest, (1984)

9. Suărăşan, I., Budu, S., Biluca, S.: The influence of the frequency upon the corona discharge. Ann. Fac. Eng. Hunedoara, ISSN 1454–6531, pp. 109–112. Hunedoara, (2000)
10. Suărăşan, I., Budu, S., Oros, O. D., Morar, R., Ghizdavu, P.S., Ghizdavu, L., Muntean, I. O.:The efficiency increase of equipment for treatment in high intense electric fields with abundant ozone generation. In: International Conference on Ozone & Related Oxidants in: Advanced Treatment of Water for Human Health and Environment Protection. Brussels, Belgium, May 15th–16th, (2008)
11. Suărăşan, I., Mudura, M., Budu, S., Oros, D., Mischian, A., Morar, R.: Ozone and High Intense Electric Fields—Possible factors for wastewater cleaning. In: International Conference on Ozone & Related Oxidants in: Advanced Treatment of Water for Human Health and Environment Protection. Brussels, Belgium, May 15th–16th, (2008)

Technology and Education

Integrating IoT in Educational Engineering Application Development - an Emerging Paradigm

I. R. Nicu(✉), A. I. Nicu, and Anca Constantinescu-Dobra

Technical University of Cluj-Napoca, Cluj-Napoca, Romania
razvan.nicu@staff.utcluj.ro, Anca.Nicu@ethm.utcluj.ro,
Anca.Constantinescu@enm.utcluj.ro

Abstract. In recent years, due to the pandemic conditions caused by COVID, digitalization has become mandatory for the development of teaching activities in optimal conditions. A new paradigm for smart education has appeared not only in the engineering field but also in other educational fields: the obligation to interconnect innovative IoT solutions (sensors, open-source electronic devices such as Arduino or Raspberry pi) with classic engineering solutions to develop smart projects. In the digital university, access to technology reduces costs and risks, improves working methods, increases the visibility and skills acquired by future graduates who will enter the labour market. Through a practical and methodological approach, we will analyse the advantages and disadvantages of using IoT in the educational process for the development of engineering skills.

Keywords: IoT · Smart education · Engineering · Connected devices · E-learning

1 Introduction

"Ashton's original definition was: 'Today computers—and, therefore, the Internet—are almost wholly dependent on human beings for information. Nearly all the roughly 50 petabytes (a petabyte is 1,024 terabytes) of data available on the Internet were first captured and created by human beings—by typing, pressing a record button, taking a digital picture, or scanning a bar code. Conventional diagrams of the Internet... Leave out the most numerous and important routers of all - people. ...... If we had computers that knew everything there was to know about things—using data they gathered without any help from us—we would be able to track and count everything, and greatly reduce waste, loss, and cost. We would know when things needed replacing, repairing, or recalling, and whether they were fresh or past their best. The Internet of Things has the potential to change the world, just as the Internet did. Maybe even more so."[1].

Extrapolating the definition that Ashton gave in 1999 and combining it with the environmental conditions that we had to live in the past 2 and half years in the academic community and in real life one can say that IoT played a key role in sustaining and

S. Vlad and N. M. Roman (Eds.): MEDITECH 2022, IFMBE Proceedings 102, pp. 137–142, 2024.
https://doi.org/10.1007/978-3-031-51120-2_15

development of education not only at Technical University of Cluj-Napoca where we are today but also in all levels of education, in industry and in human communities all over the world. Bogdanovic, Z. and all proposed in [2] a "skeletal type" course structure that included first programming, microcontrollers, web (design and/or web services) and mobile application development.

The feedback received during the TUCN presentations – the educational offer at the University Fairs or at the high school level, held on-site before 2020 or online during the pandemic years led us to conclude that future engineering students are eager to learn programming languages, how to use sensors, actuators and IoT in active learning/e-learning techniques related to their engineering application development work.

In TUCN, in the past years IoT helped both teachers and students to continue the smart teaching/learning process. Because of the emerge of Internet of Things, the Smart education paradigm is the new way to educate engineers due to the new skills that had to be developed by the engineers to meet the society requirements for the new type of jobs. Thus, led the university to adopt new teaching methods and adjust the curriculum for the students to be prepared for meeting the industry needs. Both teachers and students benefited from both on site teaching methods and online and the obtained results were encouraging – more than 65% of the TUCN alumni found jobs at their qualification level and 80% of the 2020 alumni are employed in Romania. The statistical data is available in the Annual Rector's Report for 2021 [3].

With help of IoT one can manage things efficiently. UTC-N is having IoT - support infrastructure, smart campus with smart facilities, labs, and buildings. The Virtual Campus developed at UTCN level and the implemented IoT facilities led to a smooth transition from the onsite to the online environment.

Muhammad Kashif Saeed [4] et. All explained the challenges in implementing the IoT in universities but also the benefits gained by academic staff, students and administrative staff.

IoT in educational engineering development

Conventional/traditional methods of education in course classrooms are no longer the most proper channels for ensuring the transmission of information to students due to the rapidity with which technological development played an enormous role into our life. From simple applications developed for wearable devices to modern interactive devices equipped with small sensors using IoT for transmitting different parameters smart phones or other smart gadgets, the educational sector needed to be up to date.

The imposed conditions between 2020 and 2022 forced the educational sector to change the educational process from onsite to online and this was really a challenge in the engineering domain. Many applications for the laboratory and seminars were developed using IoT to ensure the competences of the BSc students. An IoT.

Materials and methods

The IoT-enhanced laboratory comprises laboratory equipment integrated with state-of-the-art IoT technology and mobile applications. Tests and simulations are conducted remotely, connecting with various instruments.

Some of the applications developed by teachers or students revealed new insights that will help the educational process development for the next generations. Students in TUCN moved progressively from using books and notebooks to tablets, laptops, smart blackboards, IoT sensors, e-learning platforms in order achieve all the competences needed when they apply for a job after graduation.

One example is presented in Fig. 1. Temperature and humidity monitoring application for neonatal care - an mHealth solution [7].

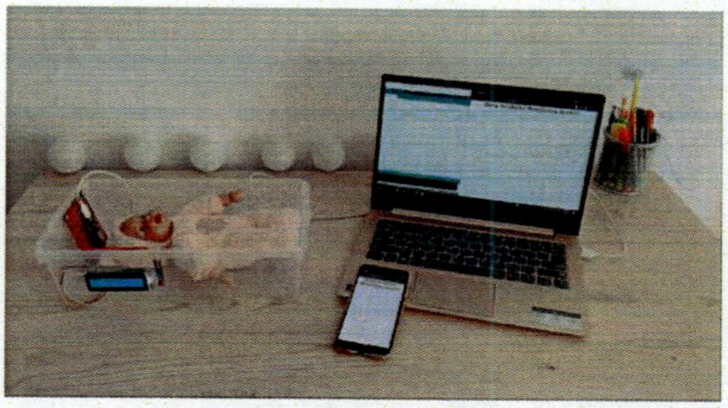

Fig. 1. Caption of the developed system using IoT for monitoring biomedical parameters.

This application uses IoT elements to transmit data in real time for visualization of the parameters in real time on a smart phone or a computer. The baby incubator monitoring systems is a real help for the medical assistants due to the temperature chart that can be visualized on a monitor/smart device or a humidity chart (see Figs. 2 and 3).

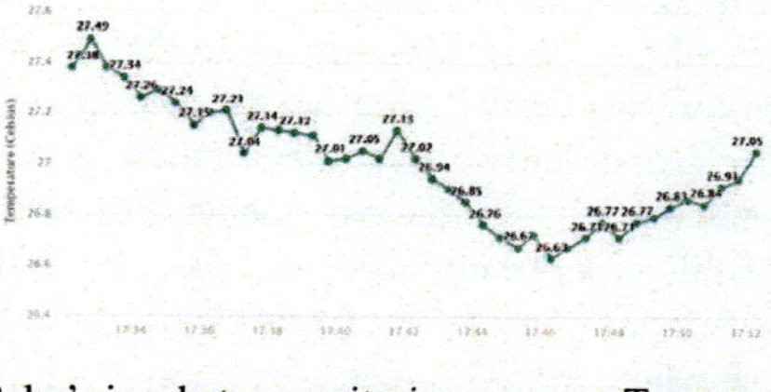

Fig. 2. Baby's incubator monitoring system - Temperature chart

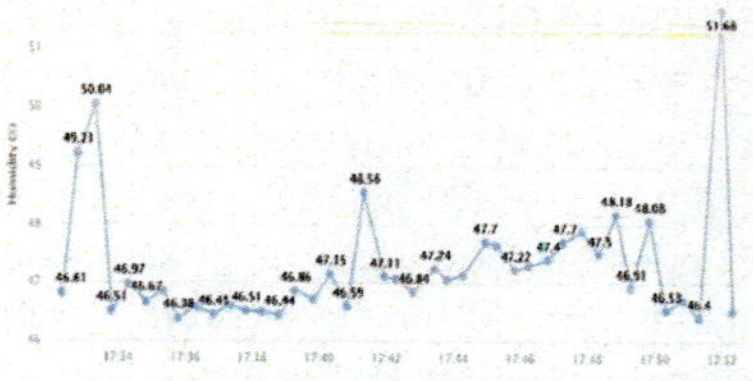

Fig. 3. Baby's incubator monitoring system - Humidity chart

All the obtained data were validated by monitorization of the parameters using conventional equipment. The didactic example is integrated in the IoT category, and at the medical level it represents an mHealth solution. Creative use of versatile new health information and sensing (mHealth) technologies have the potential to reduce the cost of healthcare and improve new-born health in numerous ways.

A low-cost solution that allows avoiding certain critical situations in a neonatology salon is that, through notification, the doctor is alerted in time, thus being able to make the right decisions. Versatile and flexible architecture that can be improved later by adding other elements.

Another didactic example is how a TV can be transformed from a non smart into a spart TV by using a Raspberry PI system (Fig. 4):

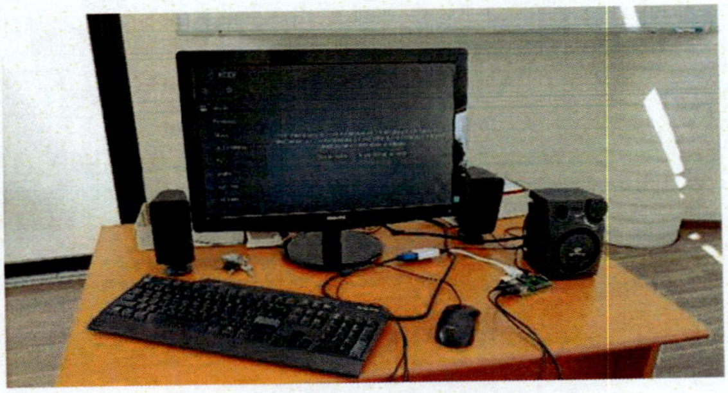

Fig. 4. SmartTV with Raspberry PI

By using IoT elements the students are taught how to format a MicroSD card using the FAT32 file system, install the NOOBS operating system on the formatted card, connect via a video/audio adapter the Raspberry Pi to the TV/Monitor, install the OpenELEC operating system for Raspberry Pi, Set- up the operating system and KODI media center, install and use the proper software remote on their smart phone.

After all the above steps are made by the student, with additional help offered by the teacher, some of the experiments were installation of additional modules for viewing online video and audio content or playback of static visual content (pictures) from external storage media.

There are a lot of examples developed for didactic purposes depending on the field of study (robotics applications that use the LabVIEW graphical development environment, which together with the LEGO Mindstorms NXT or EV3 platforms, as well as software libraries developed by the community, are used to monitor and control the resources available in the educational set (controllers, sensors, motors, etc.) through configuration and development of virtual tools specific to each task). All these applications helped the students to better understand the theoretic phenomena, and teachers to develop specific applications for the theoretical for the theoretical part transmitted in the courses using modern techniques using modern techniques.

Issues and challenges.

"Success depends on ensuring the integrity and confidentiality of IoT solutions and data while mitigating cybersecurity risks." The beneficiary of the IoT solutions must also understand the cybersecurity risks when they are adopting this type of solutions. There are many factors to consider and in Fig. 5 potential security weaknesses are presented with respect to the developed application.

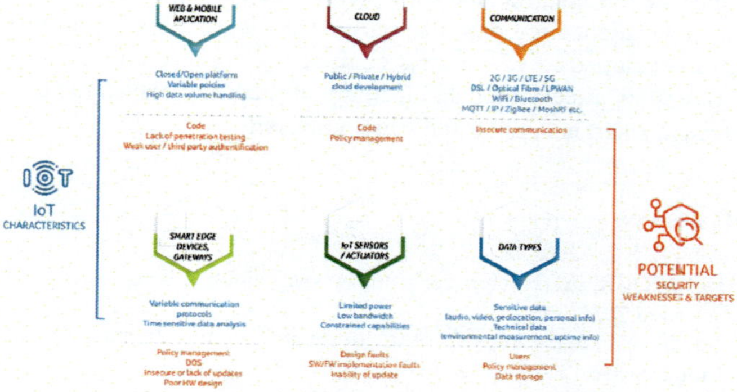

Fig. 5. Risk assessment

There is a digital security risk that one is exposed to when working with IoT systems. But understanding those potential security weaknesses could lead to a better protection strategy and build confidence in integrating such applications into the modern teaching methods. This is why there are experts in this field that can guide users in choosing the proper security mechanisms to be implemented depending on the developed application used.

Although IoT makes the classroom environment smart due to exceptional development of global computing (cloud computing, big data) to achieve the effective in integration of IoT devices within a campus environment, educational institutions may encounter several challenges: the use of e-learning management systems (like Moodle), lecture recording and web streaming generates a big amount of data that needs to be handled during online courses; lack a clear strategy for cost-sharing when it comes to the entire IoT infrastructure, often constrained by budget limitations that cand be addressed by innovate in the realms of finance, IT infrastructure and services [8–11].

Conclusion

In sustaining our findings after analysing many related topics in terms of effect of using IoT in engineering application development, and in the educational process in universities and more specific in TUCN, there is a survey regarding the role of IoT in development of education published by Rihhab Sami Abd-Ali et all. in 2020 [5]. Although the educational system suffered from many restrictions imposed by the COVID conditions, **Smart education** still plays the key role for the 21-st century. It integrates not only finding the smart teaching and learning methods and applying them.

The adoption of IoT devices in the field of education is a burgeoning trend worldwide, offering a fresh and inventive approach to both teaching and classroom management.

A variety of tools are employed in this context, with some of the most frequently utilized IoT devices in educational settings being: interactive whiteboards, eBooks, tablets, attendance tracking systems, clasrooms sensors, security cammeras etc.

The present paper reveals a small part of the effort made at TUCN level towards meeting the new requirements for continuing the educational process by integrating the IoT into the teaching methods in a period when all academic instutions had to switch almost over night from onsite to online teaching methods. The diversity of IoT applications developed as educational engineering application offered the perfect solution for continuing the teaching and learning process and played the key role in building an innovative smart education and smart university.

References

1. RFID JOURNAL Homepage, https://www.rfidjournal.com/that-internet-of-things-thing, last accessed 2022/10/1
2. Bogdanovic, Z., Simic, K.: A platform for learning Internet of Things. In International Conference e-Learning, (2014)
3. Annual TUCN Rector's Report for 2021, https://www.utcluj.ro/media/page_document/463/Raport_Rector_2021.pdf, last accessed 2022/10/2
4. Muhammad Kashif Saeed, Shah A.M., Mahmood ul H., Khan J., Babar N., Usage of Internet of Things(IOT) thecnology in the higher education sector. Journa Enhineering Sci. Technol., **16**(5) 4181–4191 (2021)
5. Abd-Ali, R.S., Radhi, S.A., Rasool, Z.I.: A survey: The role of the Internet of Things in the development of education. Indones. J. Electr. Eng. Comput. Sci. **1**(19), 216–221 (2020)
6. Popusor, A.: Temperature and humidity monitoring application for neonatal care—an mHealth solution, BsC thesis, (2021)
7. https://www.thalesgroup.com/en/markets/digital-identity-and-security/iot/iot-security, last accessed 2022/10/1
8. Ahmed, V., Alnaaj, K.A., Saboor, S.: An investigation into stakeholders' perception of smart campus criteria: The American university of Sharjah as a case study. Sustainability **12**(12), 5187 (2020)
9. Tegta, O., Khurana, R., Kaur, R.: Placement question bank: Android informer. Bachelor Degree. Department of Computer Science and Engineering and Information Technology, Jaypee University of Information Technology Waknaghat (2016)
10. Dong, Z.Y., Zhang, Y., Yip, C., Swift, S., Beswick, K.: Smart campus: definition, framework, technologies, and services. IET Smart Cities **2**(1), 43–54 (2020)
11. Tianbo, Z.: The internet of things promoting higher education revolution. In: Fourth International Conference on Multimedia Information Networking and Security. Nanjing, China, 790–793 (2012)

Post- COVID19 Conclusion Regarding the Education in a Technical University in Romania. How Does Stress Influence the Educational Process

Cîrlugea Mihaela(✉) and Farago Paul

Technical University of Cluj-Napoca, Cluj-Napoca, Romania
Mihaela.Cirlugea@bel.utcluj.ro

Abstract. A survey lasing for about 20 months is presented regarding the e-learning implemented during the COVID19 crisis in the Technical University of Cluj-Napoca, Romania. The study was made on undergraduates in years 1–4 of study and master students, in engineering, where the authors are teaching. The conclusions show that students had different opinions, the most stressed were the students in years 1–2 of study, those in years 3–4 had an average percent of stress, while the master students showed more maturity and experience. Also as an unexpected conclusion, it would be beneficial for the students that the educational structure should change into a mixed onsite-online, divided into first two years of study and years 3–4 of study and a different structure for the master students. At present, all students learn in the same study formations and are all treated equally (curricula, teaching material), independently of the year of study.

Keywords: Education · e-Learning · Stress · Anxiety · Students · Engineering · MSTeams platform · Online versus Onsite · Post-COVID

1 Introduction

Because of the COVID19 crisis, emergency online learning had to be implemented, without warning, overnight, independently on the technical conditions and the limits of all users, a virtual environment for learning had forcibly to be created[7, 8]. E-learning is a pretty new area for some universities but something common for others. In distance learning, as it was the case of universities in our country, Romania, or in other countries, like for example in Malaysia or Africa [8], where the open and distance education e-system was on purpose organized in that direction [1], curricula, teaching methods, assessments, infrastructure were from the beginning thought in that direction so that in time, a routine and almost a tradition was developed, providing a flexible and consistent e-learning virtual structure. In other universities with a long tradition of the classic onsite, or face-to-face teaching, the appearance of the COVID19 crisis and the imposition of the lockdown with sudden online classes, brought confusion and panic amongst all the people involved, from the university management structure and communications

S. Vlad and N. M. Roman (Eds.): MEDITECH 2022, IFMBE Proceedings 102, pp. 143–153, 2024.
https://doi.org/10.1007/978-3-031-51120-2_16

and virtualization collective, to each teacher and student. Like all changes in the history of humanity, this crisis had to be understood, overcome and tools adapted as soon and as good as possible. In some Slovak universities, the social networks were, with success!, strongly used for advertisement and distribution of important information among students [2], proving that, online marketing is crucial to new media, a communication tool naturally used by Millennials. The issues that appear in the sudden online teaching activities were sometimes similar, sometimes different regarding the university profiles and the communication tools involved. In our case, we determined that not all years of study, undergraduates or master, need the same teaching approach. And also what came clearly, that a lot of stress was envolved during the two years of COVID crisis, jeo-pardizing the heath and the educational process of both, the teachers and students. The present study was done in a technical university with a tradition of over 100 years, medical-social aspects were studied, like the educator-student relationship [4] and the psychic stress and the ability to adapt or not, in case of both the educators and students [5]. The adapting skills of each of us were important, main thing, all the people envolved were trying to do their best to sustain the new situation.

2 Moving into Virtual

2.1 The Online Teaching Platform. Impact on the Participants

An infrastructure has been created to facilitate the teaching content delivery and also the student participation to the online classes [8]. In our case, the Microsoft M365 platform was used, a robust and versatile tool with more advantages than drawbacks. M365 allowed the simultaneous access of hundreds participants to a group, thousands of participants in various simultaneous meetings and permitting a great cloud space for do-cumentation storage, great tools for teacher-student interaction, simulating the blackboard, the notebook and allowing easily access and uploads of homework and assessments. There were times when the platform was used for totally online education or for mixed-blended teaching. This was useful because the employees had board meetings or councils, all the participants in classes, teachers or students, could easily enter various classes or online events, without losing any time for moving from one place to another. Theoretically, all participants could easily interact and virtual classes could become similar to those in real-life. All the students could simultaneously write on screen or solve a problem. Students could be evaluated during a class. Theory and si-mulations can be simultaneously and parallel illustrated.

Documentation was easily uploaded, allowing a huge amount of data to become instantaneously accessed by the students. Even now, when the COVID restrictions are removed, the documentation is stored online on the platform. Students upload homework, allowing easy loading and easy reading for users on both sides. The homework and the curricula documentation are stored on the platform in an organized way, thing that wouldn't be possible with physical projects or documents sent in emails.

The lists of the attending persons to a meeting can be created and saved, lists that contain the exact moment when anyone entered or left. This is an aspect that induced stress in some students, because of the permanent sensation of being watched and because of the stress that they might enter late and each second is noted.

One drawback of the platform appears when dealing with other operating systems than Windows, or with browsers that are not, or not entirely supported. It can happen that users have trouble with Apple laptops, or they have to use virtual machines in case of primarily working in Linux. For students that could be an inconvenience if they preferred other operating systems than Microsoft and, as a matter of fact, no one could impose something like that!

Issues arouse if a user had not a proper technical device or a proper internet connection. It happened when performing real-time simulations that the results of some signal si-mulations appeared delayed or discontinuously and couldn't be followed by the students during the class teaching. It also happened that students were logged off during the class or, worse, in the middle of the online exam and the teachers had to find correct solutions for the situations. These cases, especially the log off during the exams, were also stress and anxiety inducing factors for the students.

Teachers had to revise their whole documentation, their education strategy, to adapt to the needs of the generations, in every and each aspect. They also tried to involve affectively the students so that they show more interest in study and learning [10, 12].

2.2 Psychological and Physiological Conclusions

If the use of the platform was welcome by young educators and most of the students in the beginning, the teachers over 35 were experiencing some stress. The stress was generated because they had to change mostly of the structure of their teaching documentation and had to spend from 8–10 h per day in front of the computer, having consequences like eye strain, headache and weight gain.

Some technical issues caused also stress to all participants, such as browsers that weren't entirely supported in Windows, the lack of a strong internet connection, students that were logged off during the class or during an exam. During the exam control could also miss, also the risk of cheating could increase, as noted in study [3].

In case of teaching, the lecturer does it usually one way, students remain passive, they don't answer questions and don't interact [3], though it should be generally a "collaborative learning". After some months, the student's stress increased, because they realized that during some curricula they couldn't pay attention while online and were not able to learn or had issues in understanding the documentation.

Another drawback was the absence of emotion and of socializing, students were not interested in some curricula and neither in meeting the "guy behind the voice" online, from the educator's perspective, students were depersonalized, becoming some names and numbers on the screen.

After taking the survey regarding the stress and problems due to online education, from the student's point of view, the opinions and needs could be grouped into undergraduates in the first two years of study, students in years 3 and 4 of study and master students, which are, in majority, already hired.

The opinions presented in this chapter are a summary report. The subjects are students from the Technical University in Cluj-Napoca, in engineering sections where the authors teach. From 336 students in years 1 and 2, a percent of 89,7% took part in the study; from 274 students in years 3 and 4 a percent of 71,5% took part in the study; from 52 students in master, a percent of 96,1% were willing to take the survey. The answers are reported in Table 1.

Table 1. Student feedback for online education, years 1–2 and years 3–4.

Feature	Students feedback years 1–2 [%]	Feature	Students feedback years 3–4 [%]
Headaches, blurry vision	93,1	Depression	68,3
Depression	89,7	Interest in curricular activities	67,4
High pulse/tachycardia during exams	85,3	Headaches, blurry vision	56,9
Missing human interaction	79,9	Participating to debates, discussions	54,8
Eagerness for study	78,2	Anxiety	49,7
Anxiety	73,2	Eagerness for study	47,5
Insomnia	72,4	Good management of the learning time	46,3
Frequently catch cold /allergies (low immunity)	69,1	Pleasure in participating to the classes	45,1
Fear, mistrust regarding the educator	67,4	Enthusiasm in presenting their work and projects	42,4
Interest in curricular activities	33,3	Attention in attending classes for hours	39,1
Pleasure in participating to the classes	27,7	High pulse/tachycardia during exams	38,9
Good management of the learning time	25,5	Frequently catch cold/allergies (low immunity)	37,3
High pulse/tachycardia during classes	22,1	Insomnia	32,2
Participating to debates, discussions	21,4	Fear, mistrust regarding the educator	23,7
Enthusiasm in presenting their work and projects	15,2	High pulse/tachycardia during classes	15,1
Attention inn attending classes for hours	14,7	Missing human interaction	12,4

One can see that, if for the students in years 1–2 the stress, anxiety, insomnia, depression and other factors were the highest, so that the learning process was deeply influenced, fact that was visible also in their grades. These students obtained better grades in on-site exams than the grades in online exams. The on-site teaching was vital, because they needed to acquire basic notions and felt more secure collaborating with a real person in the classroom, sensing a closer relationship to the teacher, in the manner of a friend or a parent that could guide them. The stress of the students can be diminished if the educator is compassionate and caring [4], paying attention to their needs, having to accommodate to the knowledge and mental possibilities of each group, because generations are different and educators need to be there for student's growth and self-discovery [4].

A major disadvantage was that the students couldn't stay focused for hours, during all lectures. They could be easily distracted and not being able to answer even simple questions. The lecture, traditional on-site, didn't always function well online as the primary teaching method, shorter lectures with application questions and group work were instead preferred[8]. Sometimes they had to spend up to 12 h a day in front of the screen. The students mentioned also the technical issues that made e-learning harder. These students, being younger and unexperienced with independent learning, were the most stressed. But in their case, *the curriculum is the most rigid, containing basic knowledge, that you have to learn, there is not much place for creativity, discussions and debates.*

The students in years 3–4 showed average scores in almost all features, they were stressed but not necessary because the online classes but because they also started working and have some jobs. They knew the educators as persons, so they knew what to expect in exams and what the requirements generally were. A positive aspect when being online was that they could be at home or in any place, eat at home, not spending money for campus, travel and supplementary food. Also a good thing was, for all students, that suddenly the documentation was richer, better structured, all in electronic format, easily to be accessed and all in one place. There was no need for visiting libraries and borrowing books. They complained that during e-learning they got more projects and homework, instead of spending each 2 h onsite in the laboratory, they had to work at home longer for their homework. Though it was easier for them to prepare the projects and to manage their working and learning time. For years 3–4 the curricula is more specialized and thus the students have more interest in learning a specific knowledge and doing a specific research.

In case of the master students, they also had headaches, depression and blurry vision, because of the long time spent in front of the screen, as indicated in Table 2, because they had to work during the day and attend classes in the afternoon. Though, they had more fun and enthusiasm in researching and working for school, in discussions and everything the teachers would share with them. The master students have all the basic curricula already learned and are more interested in learning and discovering new and fresh things. Also their projects could be focused almost integral on creativity and on their research interest, so that the enthusiasm during classes, debates and projects presentations was bigger.

So if for the younger students the mixed learning or the onsite learning is way more useful and socially necessary, in case of the students in the 3rd and 4th year of study, graduates and master studies, who mostly have a job, the needs differ. The latter prefer in a great majority the online education, because they don't loose hours in traffic, they can connect to the classes maybe even while being at the job, they can freely discuss online during the lectures because they know their teachers already and they are more interested in learning something new and interesting than in spending time for sociali-zing. For the older students it is easier to participate to online lectures also because they have the knowledge basis and can easily understand.

Table 2. Student feedback for online education, master.

Feature	Students feedback master (%)
Enthusiasm in presenting their work and projects	95,2
Participating to debates, discussions	89,8
Good management of the learning time	82,6
Attention during classes for hours	78,7
Pleasure in participating to the classes	75,5
Interest in curricular activities	72,1
Frequently catch cold/allergies (low immunity)	33,3
Depression	25,4
Headaches, blurry vision	23,1
Insomnia	23,1
Eagerness for study	17,2
Missing human interactions	15,7
High pulse/tachycardia during exams	12,4
Anxiety	9,1
Fear, mistrust regarding the educator	3,3
High pulse/tachycardia during classes	1,1

Also it is possible that their job is related to some curricula so they also have some prior knowledge. Besides this, in comparison to the younger students whom the tea-chers have to tell each step they have to take in creating projects, the older students are more happy when they can do homework or projects that envolve creativity, freedom regarding the chosen subject, maybe an trans-disciplinary theme, where they can use their creativity, their basic concepts and notions and build with them, each student can learn new information in an area they are particularly interested in, developing the projects in the amount of time they want and developing in any direction they find inte-resting; of course with the mention that the project is somehow connected to the related curricula.

From the educator's perspective, there should be a correlating, bidirectional connec-tion between the teaching and the learning process. Though when working with all the people envolved in the educational process, a totally accord is impossible.

2.3 Pedagogical Aspects

The Ternary Education Model

We developed a ternary model for the analysis, illustrated in Fig. 1, namely the **"Student-Teacher-Curricula"**. The **student** is the client and the main active character of the educational process, online or onsite. Therefore the student occupies the central place of the model, with his needs and demands. Then, the **teacher** as also a human and active element is important, providing the environment and the right circumstances for learning. And last, but not least, the **curricula type**, seen though as a passive element, is crucial whether the education type is appropriate for online or onsite, or mixed.

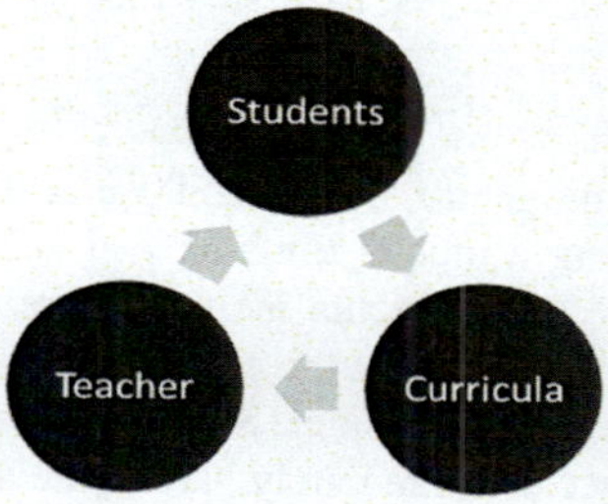

Fig. 1. Ternary education model

The **teacher** is the one that has to be the binder between student and curricula, with his experience molding the curricula, adapting it to the necessities of each generation, because not all generations are the same, some are more curious, some are more eager to learn new things, others are more inertial or more shy in the social interaction. In the present case, passing from on-site classes to online, the teacher had, in the first place, to adapt their teaching methods, the documentation, the assessments, the exams to the present imposed circumstances. Keeping in mind that teachers are human, with different training, different ages and experience, each of them did their best, some of them rose to the student's expectations, some didn't. In each case, they all did their best, in a positive, constructive effort.

The third and passive element of the ternary model is the **curricula**, here being mentioned the fact that this model and partitioning works for our technical university, in case of the engineering and economics profile, where some specific subjects are taught after two years of teaching online only or mixed online-onsite, some conclusions can be drawn. Our university has a technical engineering profile, where the curricula can be divided into 3 groups as indicated in Fig. 2, each reacting different to the learning process. The 3 types of curricula we called **theoretical**, **programming** (code) and **mathematical** (problems).

The **theoretical group**, includes curricula like economics notions or logistics, enginee-ring history, economics in engineering, or other lessons containing a great amount of text and the exam consists in understanding and reproducing some texts. This group is suitable for e-learning, though the course can become boring and unilateral.

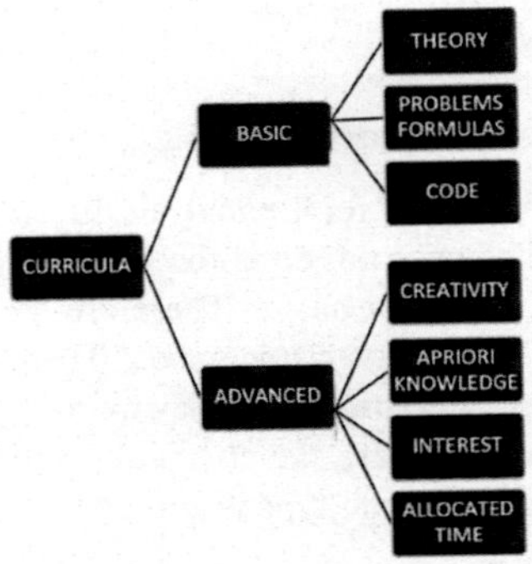

Fig. 2. Curricula classification, the basic suited for years 1–2, the advanced for years 3–4 and master studies

The **programming group**, has about 90% of the documentation referring to **code**, commands, developing a unique thinking and abstraction mode, as in Java, C + +, MatLab, VHDL etc. The curricula included here are very well suited for the online teaching, one can parallel present the course-lecture part and immediately, on the same screen show some concrete examples. So, the lessons is maintaining awake the student's interest and also they can immediately participate and verify each command. Verifying if the teacher writes the correct code can be fun for the students and involve them in a plea-sant manner in the learning process. Students can also collaborate during the online classes and the projects are easier presented online. So this type of curricula is the most suited for online approach.

Verifying student's projects is much easier online! All these commands are harder to be followed and understood while in class and also harder to verify the code for each student separately, during laboratory or seminaries.

The **mathematical** group, containing **formulas, algorithms** and **problems**, like mathematics, statistics, but also electronics and circuits or physics. The online courses are for the students almost impossible to follow, the student's attention is rapidly and frequently lost and cannot be kept without collaboration in solving problems. Because they deal with algorithms for solving problems and exercises, as well as understanding some phy-sical phenomena, the teacher-student interaction and seminaries are highly recommended, especially because most of them occur during the first two years of study. Here the teacher-student interaction and seminaries are highly recommended and necessary, therefore this group is suitable for onsite learning.

Having this study made, our conclusion is that the academic year could be reconstructed in a more efficient way, suited better for the needs of the students.

We propose that the 14 weeks of teaching, during the semester, to be split into modules, during about 1/3 of the semester the online programming modules to take place, another about 1/3 of the semester the theoretical and the other 1/3 part of the semester to contain modules with mathematical curricula. If the years 1 and 2 do alternate in this approach, there is a plenty space for classrooms. We would recommend that the 1st year to commence with the theoretical curricula and a mixed approach, so they get better acquainted and get used to the both systems of learning. In the middle of the semester to learn the mathematical parts, that are more difficult, and in the end the programming. For the second year they can commence with the mathematical curricula, which in the 2nd year are very important, then continue with the programming and in the end with the theore-tical. In the superior years of study, theoretical curricula are seldom and have not a great contribution to the final grade, so they can be left at the end of the semester.

An advantage of learning in modules is that, at once, the student focuses on 2 maybe at most 3 curricula at once. Another is that, that there is no need for revisions if the lessons occur closely in a short amount of time. The students have the previous lessons information freshly in their minds and the lessons can continue more efficiently. Then, after ending the module, the students could even sustain the exam for that subject, so even if the semester is not ready, they can peacefully concentrate on other curricula, homework and projects.

In case of the last year of study and master studies, they can attend either fully online or mixed online-onsite learning, depending on the agreement and needs between the students and the teachers. For these students, their needs differ drastically because they are not only hired, but most of them can have already families and some of them can also work in different places than where the university is and thus they have to make a tremendous effort in order to accomplish all their tasks.

Our reported findings can be visualized on the feature comparison graph in Fig. 3.

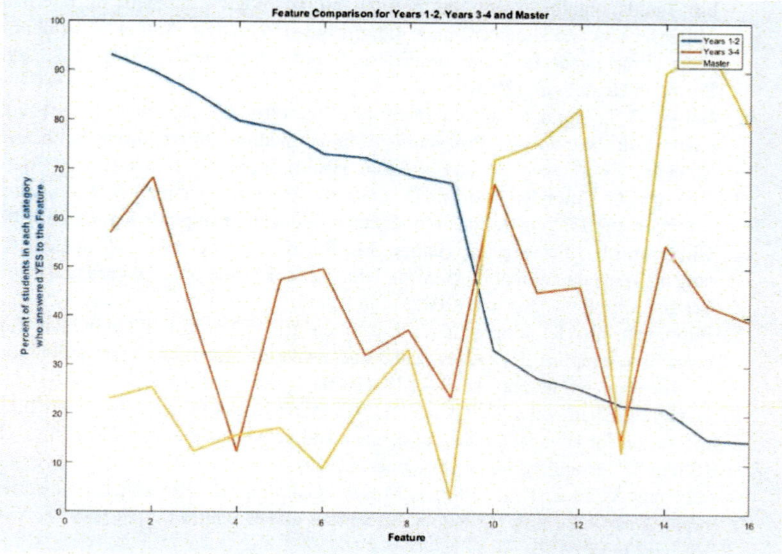

Fig. 3. Features comparison for years 1–2 versus years 3–4 and versus master students

3 Conclusion

Regarding the medical aspect, the survey showed that in the beginning, the teachers were indicating a high level of stress, because they suddenly had to change their teaching methods and documents, keeping them in front of the laptop or computer up to 8–10 h per day. The stress was higher for the educators older than 35. In the second year of study during pandemics, the higher stress levels moved to the students, on one hand because they were not able to understand the lessons as well as in the classroom and on the other hand because the long term lack of communication and socialization and also the various ways of examinations were causing them upheaval and anxiety. For the teachers, students were seen on screen as names or numbers, and for the students, educators were coercion instruments. The missing of the human factor and the lack of socializing were causing major stress and health problems. Besides the psychical factor, stress can lead to unhealthy habits like unhealthy eating, not sleeping or res-ting properly, smoking or even drinking. Unhealthy habits can have effects like a high blood pressure, high cholesterol, tiredness, being able to cause heart and circulatory diseases or even heart attacks.

References

1. Ajani, A.S., Alade O.M., Ajani, O.S., Alabi, O.J. : Development of a mobile multimodal bio signal instrument for simultaneous measurement and analysis of four clinically relevant bio signals, obtained from both normal and pathological subjects, In: International Journal of Biosensors and Bioelectronics, **4**:3, pp.148–157, (2018) Author, F., Author, S.: Title of a proceedings paper. In: Editor, F., Editor, S. (eds.) Conference 2016, LNCS, **9999**, pp. 1–13. Springer, Heidelberg (2016)
2. Hamel, B.S.: Breakdown time analysis in the effort to maximize medical equipment productivity in hospital, In: Proceedings Muhammadiyah International Public Healthcare and Medicine Conference, Faculty of Public Health, Jakarta, 1(1), (2021)
3. Corciova, C., Fuior, R., Andritoi, D., Luca, C.: Assessment of medical equipment maintenance management, In: "Operations Management", Intech open publisher, pp.1–15, (2022)
4. Ghasemi, M., Mazaheri, E., Hadian, M., Karimi, S.: Evaluation of medical equipment management in educational hospitals in Isfahan, In: Journal of Education and Health Promotion 11(3), http://www.jehp.net, (2022)
5. Piipponen, K.V.T., Sepponen, R., Eskelinen, P.: A Biosignla instrumentation system using capacitive coupling for power and signal isolation, In: IEEE Transactions on Biomedical Engineering, **54**(10), pp. 1822–1828, (2007)
6. Heuer, S., Chamadiya, B., Gharbi, A., Wagner, M.: Unobtrusive in-vehicle bio signal instrumentation for advanced driver assistance and active safety, In: IEEE EMBS Conference on Biomedical Engineering and Sciences, (2010)
7. Kiranyaz,S., Ince, T., Chowdury, M.E.D., Gabbouj, M.: Bio signal time-series analysis, In book: Deep Learning for Robot Perception and Cognition, pp.491–539, Academic Press, Elsevier Inc. (2022)
8. Li, H., Wang, J., Zhao, S., Tian, F., Yang, J., Sawan, M.: Real-time Bio signal recording and Machine-Learning analysis system, In: IEEE 4th International Conference on Artificial Intelligence Circuits and Systems (AICAS), pp.427–430, (2022)
9. Ghavifekr, S., Afshari, M., Salleh, A.: Management strategies for E-Learning system as the core component of systemic change: a qualitative analysis. Life Sci. J. **9**(3), 2190–2196 (2012)

10. Cenkova, R., Steingartner, W.: Use of internet social networks in academic environment. J. Inf. Organ. Sci. **44**(2), 275–295 (2020)
11. Bose, F.: Development and challenges of teaching law and economics online. Law Teach. J., April 2021, pp.1–20
12. Lund Dean, K.: Too much of a good thing: Escalating developmental needs in the educator-student relationship. Acad. Lett., April 2020, Article 495. https://doi.org/10.20935/AL495
13. Yeigh, T., Lynch, D.: Is online teaching and learning here to stay?, Academia Letters, November 2020, article 24, https://doi.org/10.20935/AL24
14. Pimentel, E.: Remote emergency education is not virtual education. CEVAD Universidad Central de Venezuela, (2020)
15. Oladele Owolabi, J.: Virtualizing the school during the COVID19 and beyond in Africa. Adv. Med. Educ. Pract., Dovepress, pp.755–759 (2020)

Development of a Repository of Technologies and Tools to Improve Digital Skills and Inclusivity in Education, Based on School Gardens

Laura Grindei[1](✉), Sara Blanc[2], José Vicente Benlloch-Dualde[2], Nestor Martinez Ballester[3], and Urška Knez[4]

[1] Technical University of Cluj Napoca, 400114 Cluj Napoca, Romania
Laura.Grindei@ethm.utcluj.ro
[2] Universitat Politècnica de València, Valencia, Spain
[3] Colegio La Purisima, Fundacion Educativa Franciscanas de La Inmaculada, 46018 Valencia, Spain
nestormartinezba@alu.lapurisimavalencia.com
[4] Osnovna šola šmartno Pod šmarno Goro, C.V. Gameljne 7, 1211 Lj. Šmartno, Slovenia

Abstract. This paper presents the development of a repository of technologies and tools designed for improving digital skills and competences of school teachers and students, and to promote an inclusive education by using real-life applications in ecological school gardens. The repository was developed within the eSGarden—"School Gardens for Future Citizens" Erasmus + project, which started as a strategic partnership in the field of education, in the frame of the Erasmus KA2 Supporting Innovation Action. These tools and technologies together with examples of learning activities developed in eSGarden project partner schools are facilitating a more inclusive and interactive learning environment and they are raising awareness of the technology impact on everyday life, health, and sus-tainability. The development of this repository was realized during the project through creation of eBooks and video tutorials describing the setting-up of a school garden where children will learn about healthy food and sustainable growth, guidelines concerning the use of IoT for monitoring different parameters from the garden through a new mobile app designed for schools, strategies for coding and examples of learning activities that were performed in primary and secondary schools based on these technologies.

Keywords: ICT tools and technologies in education · Digital skills · School garden-based education · IoT · Inclusive education · Immersive tools

1 Introduction

Nowadays, schools worldwide use a variety of ICT ("Information and Communications Technology) tools to create, disseminate, store, and manage information, to interact and communicate with students in teaching activities. The potential of using technology

S. Vlad and N. M. Roman (Eds.): MEDITECH 2022, IFMBE Proceedings 102, pp. 154–162, 2024.
https://doi.org/10.1007/978-3-031-51120-2_17

and ICT tools in education is very high, but it is also challenging for schoolteachers. When schoolteachers are digitally literate and trained to use ICT tools and technologies, this educational approach can improve students' problem-solving skills, provide creative and individualized support for all students, and challenge students to acquire more information and expertise in a multidisciplinary context for finding solutions to deal with ongoing technological change in society and environment.

The paper presents the results of the eSGarden project from the perspective of tools and technologies integration in primary and secondary schools' education with the goal of facilitating a more inclusive and interactive learning environment while raising awareness of the technology impact on everyday life, health, and sustainability.

The eSGarden project represents a collaborative educational Erasmus + project between schools and universities, that was initiated for transferring knowledge from the partner universities to primary and secondary schools, in terms of digital skills and competences, to improve the teaching activities and to provide a more inclusive environment based on school gardens activities.

Teaching activities performed in the schools' gardens promote values for school children that will become future citizens towards respect for the environment and responsible behavior, while raising awareness for sustainable production of healthy food. Setting up and monitoring school gardens could inspire children from primary and secondary schools to use technologies and innovative tools to perform learning activities in all domains including science, math, literature, arts, and crafts [1].

The eSGarden project started in 2018 and has been implemented during a period of three years till 2021 and extended for six months till 2022, due to pandemic. As partners in the project, three universities from Spain, Portugal and Romania were involved: Universitat Politècnica de València, Spain, Universidade do Porto, Portugal, Technical University of Cluj-Napoca, Romania, and four schools from four countries: Colegio la Purisima Franciscanas, Valencia, Spain, Agrupamento de Escolas de Paredes, Porto, Portugal, Osnovna sola Smartno pod Smarno goro, Lujbljana, Slovenia, Directorate of Primary School Education, Preveza, Greece, and two private companies from Spain: TB Agrosensor S.L.,Valencia, and Fundación CajaMar Comunidad Valenciana.

2 Repository of Resources for Schoolteachers

The repository of resources for teachers from primary and secondary schools was developed within the eSGarden project as an educational platform and it is available at the following address: https://esgarden.webs.upv.es/ [2] with public access. It integrates video tutorials, eBooks and guidelines for using technology. In addition, a MOOC course was developed with restricted access for project partners and hosted at the Universitat Politècnica de València, Spain. The repository is structured in several sections concerning the: Design and management of school gardens, IoT in school gardens, School Climate and Inclusion, Examples of learning activities base on school gardens, and Digital tools for education and will be presented below.

2.1 Section 1: Design and Management of the School Gardens

This section includes video tutorials and eBooks for the design and management of the school gardens with practical information and guidelines for their setting up, from preparation of soil, selecting and planting seeds, irrigation, creating compost to using IoT and technology for monitoring them.

Two eBooks in English and Spanish were developed within the eSGarden project as support for teachers from schools to set up their own school gardens, including chapters on finding school garden location, infrastructure needed, crop choice & seedling nursery, nutrient requirements, manure and composting, planting & semi-protected systems, crop care, water supply and water requirement calculation, health and healthy nutrition.

The eBooks are available online with public access and represent a very useful tool for all schools that wish to use this approach in teaching, taking in consideration that school garden enables children to directly experience the sowing, planting and cultivation of plants in natural fields, thus combining theory and practice in everyday lessons and other educational activities.

Practical activities in the school gardens offer students the opportunity to acquire skills to achieve a better quality of life through healthy eating, not only for themselves, but also for their family and community. Many physical, art, science or STEM activities can be realized in the school gardens.

The school gardens are also very useful resources for interdisciplinary work or projects in different topics including Environmental Education, Health Education, Education for Coexistence, Literature, Geology, Geometry, and Arithmetic [1].

2.2 Section 2: IoT in School Gardens

This section provides information on how to use and install IoT devices in a school garden, how to use cloud technology to store data and how to send information to a smart device such as a phone or tablet using an app (Fig. 1).

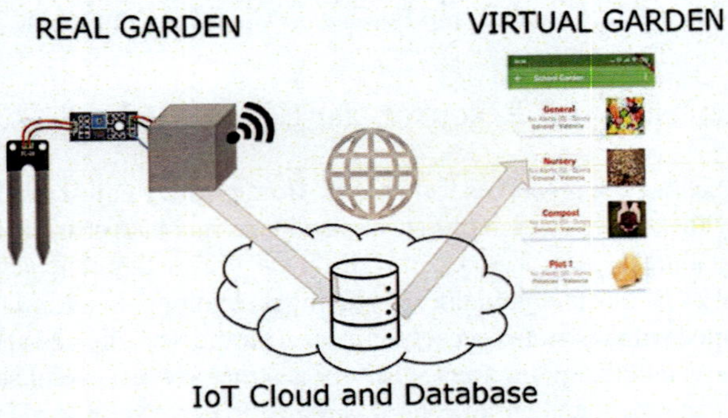

Fig. 1. Data transfer in the virtual garden platform

Within the eSGarden project, hardware kits for monitoring the gardens were acquisitioned for each partner school and were installed in their school gardens and the repository offers information on setting up all devices, configuring the database in the cloud and programming guidelines. An educational app for monitoring the gardens from mobile devices was designed and implemented with free access for teachers and students from schools who want to use these technologies in different learning activities.

Physics, mathematics, biology, science, informatics and other competencies can be achieved through practical activities based on data obtained from the school garden. Several parameters can be measured with a weather station installed in the garden, like temperature, humidity, and others, that affect both the growth cycle of plants and the human health. There are also several ambient parameters that can be measured with a weather station, parameters that affect both the growth cycle of crops and human health. Many creative teaching activities and DIY projects can be developed in the classroom related to this technology.

In Fig. 2 are illustrated the three stages of setting up the real and virtual garden using IoT devices which were presented to teachers and students from partner schools. The virtual gardening platform was designed to integrate different sensors for monitoring temperature and humidity using professional sensors used in agriculture and it is based on educational easy-to-use off-the-self kits such as Arduino boards or Micro::bit [3, 4]. Information on using ARDUINO boards and different sensors is provided too.

Numerical data is collected by the system through a friendly user interface designed for children, including information regarding plants and vegetables selection, suggestions for watering the plants, proper time for harvest, and suitable treatments.

In order to support teachers on administration and management of the gardens, a library of resources was integrated in the virtual platform, specific for each type of plot. The eSGarden virtual platform provides support for teachers to raise children awareness on gardens' sustainability, on the importance of growing and consuming healthy vegetables while using the input data to design new creative learning activities in a variety of course topics and for all ages.

Thus, the children's learning experience improve several skills and competences in the European DigComp framework: "information search and retrieval, communication and collaboration in digital environments, safety in digital environments, creation of digital content, problem solving" [5].

2.3 Section 3: School Climate and Inclusion

Acknowledging the key role of educating young people for a digitalized world, this section of the repository presents a collection of technology and tools useful for the development of digital competences appropriate for teaching staff and children, and information on the pedagogical use of technologies with the goal of making learning and teaching more efficient while widening access to education for all students.

This section integrates a video tutorial realized for teachers on school climate and inclusion. Inclusive education is focused on developing and designing schools, classrooms, educational programs and learning activities so that all students can study, participate, and interact together.

Inclusive education must ensure access to quality education for all students by effectively meeting their diverse needs in a way that is responsive, accepting, respectful and supportive. Thus, the tutorials included in this section promote the use of digital

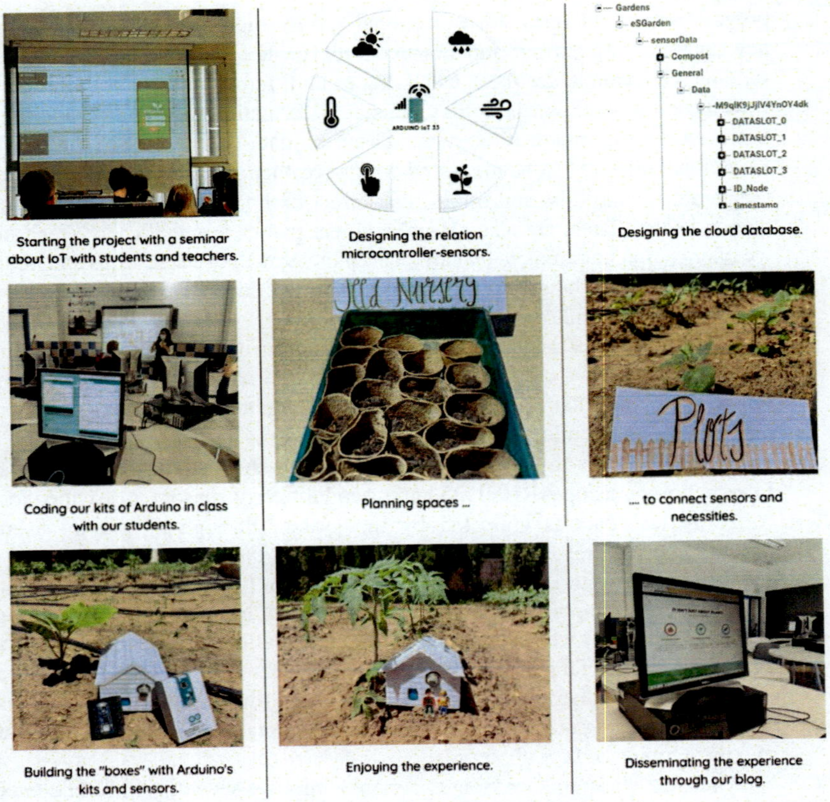

Fig. 2. Three stages of setting up the real and virtual garden

tools to support students by addressing a diversity of needs, such as learning difficulties (addressing dyslexia, dysgraphia, dyscalculia), visual impairments (for low vision, blind, colourblind or other visual disorders) hearing impairments (such as deaf, hard of hearing, etc.), mobility impairments, neurological (autism, ADD/ADHA) or mental diseases (anxiety, depression, OCD).

The repository includes information for schoolteachers for using the immersive reader to implement efficient techniques that improve learning abilities of children with special needs. These text decoding solutions offered by immersive reader tool is very useful for children with learning difficulties such as dyslexia, dyscalculia, visual and hearing impairments and for other learning difficulties. The tutorial offers examples of using this tool with Microsoft Word, and One Note for improving children reading, pronunciation, grammar knowledge, speaking and communication abilities using translation in sixty languages. Examples of using this tool for browsing the web or access text and mathematical formulas in Microsoft Form quizzes and assignments were provided, as they can inspire teachers to support children with specific learning needs in their evaluations.

Other examples presented in this section tutorial are related to Microsoft Whiteboard for classroom collaboration and Microsoft Office Lens App which is useful for students in reading and translating content from scanned text, images, and whiteboards.

The tutorial includes examples on other specific tools useful for dictation by students that for example can't use their hands to write papers and transcribe lectures into notes, and real time translation tools. The tutorial includes information on using the Math Assistant from OneNote for Windows and OneNote Online which can be a very useful tool to assist students with dyslexia who have difficulties reading math problems or students that experience focusses issues or have dyscalculia. This tool can be very useful for teachers during their lessons because it helps students in writing equations, transforming handwriting in text (Ink to Math option), hearing math solver's step-by-step solutions for easier comprehension and visualising graphics.

Information on safety in digital environments is also presented in this section of the repository, offering information for teachers regarding the tools and knowledge that can be used for protecting information and cyber safety practice, children security (cyberbullying, etc.) on Internet.

3 Success Cases: Learning Activities

The repository developed in the frame of the eSGarden project also includes several success cases developed as learning activities through the three years of the project.

3.1 Learning Activity: "Intelligent Weather Station"

An example of learning activity presented in the repository entitled "Intelligent weather station" was realized through a collaboration between two project partners from university and school and its strategy of implementation is illustrated in Fig. 3.

Different stages of implementation for this intelligent weather station are presented in Fig. 4.

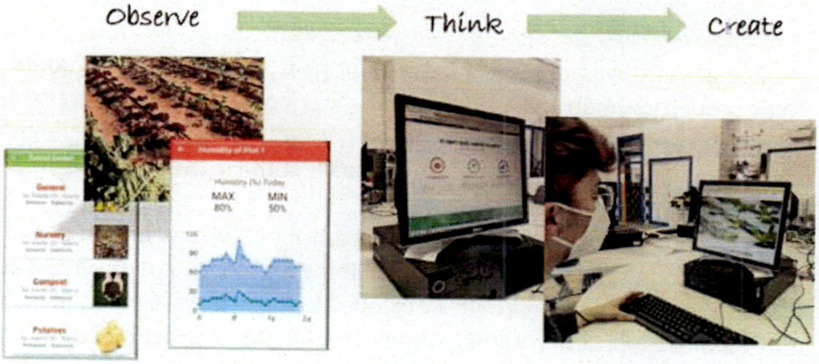

Fig. 3. Strategy for implementation of the Intelligent weather station project

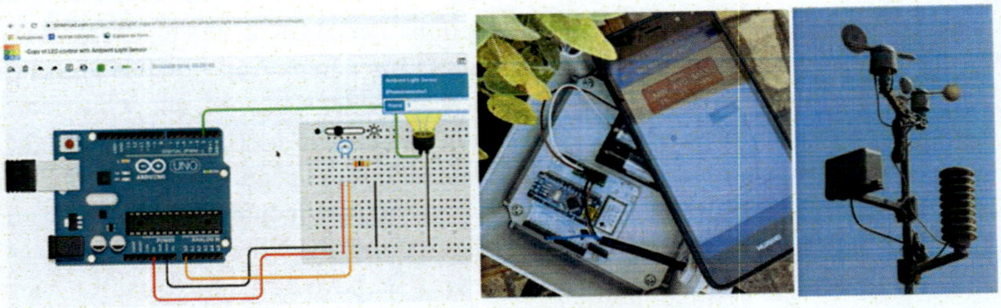

Fig. 4. Implementation of the inteligent weather station

3.2 Learning Activity: "Water is Life"

One of the success cases illustrated in the repository (Fig. 5) is represented by a learning activity entitled "Water is life" which was based on exploring information regarding water connected with climate change. Using garden-based activities in schools the children raise awareness regarding efficient water consumption and gain experience concerning the importance of water for plants, people and environment. Children are therefore encouraged to learn, think about and find creative solutions for effective water management.

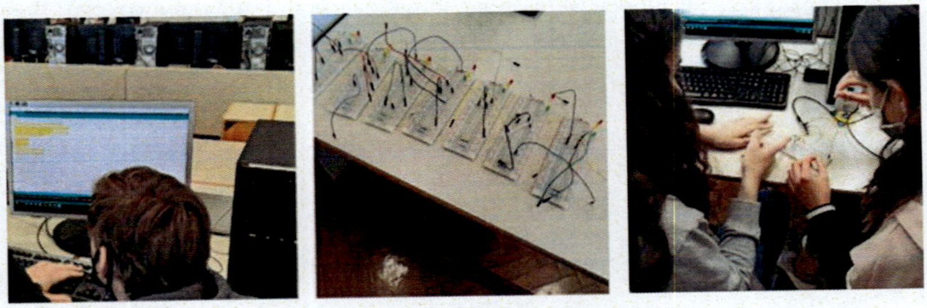

Fig. 5. Implementation of "Water is life" learning activity

The activity was implemented as a project for children that could explore specific water properties, solutions for efficient water consumption, natural soil filters of water, but also on creating sketch notes, posters & collaborative digital content, gaining informatics knowledge and skills, learning basic coding, using 3D printing and working in groups.

The methodology used for all the learning activities is based on blended learning approach including individual and collaborative learning in project-based projects.

The main competences to be developed in these learning activities are mutual respect and collaboration, active participation, creativity and critical thinking, efficient use of all natural resources, reduction of waste, recycling, multilingual communication, internet safety, copyright information concerning digital content, programming languages, etc.

The repository was published on Internet with free access and the Fig. 6 presents the analytics for the period: June 2021 till September 2022 showing a real interest from educators and students for school garden based education. Figure 7 presents the Google analytics statistics for the users accessing the eSGarden website after the end of the project.

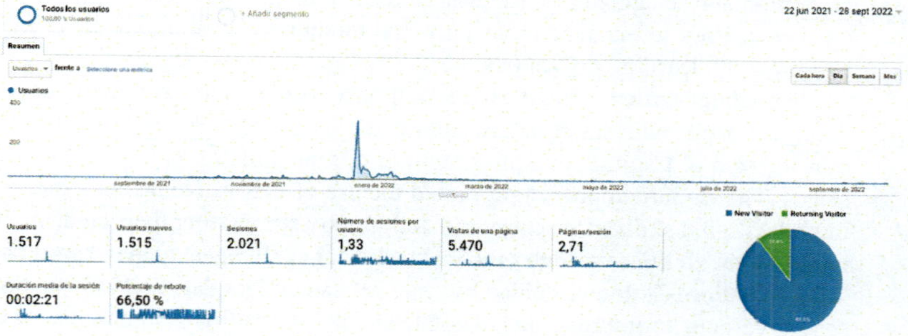

Fig. 6. Google analytics for the eSGarden project website for: September 2021-September 2022

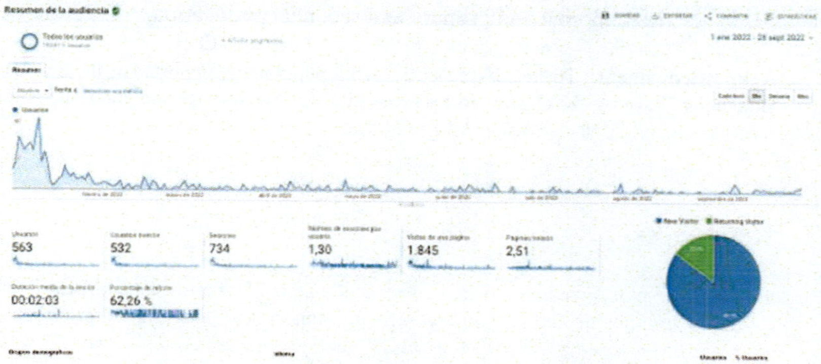

Fig. 7. Google analytics for the eSGarden project website for: February 2022-September 2022

4 Conclusions

School gardens can contribute to first levels of children education, as a foundation for integrating multidisciplinary learning and representing a valuable resource for their future carriers and personal life, while school teachers benefit from a creative environment forteaching activities, offering opportunities for school and community interaction and a powerful resource for the whole school community [6].

The repository developed in the frame of the eSGarden project represents a valuable resource for teachers from schools for setting up school gardens and connect them through innovative technology to a virtual environment transforming basic observation into garden monitoring. The data and information collected allow teachers to develop educational resources based on physical school garden and the virtual platform, with many applications outside the classroom. The information gathered on technology and tools provided in eSGarden repository represent a basic support for increasing the motivation to obtain more digital skills, knowledge and expertise regarding environment protection and sustainability. Relevant tools and technology are integrated in the developed repository to enhance inclusivity and to support widening access to learning for children with learning difficulties.

The school gardens offer the base for different educational activities combining technological needs with traditional teaching and focused on environmental sustainability, transmission of tradition and promotion of digital skills for children from early school stages. The eSGarden project promoted the use of innovative technologies and tools to improve digital skills of teachers and children by stimulating their creativity and working in group abilities through practical technical challenges, games-based projects, and self-evaluation. Children, guided by teachers can collect data and information from the school gardens to improve their knowledge about healthy food and use of technology to ensure sustainability that will make them become more responsible in the future. Therefore, one of the most meaningful results of the eSGarden project is the creation of a new open access repository that could inspire schools worldwide to adopt the garden based activities approach in primary and secondary education.

Acknowledgement. The results presented in this paper were supported by the European Commission under Erasmus+ KA2 Supporting Innovation Action, through the grant of eSGarden project, project number: 2018–1-ES01-KA201–050599.

References

1. Cárceles, J.O., Fernández G.E.A., Fernández-Díaz,M., Fernández, J.M.E.: School gardens: initial training of future primary school teachers and analysis of proposals. Educ. Sci. **12**(5). https://doi.org/10.3390/educsci12050303, https://www.mdpi.com/2227-7102/12/5/303/htm, last accessed 2022/10/02
2. eSGarden Project. https://esgarden.webs.upv.es/, last accessed 2022/10/02
3. Guide for Arduino. https://www.arduino.cc/en/Guide/HomePage, last accessed 2022/10/02
4. Microbit. https://microbit.org/, last accessed 2022/10/02
5. Vuorikari, R., Kluzer, S., Punie, Y.: DigComp 2.2: The Digital Competence Framework for Citizens—With new examples of knowledge, skills and attitudes. https://publications.jrc.ec.europa.eu/repository/handle/JRC128415, last accessed 2022/10/02
6. Austin, S.: The school garden in the primary school: meeting the challenges and reaping the benefits. Intern. J. Prim. Element. Early Years Educ. **50**(6) (2022). https://www.tandfonline.com/doi/abs/10.1080/03004279.2021.1905017, last accessed 2022/10/02

Social Media as a Teaching Tool During Pandemic. A Case of Romania

Anca Constantinescu-Dobra(✉), Carmen Homescu, Veronica Maier, Madalina Alexandra Cotiu, and Anca Iulia Nicu

Technical University of Cluj-Napoca, 400114 Cluj-Napoca, Romania
Anca.Constantinescu@enm.utcluj.ro

Abstract. Social media platforms became important communication tools for all universities during the COVID19 pandemic. As the isolation created a gap between different actors (students, future potential students, students' families, and professors), universities began to put a greater emphasis on communication through social media and social media became a bigger part of the overall communication strategy of universities. The present article aims at analyzing two prestigious technical universities in Romania, namely the Technical University of Cluj-Napoca and the Polytechnic University of Timisoara relating their social media posts during the COVID 19 pandemic. The two universities have been chosen because they are similar in size, in terms of the number of students. The methodology is based on a quantitative exploratory study and comprises a total of 28385 posts that have been analyzed based on the attractiveness to the target audience. The target audience of the analyzed universities are students, future students (along with their influencers), and professors, so their navigation habits and social media behavior needs to be investigated in depth. To leave an impact and communicate effectively post must be tailored according to the target audiences' interests. The main categories the investigated universities focus on are events, achievements, brand awareness, and partners. Yet, although they target the same audience, the way they communicate on social media presents huge differences. The results are correlated to findings in prominent literature, and they show us that the students are most active during the exam period, holidays, and Mondays.

Keywords: Social media · Technical universities · Pandemic · Communication

1 Introduction

The COVID-19 pandemic has changed the way individuals connect and communicate. Amid the emergency circumstance caused by the COVID-19 pandemic and isolation caused gap between different actors (a) students, (b) future potential students, (c) students' families, (d) professors, most communication forms between universities and their individuals also between universities and their outside audience, took place solely via de online platforms so that social media became a big part of the overall communication strategy of universities.

S. Vlad and N. M. Roman (Eds.): MEDITECH 2022, IFMBE Proceedings 102, pp. 163–171, 2024.
https://doi.org/10.1007/978-3-031-51120-2_18

Research shows that the Internet is an essential source of information for consumers worldwide (Bayraktaroglu & Aykol, 2008), hence the importance of social media in online communication is increasing. More and more people are joining social media sites and using them regularly.

According to Datareportal [8] the global population is at around 8 billion people, out of which around 5 billion stays connected to the Internet and social media through their mobile devices [11], as around 69% of them are unique mobile phone users.

2 Literature Review. Universities and Social Media

In today's world, where the Internet and the social media networks have managed to remove communication barriers [5], social media has gotten to be a basic communication tool utilized by governments, organizations and universities in their attempt to spread vital information [13]. Social media generates value based on the content created by users, while giving them the chance to communicate, portray, and self-present themselves to a wide and limited public [7]. Universities are using social media with the aim of sharing data and information about their institution, disseminating special events, communicating as well as connecting with their current and potential students, strengthening student-to-student interaction, engagement and involvement, as well as promoting student learning and academic results [15] (Davis et al., n.d.). Thus, it is mandatory for them to pay attention to the way they send these messages so that they match the commitment made by them to their audience [6, 12], as users have the capacity to select the information based on their personal interest [3]. Even though information is harder to control via social media, research show that it is mandatory for universities to be part of social media, as here is the place where their target audience resides [2].

The target market of universities is formed of youngsters pertaining to Gen Z namely people born in the year 1991 and after, that have experienced an unusual amount of technology in their education [4] so that social media became a significant part of their socializing behavior [14]. Being exposed to the internet from an early age Gen Z exhibits tough purchasing power, suggesting that universities need to manage their brands with a strong understanding of students' needs, desires and perceptions [2], as studies show that students' perception of a university brand is comparative to the brand of competitors [10].

3 Objective and Methodology

The present article aims at analyzing the communication strategy via social media postings of two prestigious technical universities in Romania, during the COVID-19 Pandemic, namely the Technical University of Cluj-Napoca (TUCN) and the Polytechnic University of Timisoara (PUT).

We chose this universities as being the most important technical—educational poles in their regions (North-Western part and South-Western part of Romania) and also of similar sizes.

A quantitative exploratory study was implemented in order to achieve the results.

A total number of 28385 posts have been analyzed based upon the fervency and interactivity with target audience during a three-month period (November, December and January of 2019 and 2020). We have chosen these months because they cover all aspects regarding university activities, including students' load with lectures, projects, exams etc.

The assessment was made taking into consideration three main directions:

- The content—by analyzing the topics
- The frequency of posts—by analyzing the time and weekday of postings
- The target segment interaction

The target audience of the analyzed universities are students, partners, prospective clients (along with their influencers), and professors, so their navigation habits and social media behavior needs to be investigated in depth.

We choose Facebook as the platform for our analysis as, compared to Instagram or other social media platforms, these is the platform were most of the interaction for our analyzed universities happens.

4 Results and Discussion

The findings of the Technical University of Cluj-Napoca (TUCN) and the Polytechnic University of Timisoara (PUT) Facebook content analysis are presented in a comparative manner. In the following subchapter, all the collected data will be presented, afterwards, the findings will be distinctively assessed by each university, and finally the comparison will be made. Moreover, the content of social media posts will be interpreted and suggestions will be made in order to increase the degree of interaction with the audience.

4.1 The Results for Technical University of Cluj-Napoca

For the Technical University of Cluj-Napoca (TUCN) the results look as follows:

- Total no. of likes within the analyzed 3-month period: 3540
- Total no. of comments within the analyzed 3-month period: 169
- Total no. of distributions within the analyzed 3-month period: 281
- Total no. of postings within the analyzed 3-month period: 53
- Most common posting day: Friday

It is worth mentioning that the numbers above are averages for the year 2019 and 2022.

Moreso, for keeping the big picture, we applied the following rules in assessing the interactions:

- Only posts with over 100 likes were considered;
- Only posts with more than 10 comments were considered;
- Only posts with more than 10 shares were taken into account;

According to these criteria, we took the day/date and time and the following conclusions could be drawn:

- Basically, all high rating posts were made by lunch time;
- All high rating posts were made only during working days (Monday- > Friday)
- For Mondays we have two good results from a total of three postings:
  - 122 likes; 1 comment; 13 distributions; time of posting 14:09 o'clock;
  - 116 likes; 40 comments (the highest number of comments on a post in the analyzed 3-month period); 5 distributions; time of posting 10:00 o'clock;
- For Tuesdays we have two good results from a total of two postings:
  - 33 likes; 6 comments; 51 shares (the highest number of shares for a post in analyzed 3-month period); time of posting 12:57 o'clock;
  - 122 likes; 1 comment; 8 distributions; time of posting 14:00 o'clock
- For Wednesday, the best result from a total of four postings looks as follows:
  - 138 likes; 25 comments; 2 distributions; time of posting 08:00 o'clock;
- For Thursday, the best result from a total of two postings is:
  - 128 likes; 4 comments; 7 distributions; time of posting 12:05 o'clock;
- For Friday, the best result from a total of three postings looks as follows:
  - 248 likes; 1 comment; 1 distribution; time 09:10;
- The total number of comments is quite high, but the conversation is not maintained or continued on the social media page;
- The most appreciated posts were the ones with an entertaining/comic/social character;

According to the findings above, the day with the highest interactions is Friday (248) 09:10 o'clock, the day with the most commented posts is Monday (40) 10:00 o'clock, and the day with the most shared posts is Tuesday (51) 12:57 o'clock. Having these overview, we can state that, on average, the successful TUCN posts are made during mornings between 8:00–10:00 o'clock or during lunch time between 12:00–14:00 o'clock.

Taking all these information into account one can suggest that, in order to increase the ratings, TUCN should post information on their Facebook page on Mondays, Wednesdays and Fridays.

4.2 The Results for the Polytechnic University of Timisoara

Based on the findings, it can be seen that Tuesday is the day of the week with the most postings for PUT. Monday and Wednesday have also a high number of postings, Friday is a day with fewer posts, Saturday had only one announcement during the analyzed 3-month period, while Sunday had two postings. It should also be noted that there are days when up to a maximum of three posts per day were made, but also days without any postings.

The most significant days and times according to the numbers of likes/comments/shares are displayed in Table 1.

Table 1. Most significant postings based on Day/ Time/ Ratings/ Comments/ Shares

Day	Time	Ratings	Comments	Shares
Monday	17:00	125	15	47
Thursday	00:27	149	18	26
	19:10	245	–	115
Wednesday	11:48	431	47	4
	14:40	114	45	12

Also, investigating the interactions for PUT announcements, the results are the following:

- Total no. of likes within the analyzed 3-month period: 2687
- Total no. of comments within the analyzed 3-month period: 152
- Total no. of distributions within the analyzed 3-month period: 273
- Total no. of postings within the analyzed 3-month period: 57
- Most common posting day: Thursday

According to these quantitative assessments we can draw the following conclusions:

- High rating posts do not follow a particular period of time;
- All high rating posts were made only during working days (Monday- > Friday)
- For Monday we have one good result out of the total postings, namely:
- 125 likes; 15 comments; 47 distributions; time of posting 17:00 o'clock;
- Although comments are high in number, communication is not continued on the social media page;
- The most appreciated posts were the ones with a formal character, such as rector election posts and the visit of different officials;

Concluding the information presented one can notice that the day with the most liked post and comments is Wednesday (431) 11:48 o'clock and the day with the most shared post is Thursday (115) 19:10 o'clock. Successful posts for PUT are those made at lunch between 12:00–13:00 o'clock or in the afternoon between 17:00–19:00 o'clock. For a growing rating, the posts must be as balanced and structured as possible, more precisely, it is preferable to make the posts during lunchtime or in the evening, but only on certain days.

In terms of frequencies, the number of posts is approximatively the same, so we can mention that each university knows how to highlight their strengths to the maximum.

In this case, of course, balancing posts is recommended. There must always be curiosity towards things/events around us, always in resonance with the field and paying attention to details. So, what harmonizes these pages, is the curiosity and also analyzing the competition, i.e., the other universities, in order to see what improvements, they could bring to their own university.

Table 2 presents the most common posting days, for the assessed 3-month period.

Table 2. Social media postings during a week. Comparison between TUCN and PUT

Days in a week	TUCN	PUT	Difference
Monday	11	12	1
Tuesday	11	10	1
Wednesday	11	11	
Thursday	7	14	7
Friday	12	7	5

The biggest disparity is registered on Thursdays, as PUT tends to post more information on that particular day compared to TUCN. Worth noticing is also the fact that the interactions during that day are weaker.

To sum up, one can observe that students are mostly active during the exam period or at the beginning of the week as they try to reconnect after the weekend. Generally, people navigate on Facebook when they need a break or to relax. Professors, being the largest group that shares information on social media, post most likely during lunch breaks or in the evenings.

Recommended posting time in order to increase impact with educational content would be in the morning between 8:00–9:00 o'clock, or at noon between 12:00–15:00 o'clock.

4.3 Social Media Content in Romanian Technical Universities

In the assessed period, PUT Facebook page had 16 videos and 6398 images posted, 25.775 page likes and 15.014 followers while TUCN had 64 videos and 20,444 images posted, 32,970 page likes and 17,23 followers.

According to the data presented in the Table 3, it can be observed that the most prominent topic for both analyzed universities is related to achievements. Therefore, TUCN has 30 posts and PUT has 18 posts on this subject, informing the target segment about accomplishments and performances at the university. The universities inform the members about new research contracts, new collaboration for education, prizes they won and members that performed better in some technical branches. Also, information related to the universities' performance at national level or worldwide is being posted. The content is crucial for the brand awareness of the university, building of trust and consolidating a positive image.

Next topics according to their importance for universities are information related to education in general but also community events designated to the target segments. These categories comprise different projects of stakeholders that are related to education, such as workshops, conferences, internships for students and professors, volunteering

Table 3. Content topics of the two analyzed universities

Content topic	TUCN	PUT
Informative educational announcement	10	6
Humanitarian announcement	2	2
Cultural /entertainment announcement	12	14
Sports announcement	1	4
Informative social/community announcement	14	10
Promotion (own page, voluntary organizations or other pages)	8	1
Articles based on students' own experience	1	0
Educational informative articles	1	2
Achievements (projects, educational, research projects, collaborative projects)	30	18
Workshop/Presentation/Workshop/Conference/Seminar	8	8
Educational and professional development contest/competition	2	4
Holiday activities announcement	10	4
Page maintenance (change profile/cover images)	2	16

activities etc. We can see a slight difference between TUCN and PUT as TUCN is being more integrated into the local ecosystem. As can be seen there are categories, where there are significant differences between the two universities, namely: events, page maintenance, promotion and achievements. An interesting fact worth mentioning is that rational announcements weight about 85% of the total postings, those with moral values, about 15% and the emotional ones are missing completely for both universities. This could be a mistake in the communication strategy of the universities because during the COVID-19 pandemic the care related to the involvement of the public in the educational act should be taken into consideration.

In the case of TUCN, posts are balanced, diversified and relevant. The most loved and appreciated content were those with an entertaining/comic character, but also the educational ones. The high interest of both students and teachers can be observed, so for a greater interaction, comments should be answered to and emotional stories shared.

PUT tries to increase the number of posts during a day and keep the interaction with the public active, by having also diversified and relevant postings. It was observed that the posts have also cultural and sportive character yet the most appreciated posts were those of organizational, administrative interest.

In conclusion, the PUT does not have an organized schedule for posting, with many postings being in the evening, at night when followers are not checking their social media accounts, compared to TUCN who tries to maintain a constant posting schedule. None of the universities provide social media postings with educational materials regarding cyber security. This is an important aspect that concerns both students and employees of these institutions as the attacks are becoming more and more violent, and those with a technical background must possess knowledge when it comes to this topic.

5 Conclusion

In conclusion, it is worth appreciating the fact that each university, subject to the present study, focuses on certain types of posts, having their own and original style. It should be mentioned that the target audience of both universities are students, pupils, parents, partners and teachers, so knowing their habits is a must in order to share valuable content. For a good impact and effective communication, one must know the audience very well and make the posts accordingly.

After analyzing the findings, some conclusion could be drawn:

- Social media platforms became important communication tools for all universities during the COVID-19 pandemic.
- The results are correlated to the findings in the literature.
- Although both universities target the same audience, the way they communicate on social media presents few differences.
- Students are most active on social media during the exam period and at the beginning of the week.
- Professors are disseminating the posts in a greater extent than students do.
- Professors having a longer working schedule, prefer to post during lunch breaks or during evenings.
- The recommended time for posting educational content in order to increase impact would be in the morning between 8:00–9:00 o'clock, or at noon between 12:00–15:00 o'clock.
- Maintaining and increasing the interaction is recommended.
- Communication with emotional character is missing completely and rational and moral announcements are prevailing.
- In case of TUCN, postings are balanced, diversified and relevant. Most loved posts are related to entertainment and education.
- In case of PUT, the posts have also cultural and sportive character but the most loved ones are those related to the organization and with administrative interest.
- PUT does not have an organized schedule for posting, while TUCN tries to maintain a constant posting schedule.

References

1. Bayraktaroglu, G., Aykol, B.: Comparing the effect of online word-of-mouth communication versus print advertisements on intentions using experimental design. İsletme Fakültesi Dergisi **8**(1), 69–86 (2018)
2. Bélangera, C.H., Balib, S., Longdenc, B.: How Canadian universities use social media to brand themselves. Tert. Educ. Manag. **20**(1), 14–29 (2014)
3. Boyd, M.D., Ellison, B.N.: Social network sites: Definition, history, and scholarship. J. Comput.-Mediat. Commun. **13**(1), 210–230 (2007)
4. Brosdahl, D.J., Carpenter, J.M.: Shopping orientations of US males: a generational cohort comparison. J. Retail. Consum. Serv. **18**, 548–554 (2011)
5. Bularca, M.C., Nechita, F., Sargu, L., Motoi, G., Otovescu, A., Coman, C.: Looking for the sustainability messages of European universities' social media communication during the COVID-19 pandemic. Sustainability **14**(3), 1554 (2022)

6. Carpenter, S., Takahashi, B., Cunningham, C., Lertpratchya, A.P.: Climate and sustainability the roles of social media in promoting sustainability in higher education. Intern. J. Commun. **10**, 4863–4881 (2016)
7. Carr, C.T., Hayes, R.A.: Social media: defining, developing, and divining. Atlantic J. Commun. **23**, 46–65 (2015)
8. Datareportal (2022) Digital 2022. October Global Statshot Report. https://datareportal.com/global-digital-overview, last accessed 2022/10/11
9. Davis, H.F.C., Deli-Amen, R., Rios-Aguilar, C., Gonzalez Canche, S.M.: Social media in higher education: a literature review and research directions. Published by the Center for the Study of Higher Education at the University of Arizona and Claremont Graduate University (n.d.). Retrieved from https://old.coe.arizona.edu/sites/coe/files/HED/Social-Media-in-Higher-Education%20report_0.pdf, last accessed 2022/10/11
10. Ivy, J.: Higher education institution image: a correspondence analysis approach. Intern. J. Educ. Manag. **15**, 276–282 (2001)
11. Kaplan, A.M., Haenlein, M.: Users of the world, unite! the challenges and opportunities of social media. Busin. Horizons **53**, 59–68 (2010)
12. Pringle, J., Fritz, S.: The university brand and social media: using data analytics to assess brand authenticity. J. Mark. High. Educ. **29**, 19–44 (2019)
13. Tsao, S.F., Chen, H., Tisseverasinghe, T., Yang, Y., Li, L., Butt, Z.A.: What social media told us in the time of COVID-19: a scoping review. Lanc. Dig. Health **3**(3), 175–194 (2021)
14. Yadav, G.P., Rai, J.: The generation Z and their social media usage: a review and a research outline. Glob. J. Enterp. Inform. Syst. **9**(2), 110–116 (2017)
15. Zachos, G., Kollia, E.A.P., Anagnostopoulos, I.: Social media use in higher education: a review. Educ. Sci. **8**(4), 1–13 (2018)

Assisted Evaluation Method as Periodic Medical Control for Professional and Regular Drivers

Barbu Braun(✉) and Drugă Corneliu

Transilvania University of Brasov, Brasov, Romania
braun@unitbv.ro

Abstract. The paper describes how a revolutionary method was proposed, developed and tested regarding the assisted testing of the visual function in the case of drivers, within the procedures of periodic medical control. The main purpose of the method is to ensure a much more efficient and objective medical control than current methods. Another advantage would be that the method could help the examiner, being clear and easy to apply. At the same time, the objectivity of the assisted procedure could drastically reduce fraud situations. Until now, researches have focused on the aspect of medical control from the point of view of visual function, but in the future they will also expand to other aspects related to periodic medical control (pulmonary function, auditory function, locomotor function, etc.). Specifically, the method consists of a staged test of the visual function from all points of view (acuity, 3D perception, chromatic perception, visual field, etc.), it being intended for both regular and professional drivers. The basis of the assisted assessment procedure was the design, programming, testing and continuous improvement of a software interface, presented as a virtual instrument within the reach of optometrists and specific medical personnel.

Keywords: Evaluation · Visual function · Interface · Testing · Medical control

1 General Aspects

1.1 Current Methods of Medical Examination of Drivers

Nowadays, generally, periodic medical control among drivers involves going through several check sections, for lung capacity, visual, auditory and locomotor functions. Each one involves interfacing with a team of doctors, specific to each section, meaning the advantage of face-to-face interaction and, usually a quick passage through all procedures. The shortcoming of these, however, may arise from the fact that subjective interpretations may appear. This could result in some people being able to drive even though they, objectively, would not meet the medical conditions, while others, even though they would actually have all the abilities, due to erroneous subjective interpretations would risk being deprived of the right to drive [1, 2].

S. Vlad and N. M. Roman (Eds.): MEDITECH 2022, IFMBE Proceedings 102, pp. 172–180, 2024.
https://doi.org/10.1007/978-3-031-51120-2_19

1.2 The Importance of Visual Function Assessment in Drivers

It is known that among the five senses sight means the most important one, about 80% of the information amount from the surrounding environment arrives visually. Consequently, it is obvious that in the strategy of periodic medical control among drivers, checking the visual function, under all aspects, represents the most important step. For this reason, until now, researches have focused in particular on the aspect of medical evaluation from the point of view of visual function [2, 3].

2 Proposed Solution

2.1 Method Implementation Issue

Unfortunately, there are many situations where, under certain circumstances, some people could obtain the right to drive from a medical point of view despite not having the necessary medical skills. On the other hand, there may situations where, due to requirement excess or erroneous subjective judgments, for small deficiencies in some tests, people who would be fit cannot obtain the right to drive. A more precise, impersonal and objective evaluation from this point of view would therefore be more than welcome [1, 3].

Thus, an evaluation based on clear, strict, some even standardized criteria is considered as a good solution. At the same time, because in present, the general trend is towards the digitization of services and computerized access to databases, the problem arose of finding a solution through which the medical evaluation, in all its aspects, could be computerized and much faster and objective [3]. Thus, until now, research has focused on the development of a method for assisted medical testing from the point of view of visual function [4, 5].

2.2 Evaluation Procedure Description

The software interface development for assisted testing was based on the theoretical foundations of a standard procedure for assessing the visual function among drivers in all its aspects.

Due to the quickly changing traffic conditions both during the day and night, it is clear that the assessment of visual function must include several aspects. In fact, many of these are also taken into account in the classic examination procedures, they being essential in driving.

Knowing that it is desirable that a complete and objective assessment procedure can be applied to both ordinary and professional drivers, the examination strategy should take into account the following aspects: distance and near visual acuity, 3D and color perception, visual field and hand-eye coordination, all being related to driving skills. However, it was considered that in order to take into account both drivers categories, there should be a differentiation in the assessment of visual function. It was considered that the same aspects should be tested for both categories, for professional drivers the criteria for passing the test should being more severe [6, 7].

2.3 Software Interface

In the first research stage, based on the considerations above, an algorithm was designed for the software interface programming and development. The design of it was carried out starting from the aspects related to the usefulness of the method; it is about how the interface should work so that it is friendly to the examiner, and also to ensure an effective and objective assessment. For this, the first issue was that the interface should be flexible, addressed to both regular and professional drivers. Besides, it was aimed that the assisted testing would allow the examiner to choose whether or not to save the data. Another skill was to allow the examiner to go through the test step by step, in its entirety or punctually, with the possibility of saving the results for each stage of the testing, in part.

Specifically, each stage of the test was designed to represent each of the aspects of visual function presented in paragraph 2.2, with the possibility of displaying the partial father-in-law for each stage separately. In Fig. 1 there is presented the way to select the category of drivers for which the test must be carried on. What was considered to be the most important was to display the final score, with the possibility of data saving, besides a final conclusion. Thus, depending on the result obtained, three types of conclusion can be drawn up: (1) the test was successfully passed; (2) the tested subject could receive the right to continue driving conditionally (i.e. wearing glasses, contact lenses, etc.) or (3) the subject is no longer fit to drive [7, 8].

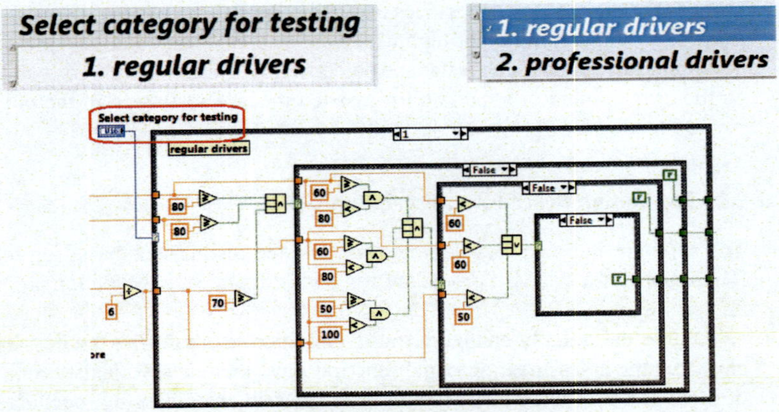

Fig. 1. Aspects of the program routine for establishing the category of tested drivers

Next, the program routine regarding the option to save the final results was carried out. For this, a Boolean input variable was defined as a virtual button, through which the examiner can check or not this option. Related to this, a True-False structure was used, which, in turn, includes another sequential structure, for point-by-point saving of all data specific to each stage of testing. That structure was programmed to work only for the True case (ie, for checking the save data option) (Fig. 2).

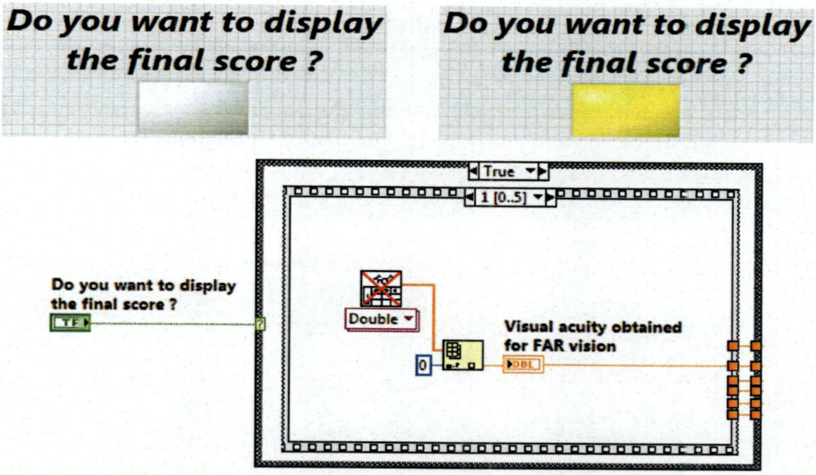

Fig. 2. Program routine for saving the final results option

Below, it is broadly presented how the program sequences specific to each test stage were built, in part.

For the first stage, visual acuity, close vision evaluation, a virtual button was used to start this stage, also a button similar for the option to save data specific.

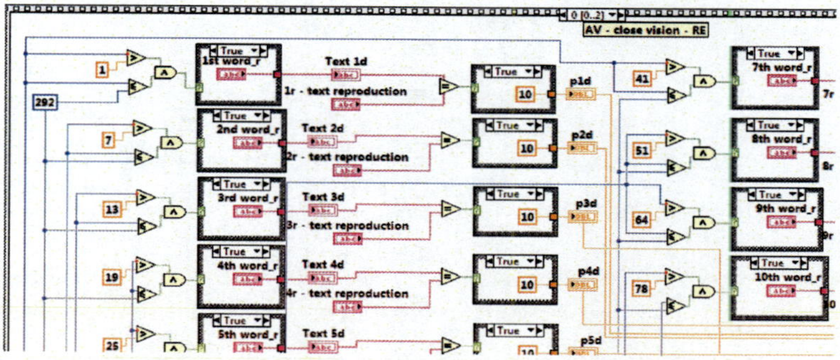

Fig. 3. Example meaning the program sequence for right eye testing

The algorithm for this first stage assumed that testing should be done in three sub-stages: testing on the right eye, then on the left eye, and then in binocular vision. For this, a sequential structure with the three sequences was used, each one including 10 iterations. These refer to 10 text messages that the evaluated person must identify correctly, depending on this receiving a partial score. Figure 3 presents one of the three sequences, namely for the right eye (RE) testing. Similarly was proceeded for the next testing step, meaning the visual acuity in far vision.

For the 3rd stage (3D view), the procedure was the similar when programming the specific subroutines for starting the test and saving the data. Particular to this stage was a program routine that involved the use of a sequential structure with 10 sequences, for each of which using six virtual buttons as input Boolean variables and another six buttons as output Boolean variables (Fig. 4). The first row of buttons refers to the answers the test taker has to give based on what he sees in the 2nd row of buttons. More precisely, it must specify which of the buttons are more prominent.

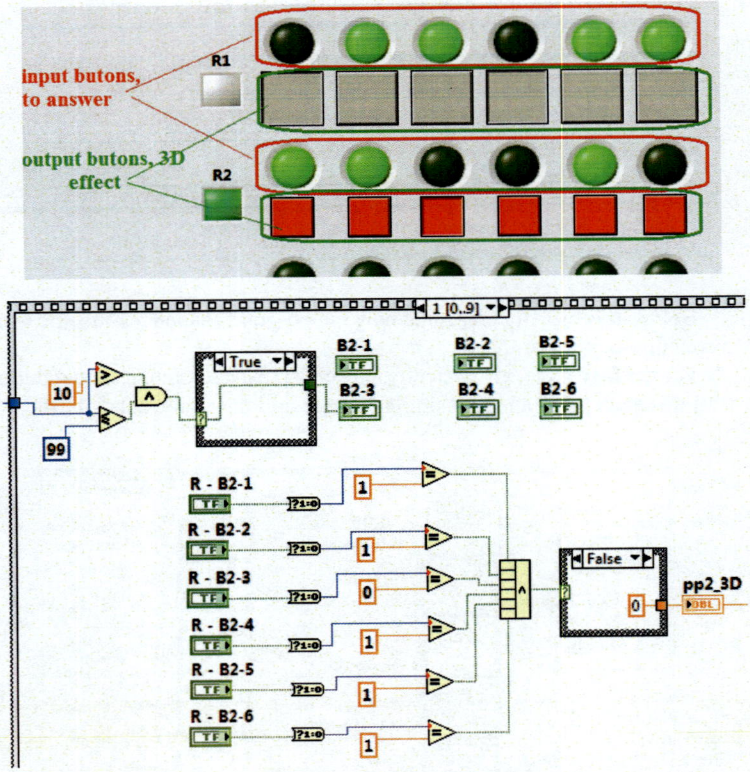

Fig. 4. Aspects of stage scheduling for 3D vision testing

The 4th stage, the programming algorithm involved the use of another sequential structure with three specific sequences (right eye, left eye, and binocular). Each one contains 144 Boolean input variables, in the form of buttons that form a background matrix on which to project a current number to be displayed. it must be recognized by the person tested, and if the number was identified then the partial score is awarded. an example can be seen in Fig. 5.

The 5th stage means the visual field and, for this, a virtual button has the role for a fixation point by the tested subject. In contrast to this, other LED buttons were used,

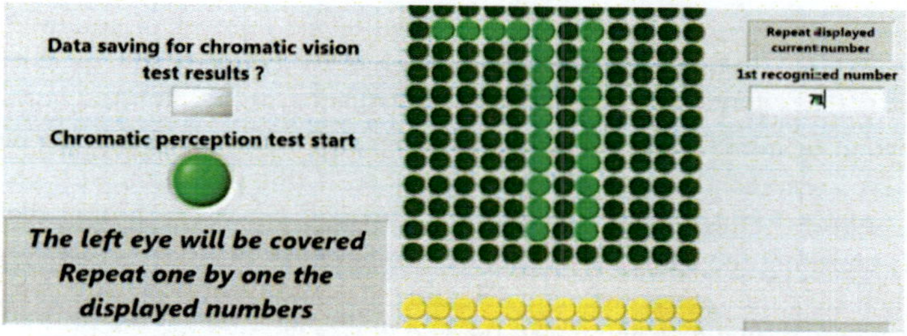

Fig. 5. Example of how color vision testing is done.

as Boolean output variables, lighting up one by one, in a certain order, unknown to the investigated person. Their location on the display was established randomly, around the fixation point, the important being whether or not they can be observed when they light up, fixing on the central button. As programming, an While-Loop structure was used, including three sequential structures, one for testing on the right eye, one for the left eye and one for binocular vision. Each structure was intended to contain 10 successive sequences, as an algorithm for programming the successive events of stimuli turning on, this being related to the current number of origins of the specific iteration of the While—Loop running structure.

The last stage refers to the assessment of hand-eye coordination, for which, in the same idea three subroutines are programmed. For each subroutine, three virtual buttons were used, one as an output variable, the other two as input variables. The output variable button, in the test cycle, has the role of the stimulus, having a ring shape, which, when the subject sees, he must react. The subject's reaction involves pressing one of the other two input variable buttons, more precisely if he presses the button located in the center of the stimulus, then his reaction is correct (he saw the stimulus and correctly pressed the confirmation button). However, there is also the case where the subject can see the stimulus, but does not react properly, that is, he can mistakenly press the other button, the background button. The 3rd situation is where the subject has no reaction, because he didn't even see the stimulus when it came on (Fig. 6).

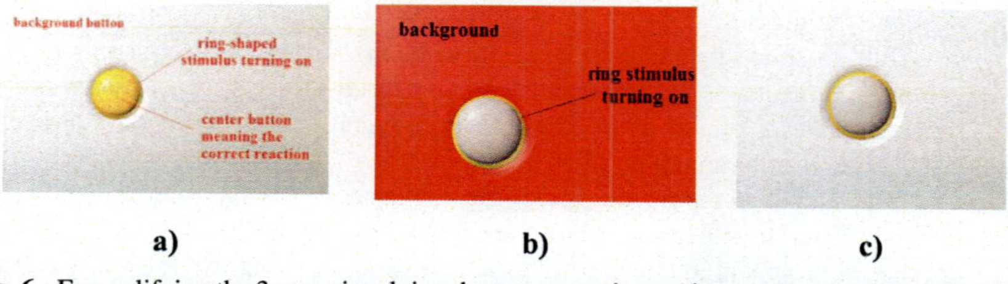

Fig. 6. Exemplifying the 3 cases involving the test person's reaction: **a** correct reaction; **b** wrong reaction; **c** loss of reaction

The algorithm specific to this stage was designed so that, at the end of the cycle, it is possible to count how many correct answers, how many wrong answers or how many missing answers the subject gave, related to the number of stimulus displays. Thus, depending on these results, the partial score for this stage can be calculated. For this, the buttons as Boolean variables were defined within a While-Loop structure, these, generating a vector of Boolean values (logical 0 and 1) regarding the number of correct or incorrect reactions, as well as the number of stimulus turning on.

About the interface using, the examiner would have to go through the following steps: (1) choosing the category of subjects (ordinary or professional drivers); (2) choosing whether or not to save the data; (3) going through the tests step by step, with the option of saving partial data and observing and finally interpreting the results.

3 Results and Discussion

The research stage that followed the software interface development focused to test five subjects, both female and male, three of them being regular drivers and the other two being professional drivers. The people selected for testing were classified into three age categories, the 20 to 30 year old group, the 30 to 40 year old group and the 50 to 60 year old group. The reason for choosing subjects from several age categories was to observe to what extent they can adapt and accept a computer-assisted assessment.

It should be mentioned that three of these subjects, at their last ophthalmological consultation, were considered Emmetropic subjects, and the other two had ametropia of various degrees, they wearing glasses. Upon evaluation of the three emmetropic subjects, they passed the test successfully, two of them being regular drivers and the third being a shooting driver. When testing the other two visually impaired subjects, the results were very different. For the person with low myopia (–1.5 DS), there were no problems, he passed the test, obviously the person in question was wearing distance glasses during the assisted test. The other person with refractive diseases was recorded as having a Myopia of –4.75 DS, associated with an astigmatism of –1.25 DC (Axis at 175°) on the right eye, respectively a myopia of –3.5 DS, associated with an astigmatism of –0.75 DC (axis at 160°) on the left eye. However, it should be noted that the person in question had his last medical check-up more than two years ago, and he had been wearing the corrective glasses for three years. In the case of this person, being classified as a regular driver, obtaining an overall score of 63/100 points, the final verdict was that he will be able to obtain the right to drive again on the condition that he must undergo a new eye test and change the glasses.

Table 1 shows the results when testing the first 2 subjects (both emmetropic). Table 2 shows the results of the testing of the other three subjects, two of them are wearers of glasses, and for one of them an ophthalmological consultation and a new prescription of glasses is recommended [6].

The 1st subject is regular driver, while the second is shooting driver.

Third and fourth tested persons are regular drivers and the last one is shooting driver. It should be specified that the 5th tested subject (shooting driver) wears glasses [6].

From the point of view of conducting the tests, the following can be stated: The examiner was a graduate student of the Optometry specialization from Transilvania University in Brasov.

The tested subjects were generally open to the idea of step-by-step assisted evaluation, a small exception being in the case of the 3rd subject, who is the oldest (57 years

Table 1. Detailed results for the first two tested persons

Testing stages	1st subject	2nd subject
Visual acuity (near vision)	93.33	86.67
Visual acuity (far vision)	90	90
3D vision	100	100
Chromatic perception	90	90
Visual field	63.33	67.33
Hand-eye coordination	88.33	66.67
General score	**87.5**	**83.45**

Table 2. Detailed results for the other three tested persons

Testing stages	3rd subject	4th subject	5th subject
Visual acuity (near vision)	70	70	86.67
Visual acuity (far vision)	76.67	43.33	76.67
3D vision	100	78.67	90
Chromatic perception	86.67	66.67	83.33
Visual field	66.67	55	80
Hand-eye coordination	66.67	65	95
General score	**77.78**	**63.11**	**83.33**

old), however, once it was clarified by the examiner what the evaluation consists of agreed to be investigated. In the same vein, all the subjects did very well in terms of what they have to do during the assessment, the examiner having an important role here too.

Unfortunately the testing of this new evaluation method, until now, could only be done through these five subjects, one of the main causes being the pandemic situation of the last period.

An advantage of the proposed method may also be that it could also be extended to test aircraft pilots. In addition, the evaluation method could be widely accepted and implemented in several approved medical practices, which perform periodic medical checks for the renewal of the driver's license.

As a future direction of research, the expansion of this method is considered for other steps required for a medical visit, such as for example testing hearing or locomotor function.

4 Conclusion

The proposed method proved to be practical and objective, moreover, generally accepted by optometrists as possible examiners. In order for it to be approved and applied on a large scale, it should obtain the agreement of medical associations, in accordance with all laws and regulations in the field of automotive medicine.

Acknowledgment. The research described in the paper was largely due to the contribution of Optometry graduate students, 2021–2022 promotion, within the Diploma Project, the practical activity being carried out in the laboratories of Transilvania University.

References

1. Owsley, C., McGwin, C GJr.: Sight and driving. Vision Research, no. 50 (2010)
2. Vision standards for driving in Europe, A Consensus Paper (2017)
3. Craig, S., Marsden, J.: Driving and vision. Intern. J. Ophthal. Pract. **2**(5), 2016–2222 (2011)
4. Peregrina, C., Perez, M., Colar, C., Tena, M.: Influence on vision on drivers. A pilot study. Intern. J. Environ. Res. Public Health **18** (2021)
5. Salvia, E., Petit, C., Champely, S., Chomette, R., Di Rienzo, F., Collet, C.: Effects of age and task load on drivers' response accuracy and reaction time when responding to traffic lights. Front. Aging Neurosci. **8**, 45 (2016)
6. Bucsa, I.: Design and development of a tool for the assisted verification of visual acuity in the case of professional drivers and aircraft pilots, Diploma Project, Coordinator: Lecturer Dr. Eng. Braun, B. (2021)
7. Baritz, M.: Visual memory, an integrated mechanism in the information transfer from the vision process to constructive perception, using "serious games", 14th e-Learning and Software for Education Conference eLSE 2018, Bucharest, Romania (2018)
8. Baritz, M.: Poor vision and glasses prescription. Transilvania University Publishing House, Laboratory manual (2018)

Advanced Computer Science Approaches in Alternative Education

Mircea-F. Vaida(✉), Petre G. Pop, Ligia D. Chiorean, and Cosmin Striletchi

Faculty of Electronics, Telecommunications and Information Technologies, Technical University of Cluj-Napoca, Cluj-Napoca, Romania
mircea.vaida@com.utcluj.ro

Abstract. Modern society needs specialists able to adapt to the increasing complexity of developed technologies. The training of these specialists from the basic level to the one that allows advanced research in the field of computer science is much easier to be achieved in a simple, gradual way and with common sense associations. The spiritual level of the specialists allows them much more complex approaches using technologies such as artificial intelligence, machine learning, cloud computing and security, big data, etc. The paper analyzes from a technical and a psychological perspective based on oriental spirituality, concepts, and methods regarding the formation of effective collaborative working teams. Teaching of basic programming notions as structured, modular, object-oriented programming and passing to functional programming, aspects-oriented programming, parallel and multicore programming, etc. in an advanced stage are easier to be introduce with intuitive associations to understand the principles and the depth of the activity carried out. The aspect related to globalization is introduced through associations with the notion of the cloud and a mechanism that refers to centralization/decentralization in programming and the introduction of concepts related to swarm communication and programming. Many of the concepts introduced can be closely related to psychological aspects that are easy to understand and used.

Keywords: Computer science · Programming education · Spirituality

1 Introduction

Modern human society is characterized by a competitive process often taken to extremely high limits. The desire to obtain software products in the field of computer science implies, during this period, working in heterogeneous teams that can be created using principles introduced in psychology, such as the MBTI (Myer Briggs Type Indicator) based on Jung's psychology. The first part of the paper will summarize basic elements concerning collaborative teams' creation.

The process of software developing often involves stressful activities performed in the shortest possible time, which leads to pressure on the members of the working team. That's why the process of training IT (Information Technology) specialists that does not only pursue immediate material goals but also an educational one, must be thought from the introduction of basic notions that are easy to understand, to advanced approaches that

S. Vlad and N. M. Roman (Eds.): MEDITECH 2022, IFMBE Proceedings 102, pp. 181–192, 2024.
https://doi.org/10.1007/978-3-031-51120-2_20

will be easy to be achieved. The IT developers who use advanced technologies can thus become humans with a wide, spiritual openness, compared to the routine developers who generally works in a standardized, robotic activity. We will present a survey of some elements in the training of software developers who, understanding the notions learned in the educational process, beyond just their immediate practical utility, will develop research capacities that allow the integration of knowledge gained in the use of advanced technologies such as those related to machine learning, artificial intelligence, cloud computing and security, etc.

Starting from the close connection between psychology and oriental spirituality, especially the Buddhist one, associations will be made in this process of educational presentation of notions in the field of computer science to some oriental spiritual aspects. The typologies from Kalachakra wheel of time and the families based on Dhyani Buddhas realms are very close to computer science and psychology.

2 Creating Collaborative Teams Using Typologies

The previous activity carried out over a relatively large period, realized through articles, educational and research projects [1, 2], and software applications demonstrates a close correlation between the typologies described by the MBTI based on the Jung-Keirsey system and the one based on the Enneagram. Because MBTI is not accepted by all involved peoples in the field, [15], to improve the team creation process, it is possible to integrate other systems such as Belbin, Quest, Mien Shiang, etc., [3]. Next, we will present a synthesis of the MBTI and Enneagram systems based on our previous activity.

2.1 MBTI System

MBTI is a psychological instrument used especially in medium and big companies. MBTI it is based on Jung typologies. MBTI, [4] is a personality test that measures four aspects of people's personalities: Extroverted versus Introverted (E/I), iNtuitive versus Sensing (N/S), Thinking versus Feeling (T/F) and Perceiving versus Judging (P/J). The four pairs of opposites are focused to: Extraversion—Introversion (E vs. I) -focus attention, Sensing—Intuition (S–N) -incorporating information, Feeling—Thinking (F–T)—focus decisions, Judging—Perceiving (J–P) -relation outside world. Combinations of these aspects generate 16 different personality types.

2.2 Enneagram System

The Enneagram System is used in different contexts, business, psychotherapy, spiritual development work, art, education, etc., [3]. It considers nine typologies based on Enneagram figure (Fig. 1a). The Enneagram figure points indicate several ways in which nine principal types of human personality, called Enneatypes, are connected in a psychologically mode. These typologies are expressed by names, or by numbers. In (Fig. 1b) are presented the most used forms of these types. Each Enneatype corresponds to a distinctive and habitual pattern of thinking and emotions. The Enneatype can be determined using

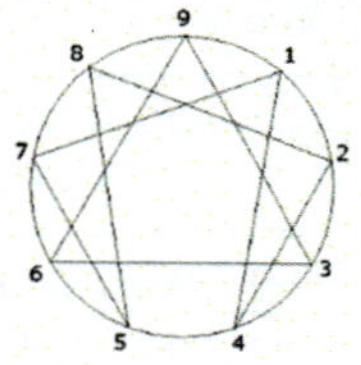

a.

1. Perfectionist, Reformer
2. Helper, Giver
3. Performer, Producer, Achiever
4. Tragic Romantic, Individualist
5. Observer, Investigator, Sage
6. Loyalist, Troubleshooter, Guardian
7. Epicure, Enthusiast, Visionary, Generalist
8. Boss, Challenger, Confronter
9. Mediator, Peacemaker

b.

Fig. 1. Enneagram system.

a RHETI (Riso-Hudson Enneagram Type Indicator) test, [4], which contains 144-paired statements, or other tests with less paired statements.

Considering Enneatypes, we may consider many strategies to define groups of working students (or any other group types as researchers) [3]. It is possible that all the nine Enneatypes to be manifested within a group, and in this case the members' evolution is more rapid. Normally we have in a group a limited number of typologies, less than 9. In this case, the unity, cohesion, and communication are very important. The aim is to create a harmonious group where members with compatible Enneatypes can easily collaborate and obtain valuable results.

Different mappings from MBTI to Enneagram can be considered to refine the typology. There is not a direct correlation accepted, but a possible correspondence is presented in [3].

The results obtained with some of our applications, as GAEM were significant, [2]. The application allows an integration process of Enneagram and MBTI tests. The application offers an automation mechanism to generate optimal groups using results from these tests. The are some situations, when the results are not concluding, and the problem is solved in a manual mode or with refinements based on other models, as Belbin, [3].

3 Computer Science, Education, Spirituality

We may consider that IS (Information Society) can be represented, on more levels [1]:

1. structural level, representing the main material or physical elements of the society (the human body)
2. compound level, representing the complex infrastructure of the society and the links among the elements considering the cognition elements (the human mind—lower consciousness)
3. energy level (usual considering the human spoken), that will connect these two levels
4. consciousness level, that is an evolution of the second level, mind as lower consciousness, and behind a "chaos" we have a universal order with adjustable and vibration sequences.

5. the enlightenment, high consciousness level, perceivable by some humans or, awareness, Selfish—Is-ness, is beyond the time and space, may be named God by a religious approach, and in this case, we don't need to consider security or other restrictions, human being detached from everything.

The initial 3 levels are represented especially by micro-electronics, computer science, communication with all technological research activity that is manifested in this period. The last two levels are specified by spirituality. We may consider the final level, that could be the potentiality in the final evolution.

Last years considered WBE (Web-Based Education) an important direction in the education process. WBE can "satisfy" the technical information process but to understand in a deeper mode the human society evolution we must also introduce the "contented" point of view based on the human personality. The virtual education carried out especially in recent years has often led to stressful situations, a lack of confidence in the students' own strengths a so-called emotional pandemic state. Emotions can be classified as positive, negative, and neutral. Recognizing the state in which the student is at various moments in the education process and finding simple antidotes to counter them offers the possibility of obtaining quick and valuable results. That is why the educational process can be easily adapted by the teacher, that has such abilities, to present the basic notions and then the advanced ones in a simple and intuitive way. Oriental spirituality can offer efficient and easy-to-integrate solutions in this regard, in case of an adequate openness of those who participate in the educational training process.

In universe the gold number (1.618034) can be considered at the base of cyclic phenomena. A proportion will be used, that will represent a harmony manifestation. Fibonacci numbers generation, Zeckendorf theorem, and gold number, gold section, gold angle are examples easy to be introduced in the teaching process in the recursively programming.

The computers evolution involves many simple and efficient ideas that belong to the common life but only some "scientists" are able to "see" and impose these ideas. To "look at" is limited in time and usually is associated with fright. To "see" is outside time and usually no scope is associated, an open state being considered.

We do not know precisely in this moment how works the human perception and how human process information to make so fast and accurate decisions. A lot of sophisticated methods are developed in this domain, but it seems that human perception is simpler and more efficient than many scientists consider and is realized from the cell level to the entire body.

Einstein says: "Make things as simple as possible, but not simpler…", so, we are able to find the simplest human language to describe the things completely and clear for students.

3.1 Human Life and Computers Architecture Evolution

A principal element considering the computers architecture evolution is to associate that the human life system is transposed in the computers architectures.

As an example, the ordinary five human senses often analyzed by psychologists, the multi-sensorial human perception, can be integrated in such an architecture, [1].

Considering a "multi-sensorial perception" based on different signals processing, some philosophical papers show that human perception could be considered as a discrete sequential environment perception with simultaneous, basic five (penta), various levels of processing or more general on 36 levels, [1].

There are some other opinions, but on consider that the visual perception which represents the more important sense for more than 90% of the common humans, do not always represent the preponderant element in this complex process of perception.

Information is considered an important key in our society. Diverse types of information must be used to obtain a consistent decision. The signal processing represents the basic technical research direction for the new information society. Teaching such a direction, students with an opened attitude can make associations with spiritual concepts from ancient civilizations, [1].

3.2 Spiritual Concepts as Possible Technical Solutions

The material life has a profound structure. A connection can be established between the material and spiritual life based on information. The information can be considered a neutral element composed by energy (+, positive, light) and matter (-, negative, dark). The information interaction is realized by signals, signs, symbols, using a minimum energy.

The holistic perspective considers the universe as an undivided or whole element. From antiquity is specified that everything can be structured in a holographic manner.

The acupuncture therapy, the iridology therapy, use the holographic concepts. In this case we may consider that in each part we have the whole. This may represent a global perspective. TCM (Traditional Chinese Medicine), Indian Ayurveda alternative medicine system, etc. are complete medical systems that has been used to diagnose, treat, and prevent illnesses for thousands of years.

The spiritual level of the "scientists" has a significant influence on the obtained results. The quantic theory specifies that it is not possible to foresee an event in an exact manner.

The human ego (selfishness) level respects the uncertainty theory of Heisenberg. Based on this theory it is difficult to obtain important results for a big ego.

In the Big Numbers theory, considering medium values, the apparent micro disorder (specific to the ego) is eliminated at the macro level (specific to the universe).

The synergetic theory may be used to understand the new order obtained. The synergetic field, that is opposite to the entropy, is upper the 3D dimension representation, and can be associated with higher formulae of the visionary scientists.

3.3 Education-Virtual Education

The physical, etheric, astral, causal, and other upper structures difficult to be perceived can offer a complex perception of the ideas.

In education, which is why live conferences, live courses, etc. have a powerful impact we have the possibility to understand in a more profound mode the new ideas using a complex connection between the participants and the high-level energies. In software

OOP (Object Oriented Programming) applications, a connection usually refers to classes and a link refers to instantiated objects.

The astral energy transfer can be realized as a snapshot with a high protection. In this case, we do not consider a local space and time, but a global one.

On the local level, we can associate the horizontal axis corresponding to the appearances and material domain, and "to have" is the specific verb. Aggregation among classes it is specific. On the global level, we can associate the vertical axis corresponding to the spiritual domain, and "to be" is the specific verb. Inheritance in software programming may be associated to this direction. The "to be" state offers a profound peaceful state, an inside serenity. In "to have" we acquire values, and in "to be", we recognize our own values.

Without "to do" no results will be obtained. That involves action, experience in any technical domain. The Professor-Students connection must be considered as a spiritual force that will offer the cohesion, the community, the serenity, the welfare.

The universe structure is not a simple aggregate of objects; it is considered a texture that connects the components from the micro level with the macro level, offering a high-level order.

We have nodes (that give information) and arcs used to link the nodes. In the teaching process is important to specify that the graph theory is a very useful to understand, design and use such an order.

4 The Human Language and Programing Language Concepts

The expression is a creation action thanks to the potential action that became a manifestation. The naming power is an element that offers a subtle domination. We may consider that who offers a name, must resonate with the essence of the name element. In programming languages, the naming process is used from variables, functions, constants names, etc., to the new concepts like contextual naming, or naming and localization. As examples, JNDI (Java Naming and Directory Interface) as Java API (Application Program Interface), Naming Space in C++ and C#, packages in Java language, etc.

Any language is composed by the lexical part (vocabulary—specifying the semantics) and the grammar (the rules—specifying the syntax). A language is a natural or artificial system composed by signs, signals, and symbols. Letters and phonemes offering an image of the micro and macro universe express the language. Each letter, or specific phoneme, corresponds to a vibration frequency and it is possible to associate different parts of the human body to it.

It is known that the alternate therapy based on sounds [16] (vowels, mantras, etc.), images, videos etc. and the power of the name are rediscovered nowadays.

The spoken language is the language considered by a collectivity, there being a strong connection with the thinking. The words, sentences, phrases are used to express what is needed.

The human language is considered a sequential one, and we make an order inside our thinking with the language.

Chomsky specified that the language structure be given by:

- significance, the profound meaning,
- order, the superficial structure.

Inside the universe logos, we have some language forms.

The discursive form of the logos, the current human speech is expressed by creation words being a uni-polar language.

The soul language is not expressed by words, being usually expressed by symbols and archetypes, and it is a multi-polar language.

4.1 Computers Languages Elements and Evolution

The computers languages evolved from the assembling languages based on mnemonics, to some specific structured languages, object-oriented languages, formal languages, dedicated frameworks as languages, etc.

The NLP (Neuro Linguistic Programming) is a psychology theory that tries to discover some efficient thinking and communication techniques if is used in a benefic mode. The aim is to create dedicated patterns that will correspond to the obtained performances in each domain.

The software patterns are reusable solutions used as a new orientation to develop software applications. The design patterns methodology offers an additional benefit for less experienced programmers.

It is possible to use constructive ways of organizing the software with patterns. It is also possible to use other patterns that are not constructive, named anti-patterns. The anti-patterns can cancel out the benefits of patterns.

The intelligence comes from inter and ligo, that means to practically link different things. The intelligence may offer harmony among mind, soul, and body. In this case, the intelligence is positive. The intelligence can be also demoniac. A good example at this moment is to use the intelligence to develop software "viruses" that can destroy a computer, a mobile device, etc. The wisdom will be always a positive concept.

In programming languages, and not only, if the experience is well oriented, one may understand that "Experience gives programmers wisdom". So, it is very important to understand the real and positive experience.

4.2 Basic and Advanced Software Programing Methodologies

The basic software methodologies used to develop dedicated applications are, structured, object oriented, formal methodologies, etc.

To explain to students recursively programming that comes naturally from the mathematics (recursion), Hanoi Tower (Lucas or Brahma) problem is an example able to introduce recursion, programming methods (divide et impera), big numbers and some spirituality, [6, 7].

Hanoi tower is associated with a legend of a Hindu temple, from Varanasi (Benares). This temple has a room with three pillars containing 64 golden disks. The priests from the room are continually moving the disks, one disk at a time based on some rules.

It is considered that when the tower is complete, the world would end, $2^{64} - 1 =$ 18.446.744.073.709.551.615 movements (big numbers), [6]. In this legend Brahma is the creator, Vishnu the preserver and Shiva (Rudra) the destroyer and they are the Hindu trinity.

FP (Functional programming) (Lisp, Haskell, ML, etc.) is programming using functions, [8]. Functional programming is a declarative programming paradigm used to create programs with a sequence of simple functions rather than statements. We don't have loop instructions in FP and repetitions are integrate with recursion. FP is considered nowadays as a mechanism capable of being used for large databases, parallel programming, machine learning, etc. Functional programming leads to stable infrastructures that are reliable, fault-tolerant, and less prone to error.

The OOM (Object-Oriented Methodologies) started with the Simula project by Alan Kay and finalized with Smalltalk; nowadays the C++ 0x/1y/2z, C#, Python, Swift and Java offer the most used OO software methodologies with a lot of refinements. The simple real life can be easily represented as an OOM, and to understand the OOP it is very useful to make some connections with the human life.

The four basic principles of OOP, [9] are considered' Encapsulation, Data Abstraction, Polymorphism, Inheritance. Exception handling is considered as an additional fifth fundamental principle of OOP. Exceptions are supported in all modern object-oriented languages and are an important mechanism of handling errors and other problems in object-oriented programming.

By a simple example that involves OOM it is possible to introduce notions as class, objects, agents, encapsulation, data abstraction, polymorphism (static, dynamic by overloading and overriding), exceptions.

Inheritance when Alan Kay developed the OOP was introduced as a supplementary element that does not clear how to be used. In the software programming evolution, inheritance is a necessity at least as a reusable mechanism. Inheritance is useful and economical. It can reduce code duplication.

To present the interface notion and abstract classes in the inheritance context in a deeper mode we may consider Kalachakra spirituality teachings that presents human evolution on Samsara, and awakening states.

When we declare an interface (specific early Java language), inside the interface we declare a minimal set of operations that will be implemented by classes which respect the interface (implements). The classes will define the methods from the interface(s) in a specific mode (static and default methods now are able to be defined in Java interfaces).

We may explain interface programming notion using the profound Kalachakra wheel of time and the families based on Dhyani Buddhas realms [10, 11], by an association to different manifestations in specific situations. Next are briefly described the 10 realm:

1. Ratnashambhava (Ratna family)—Human realm; Poison: pride, vanity; Wisdom: of perfect equality
2. Akshobya (Vajra family)—The infernal (hell) realm; Poison: angry, aversion, hate; (snake) Wisdom: of perfect mirroring
3. Amitabha (Padma family)—The realm of hungry ghosts (pretas); Poison: desire, attachment, lust; (bird- cock) Wisdom: divine discriminating

4. Amogasiddhi (Karma family)—The realm of Ashura (anti-gods); Poison: fear, jealousy, envy; Wisdom: all accomplishing (perfect realization)
5. Vairochana (Tathagata family)—The realm of Gods (Devas); Poison: ignorance, delusion, greed; (pig) Wisdom: all encompassing (of the absolute space)
6. The realm of Animals is annihilated by reflective glare in 5 colors of owning knowledge divines (the 5 Dhyani Buddhas)

The first six realms are specific to cycles involving birth, life, death, and rebirth of beings. Above these realms are four "holy" realms beyond the cycle of rebirth. The next 3 realms, 7,8, 9 are deceptive realms possibly to go back to low consciousness levels, [12] and the next four realms are:

7. Śrāvaka realm involves a guidance of a teacher. Existence in this realm involves lifelong learning, spiritual growth, and development.
8. Pretyakabuddha realm involves enlightenment without teachers, but by realizing phenomena dependent on other phenomena. Existence in this realm entails discovering truth through observation, experience, and meditation.
9. Bodhisattva realm. Those in this realm are compassionate and altruistic and make great vows to alleviate suffering and liberate all sentient beings.
10. Buddha realm. This is the state of full and complete realization and awakening, not a deceptive realm.

An emotional pandemic state with depression, fear, and panic represents problems that nowadays the people are increasingly affected by. The main mental sufferings or poisons are ignorance, attachment, and aversion. Kalachakra wheel of time offers solutions to solve the problems considering the complementary wisdoms. Considering ignorance, Samsara and Nirvana are used in our society more because are interesting words (for restaurants, music bands, etc.) to attract general people. But Samsara has as significance from oriental spirituality a circle of sufferings, unhappiness, by running in a circle with the same experience. Opposed is Nirvana, difficult to understand, like emptiness. Nirvana can be a state of mind that makes us receptive to the potential of seeing solutions related to the evolution of all beings. Technically [13], it is possible to associate Nirvana to the cloud notion and a globalization process where we have the potentiality to integrate everything.

Considering research and advanced programming methodologies, AOP (Aspect Oriented Programming) appeared, because of some limitations of OOP. AOP offers a programming paradigm that joins many aspects together providing especially modularized code development.

The advanced technologies based on cloud computing impose new strategies in the communication and security process. Students, that represent the new potentiality in the society evolution can better understand the concepts concerning centralized, noncentralized and swarm communication in association with a „dancing" process.

Based on a PhD thesis and research activities presented in [14] and [3] we present an association that involves a philharmonic orchestra in parallel with an open dancing process. Orchestration is like a system where a conductor coordinates the musicians in an orchestra. The coordinator (the intelligent node) is the one who indicates during a concert (achieving a task) the way each musician in the orchestra (each node in a distributed system) must act (accomplish an action). Therefore, we have a centralized system.

Choreography is like a space where dancers (the nodes in a distributed system) accomplish some activities according to a set of rules that they have learned and now they collaborate to perform a dance (accomplish a task). In this situation, the system is not centralized anymore.

Swarm communication aligns with this scenario and adds a new element: the refined nodes (dancers) that are part of the system, act based on rules that they do not initially know, rules brought by smart messages that will come to each node. Metaphorically, we can see the dancers as being „inspired" and acting according to the specifications from the messages.

At the end of the task, they will return to the initial state, or they will be „inspired" again (by a new message). This represents an adaptable new approach.

Swarm communication is inspired by nature and mobile code and involves: Internal Component Modeling, Software Service Composition, Micro-Services, Asynchronous Control, Integration, Business Processes, Smart Contracts, etc. We can say that swarming is somewhere between service orchestration and choreography, with more smart messages and less intelligent service nodes.

Concerning swarm programming, the syntactic description of a swarm closely resembles the description of a class, [14].

We have in the swarm description declarations of variables (attributes) and membership functions (methods), but we have a special concept called phase. A phase is a function, but its execution is done only by calling a special primitive, even called *swarm()*. Typically, an instance of a swarm is not a single object but a swarm of objects. The concept of identity gets a new and interesting technical meaning and even a spiritual dimension.

5 Conclusions

Based on a vast experience in IT domain as research and education, in the paper are presented some software elements as computer science architecture and programming language elements able to be explained in correlation with a spiritual approach.

Students can wake up from a routine activity that usual is used as „robots" in the development process of commercial products and to use creativity and intuition for new technologies development.

Spiritual level of students can be stimulated by understanding that many software concepts are close to real life and profound spirituality. This process starts with first steps of basic programming and continues to PhD students involved in high research activity.

From structured programming with the function concept, to explain recursion and to continue with functional programming based on recursion, students will be able to easy integrate programming methods based on recursion and framework approach.

Associations of access specifiers from a class with real life actions that involves full opening (public involvement), reserved access (protection in a community) or huge restrictions (as private activity) will continue to explain static and dynamic polymorphism, distinct types of inheritance, including sealed classes introduced in some programming languages as C# and Java.

Passing from a centralized approach that was specific to many societies, and programing orchestration, to decentralized process based on choreography and swarm communication and programming. That will offer the possibility to integrate innovative technologies using artificial intelligence, cloud computing, blockchain, smart contracts, etc.

The technical education process emerged with some spiritual elements proofs the possibility to obtain high level specialists to face the new technological challenges in a detached and efficient way.

Acknowledgment. The paper is supported by the project POC/163/1/3/121403, "Innovative technology models for designing and using database applications, which will ensure complete separation of the logical data model from implementation details and running on multiple platforms, including cloud running"., managed with EU funds.

References

1. Vaida, M.F.: Technical education and brainstorming technique, Conference Information: 6th IASTED Conference on Web-Based Education, ACTA Press, Date: MAR 14–16, Chamonix FRANCE, pp: 222–227 (2007)
2. Alboaie, L., Vaida, M.-F., Pojar, D.: Alternative methodologies for automated grouping in education and research. CUBE Information Technology Conference & Exhibition, Pune, pp. 508–513, 3–5 (2012)
3. Vaida, M.-F.: Collaborative education teams' development using alternative methodologies, ICETC, 28–31 October, pp. 1–5. Amsterdam, Netherlands (2019)
4. Myers Briggs, I., Myers Briggs, P.: Gifts differing: understanding personality type, mountain view. Davies-Black Publishing, CA (1995)
5. Rene Guenon, Man and His Becoming According to the Vedanta (1925), Ed. Herald (2022)
6. Mayer, H., Perkins, D.: Towers of Hanoi Revisited. SIGPLAN Notices. **19**(2), 80–84 (1984)
7. Samuel Gan: The tower of Hanoi—a test of design, planning, and purpose. https://creation.com/tower-of-hanoi
8. Miran Lipovaca: Learn You a Haskell for Great Good! edit. William Pollock (2011). https://cupdf.com/document/learn-you-a-haskell-for-great-good.html
9. Munish Chandel: What are four basic principles of Object-Oriented Programming. https://medium.com/@cancerian0684/what-are-four-basic-principles-of-object-oriented-programming-645af8b43727
10. ***, Symbolism of the five Dhyani Buddhas. https://viewonbuddhism.org/5_dhyani_buddhas.html
11. ***, The Wheel of Life Explained. https://traditionalartofnepal.com/the-wheel-of-life-explained/
12. ***, Awaken Realms –https://tzuchi.us/blog/realms-of-existence-as-states-of-mind
13. Yongey Mingyur Rinpoche with Eric Swanson—The Joy of Living: Unlocking the Secrete and Science of Happiness (2007), Ed. Curtea Veche Publishing (2017)
14. Alboaie, L., Alboaie, S., Panu, A.: Swarm communication—a messaging pattern proposal for dynamic scalability in Cloud, 15th IEEE HPCC, pp. 1930–193 (2013)

15. David Pittenger: Cautionary comments regarding the Myers-Briggs Type Indicator. Consult. Psychol. J. Pract. Res. (2005)
16. Good, M.: Effects of relaxation and music on postoperative pain: a review. J. Adv. Nurs. **24**(5), 905–914 (1996)

Biomedical Signal Processing, Medical Devices, Measurements and Instrumentation

Low-Cost Tester for Electrical Safety of the Medical Devices

C. Drugă(✉), Ional Serban, I. C. Roşca, and Barbu Braun

Faculty of Product Design and Environment/Product Design, Mechatronics and Environment Department, Transilvania University, Braşov, Romania
{druga,ionel.serban,ilcrosca,braun}@unitbv.ro

Abstract. The paper aims to make an important contribution to the development of safety in the use of medical devices, wanting an improvement and determination of staff in medical institutions, to understand the role of periodic inspections correctly performed on all medical devices. The use of electronic medical devices in diagnosis and treatment raises several important issues for both the safety of the patient and the medical staff. Therefore, it is necessary for all those who design, build or use electronic medical devices to be aware of the effects of electric currents on the body and to take all measures to exclude any risk in the use of these devices in medical activity. As a general definition of an electrical safety tester, this is a robust, portable, easy-to-use analyzer designed to test electrical safety in medical devices. This paper has presented the stages of the process of making such a tester. This electrical safety tester presents the most important parameters of a medical device, such as voltage measured in V, current measured in mA, and as well as current and ground current measurements. The device was built at the Transilvania University of Brasov with the help of CJAM Brasov.

Keywords: Electrical safety · Tester · METRON QA-90

1 Introduction

Electrical safety is an important chapter in occupational health and safety legislation, due to the complexity of electrical equipment. This reduces the degree of danger of the activity in a medical institution and highlights the degree of applicability of security measures.

Electrical safety is seen as a very well and clearly defined concept. This concept is explained as being the minimum risk state of the use of electro-medical equipment by the individual.

This branch has come to be extremely important in the field of medical engineering, motivated by the fact that, medical equipment has advanced as well as technology, currently, engineers are needed in medical institutions, to be able to carry out the technical inspection of all devices, through periodic checks so that the patients are in safety [1].

In the medical field, there are two components closely related to each other that must work simultaneously, these being the security of medical electrical installations and the security of electro-medical devices.

S. Vlad and N. M. Roman (Eds.): MEDITECH 2022, IFMBE Proceedings 102, pp. 195–202, 2024.
https://doi.org/10.1007/978-3-031-51120-2_21

This paper aims to address some aspects with practical applicability in the medical field, study of the electrical effect on the patient, but also the presentation of the technical conditions of electrical safety of the equipment medical.

To fully understand the electrical safety tester, all the components must be studied, both hardware and software. Technical details are the most important information we can gather from a medical device because, only in this way can we exploit all the functions it has to offer and at the same time, we can achieve optimal results.

The use of medical electronic devices, both in the diagnostic and treatment area, brings into view a series of quite important problems, both when it comes to security and the safety of the patient, but also of the medical staff. Considering this to be a well-founded reason, it is necessary that all those who design, build, or are put in a position to use electromedical devices, know the effects of the electrical current so that any risk in their use can be avoided and provide patient and medical staff safety.

It is broadly defined as a concept that considers minimal risk when it comes to using electro-medical equipment near people. This refers to the limitation of electric shocks which occur randomly, of explosions, but also fires or any damage (electrical) caused both to the equipment, but especially the patient, staff, or buildings.

Considering the above aspects, one can easily justify the importance of this paper for the intra-hospital environment, highlighting the problem that exists at this moment, the desire for improvement, but also for determining a way to make the population aware of the necessary role of correct and periodic checks of all medical devices [2].

Following a critical study on the electrical safety devices existing on the market, there has been established a series of conclusions: such a tester is indispensable for any medical device that uses electric current to function and presents a series of essential characteristics necessary for strict and correct function without any medical errors following the electrical safety testing. The main characteristics found in the test devices, on which the study was carried out, are the following: portable devices should be easily transported; most contain EKG simulators.

2 Initial Tests on Authorized Testers, Practical Realization of the Device/Tester

The practical realization part started by carrying out electrical safety tests of different medical devices in two stages.

In the first stage, such tests were carried out with the help of the testers (ANADEP-03, Vici VC60B+), as shown in Fig. 1, located in the laboratory of Medical Engineering of "Transilvania University of Brașov".

Started by using the "external defibrillator and pacemaker analyzer" tester. It displays various parameters such as defibrillation pulse, energy, voltage, current, and duration of the defibrillation pulse. Defibrillator charging time and cardioversion time in synchronous defibrillation are also measured. The tester simulates the patient with a resistance of 50 Ohms.

According to the results, the energy of the defibrillator was 45.9 J, the maximum voltage was 408 V, the intensity maximum of 41.3 V, and a defibrillation duration of 3.87 ms. At the same time, the graph has a value of 0.625 ms/division.

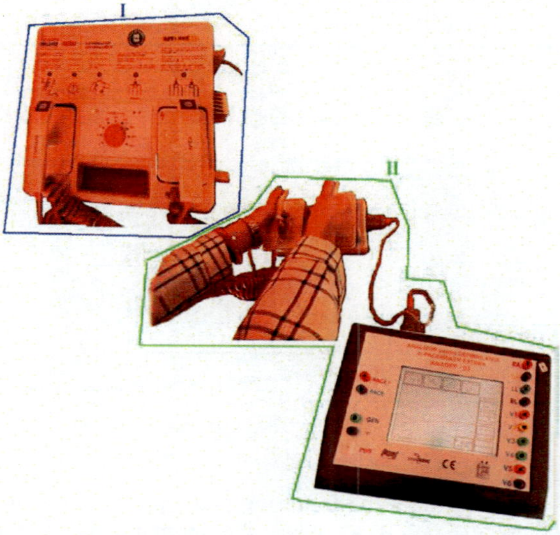

Fig. 1. External defibrillator and pacemaker analyzer (ANADEP-03): I-defibrillator; II-testing with ANADEP-03.

In the second part, the testing of medical devices in the laboratory was done with the help of the tester "METRON QA-90", located at CJAM (County Center for Medical Equipment).

The METRON QA-90 electrical safety tester was used on a syringe pump, as shown in Fig. 2. In the first stage, it measured the leakage current, the result at the time being 21 mA. Also, a series of checks were made that provide for the testing of the insulation of the medical device.

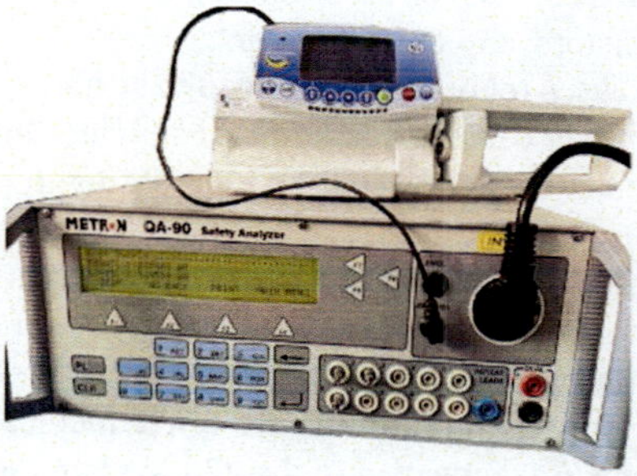

Fig. 2. Electrical safety tester. Medical device insulation testing.

The check of a secretion aspirator was tested, as shown in Fig. 3, at the end of the procedure, receiving a series of values such as received current, 230.1 V, insulation resistance, according to verification, is greater than 250 MΩ.

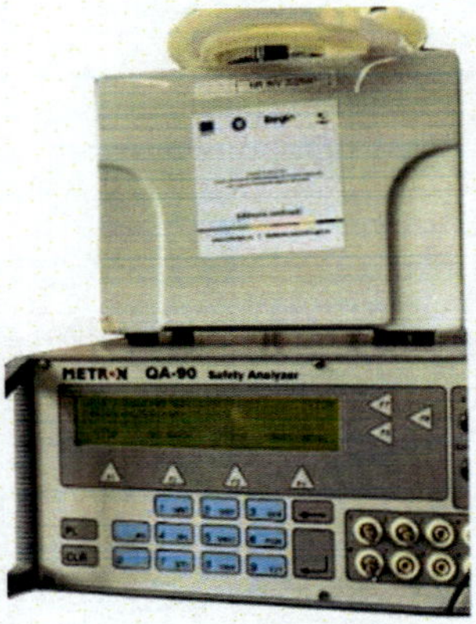

Fig. 3. Testing a secretion aspirator.

The device includes the following parts: power connector; wall outlet; switches; digital multimeter (DIGITAL type); the minimum voltage measured should be 3000 V; minimum resistance of 600 Ω; a diode of at least 1 V; buzzer; background lighting system; amplifier; prototyping board; capacitors; potentiometer; transistor; resistance; voltage riser; coil; batteries and support; relay. A block diagram scheme of components of the electrical safety tester is shown in Fig. 4.

The switches are used to select mode; display lighting/hold image; on/off chassis grounding; on/off current consumption (mA).

The batteries are supplied with a current of 3.3 V, and a current, of 12 V, is used for the measurements. This was done with the help of an operational amplifier. The 12 V is transmitted to the operational amplifier. The preamplifier has a coil through which the ground wire passes from one side to the other, through a single loop, which presents an input-output difference that it amplifies and reads.

This amplifier consists of 3 capacitors, a potentiometer with the role of frequency regulation, transistors, and three resistors.

In what follows, a relay has been added to be able to make the selections: decoupling 220 V from 12 V when the measurements are made, amperemeter-voltmeter-grounding, in order not to enter a short circuit, helping during the operation of the electrical safety tester. In the relay, only 3 positions out of the 5 available were used.

Added a switch for measuring the so-called current to the case (currents to flow from the conductors to the ground). The terminal is connected to the 220 V mains socket, and if there are current leaks, this information can be verified. If there are such leaks, the engineer must normally prohibit the use of the medical device.

The following are connected to the 220 V mains socket:

- a wire that passes through the coil, to the socket, through which the connection to the medical device can be made;
- a wire is connected to the terminal for checking the chassis grounding. With the help of this terminal there can be done additional checks;
- a wire connected to the relay;

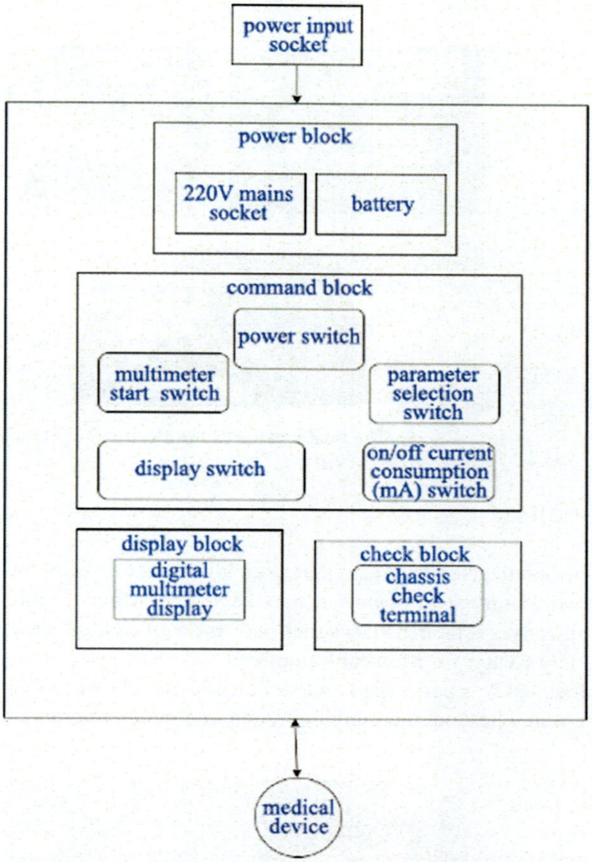

Fig. 4. Block scheme of components of the electrical safety tester

- a wire considered "extra", being spare, connected to the input socket of the device medical.

The relay has the possibility of disconnecting the 220 V current from the 12 V of the system, being connected to the following components:

- grounding button;
- current consumption button;
- operational amplifier;
- input socket of the medical device;
- mains socket and multimeter system.

The final version of the electrical safety tester, as shown in Fig. 5, is composed of the above-mentioned elements.

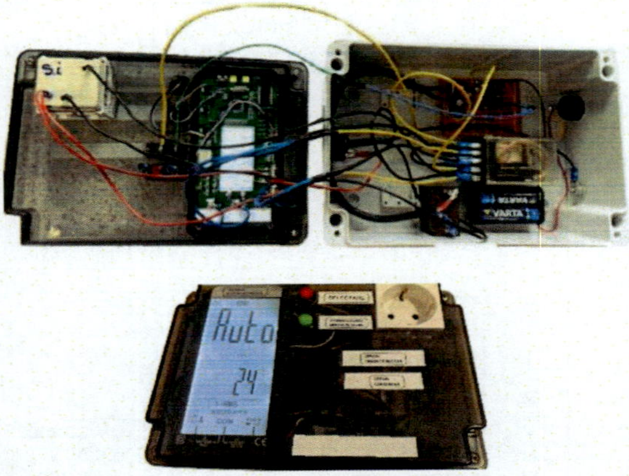

Fig. 5. The final version of the electrical safety tester.

3 Results

After the practical realization of the tester, following the verification tests of the operating parameters, its mode of operation, and the level of achievement of the device according to the objectives established. A series of tests on medical devices were carried out within the County Center for Medical Equipment.

A first test was performed on a defibrillator, as shown in Fig. 6. Parameters such as voltage were checked, measured in V, and its frequency measured in Hz.

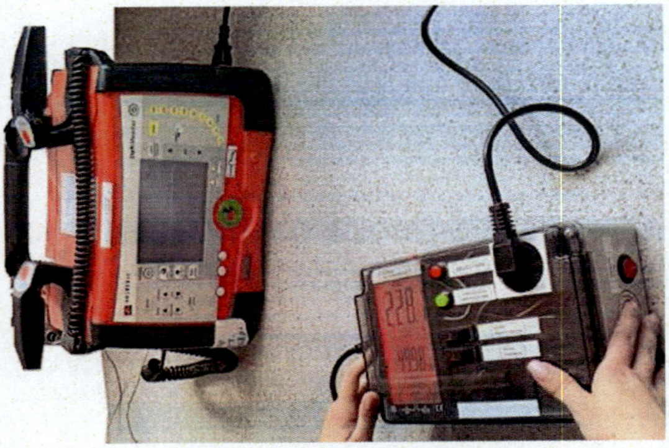

Fig. 6. Measuring the voltage of a defibrillator.

The tester also measures the environmental temperature (22 °C) and the real-time current consumption (by using a switch) measured in mA, values equal to 599 mA were obtained. Next, the tester is prepared for checking the chassis grounding, which showed a value of 59.97 MΩ.

The second part of the functional checks was carried out on a syringe pump, as shown in Figs. 7 and 8. It measured normal values showing the good functioning of the tester. The measured current values were 228 V and a frequency of 49.96 Hz.

Measured chassis grounding showed values of 60.86 MΩ and an ambient temperature of 25 °C, as shown in Fig. 8.

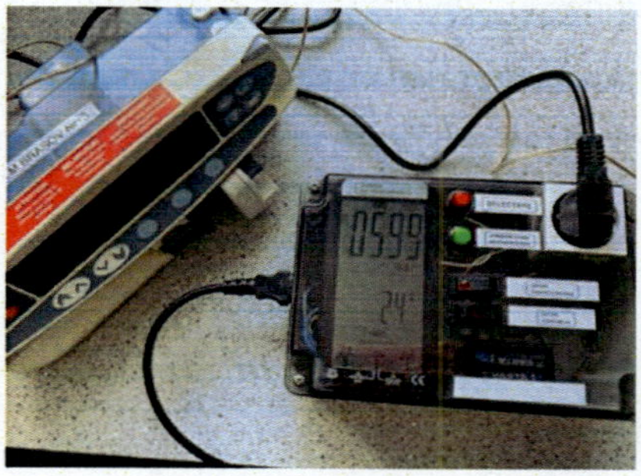

Fig. 7. Current consumption measured in mA.

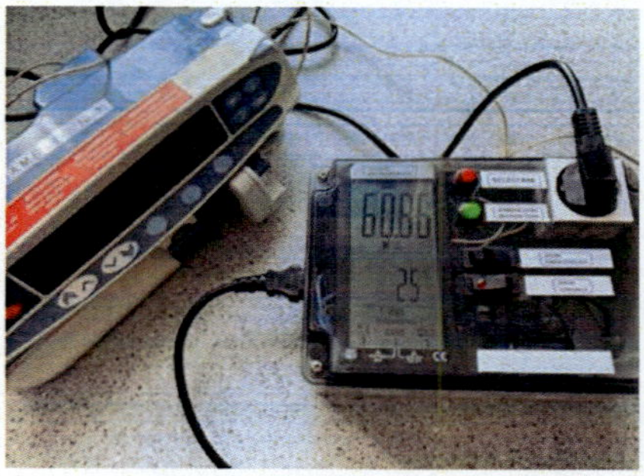

Fig. 8. Chassis grounding values.

4 Conclusions

Due to the advancement of the medical industry, electronic technologies, and the mechanical industry, the design, implementation, and maintenance of biomedical devices is in continuous development. This development led to the appearance of the most modern systems and work tools, which, in addition to other advantages, make the work of users easier. The design and construction of this electrical safety tester were aimed at improving the usability of medical devices. Thus, qualified personnel, to use the electrical safety tester, can have the certainty that following the verification of medical devices with this device, can use safely medical equipment without endangering the patient's life.

The critical study research made for the state-of-the-art testers was helpful to gather information about electrical safety, sketching the objectives, and purchasing the components. The "brain" of the tester was made of the parts of a multimeter.

The final device can be used in any test situation and in any place in a medical unit, but it was built to be used as teaching material in schools, universities, medical offices, etc.

Future directions for improvement are numerous, more parameters could be added (there are actual free slots that might be used to add new parameters).

Acknowledgement. We would like to thank, for their involvement in the development of this paper, to student Vrînceanu Andreea, and the team from the County Center for Medical Equipment of Brasov (CJAM-Bv).

References

1. Dakpogan, A., Smit, E.: Measuring Electricity Security Risk, MPRA Paper. University Library of Munich, Germany (2018)
2. Cuciurean, I.: Securitatea electrică a echipamentelor electromedicale, Disertation paper, Univ. de Medicină și Farmacie "Gr.T.Popa" IASI (2011)

Preliminaries of a Brain-Computer Interface Based on EEG Signal Classification

Evelin-Henrietta Dulf[1], Alexandru George Berciu[2(✉)], Eva-H. Dulf[2], and Teodora Mocan[1]

[1] Iuliu Hatieganu University of Medicine and Pharmacy, Cluj-Napoca, Romania
teodora.mocan@umfcluj.ro
[2] Technical University of Cluj-Napoca, Cluj-Napoca, Romania
{Alexandru.Berciu,Eva.Dulf}@aut.utcluj.ro

Abstract. Brain-computer interfaces (BCIs) are widely used nowadays in different fields. Electroencephalography (EEG)-based BCIs are especially discussed due to their applications in both medical and entertainment usage. This paper discusses some preliminaries of such BCI for wheelchair control, namely the processing and classification of EEG signals for the recognition of different arm movements using machine learning. The focus is on feature extraction, feature selection, and classification technique. The results are analyzed by different performance measures.

Keywords: Brain-computer interface · EEG signal · Artificial intelligence

1 Introduction

Brain–computer interfaces (BCI) are widely studied in recent years [1]. BCI based on electroencephalogram (EEG) signals is of special interest, being recognized as groundbreaking technology in both clinical and entertainment settings [2]. Systems based on BCI allow direct communication between a subject and a surrounding environment without muscle synergy movement. For example, BCIs have been used to diagnose cerebral diseases and to propose patient treatment using a personalised diagnostic process based on each patient's brain activity, leading to improved treatment performance [3, 4]. In addition to the use of BCI in treatment, for cases that cannot be treated due to various factors, BCI technology can replace various patient functions with the help of brain activity interpretation and artificial intelligence algorithms capable of executing the patient's desired actions. This can lead to significant improvement in a large number of people if this type of treatment is widely adopted [5]. Among BCI paradigms based on EEG signals, Motor Imagery (MI) signals take advantage of having direct social and medical impacts [6] by improving conditions of people who have lost motor skills, facilitating their independent communications with their surrounding environment [7]. Brain activity depends on the specific stimulus to which the subject under test is exposed. In particular, Electroencephalography records, non-invasively, the brain's electromagnetic activity, i.e., neurons' activity belonging to a specific area.

S. Vlad and N. M. Roman (Eds.): MEDITECH 2022, IFMBE Proceedings 102, pp. 203–210, 2024.
https://doi.org/10.1007/978-3-031-51120-2_22

The most popular method of processing EEG signals is the use of machine learning (ML) algorithms [2, 4]. A neural network is able to recognize brain energy and frequency patterns from a complex signal such as the EEG signal.

The biggest challenge in the analysis of EEG signals is the recognition, elimination, and reduction of artifacts [4]. These are the noises that contaminate the brain's electrical activity during the EEG recording. The performance of the BCI system based on EEG signals depends to a great extent on the realization of the preprocessing of these signals, i.e. on the efficient attenuation of artifacts.

The purpose of this work is to perform the processing and classification of EEG signals for the recognition of different arm movements using machine learning. The imaginary "arm movement" results are compared with the real movement in order to classify the action. These results will be later used for wheelchair control.

This paper is organized as follows. After this short introductory part, Sect. 2 presents the methods used in this work, while in Sect. 3 are presented and discussed the achieved results. The work ends with concluding remarks.

2 Materials and Methods

In order to process and classify the EEG signals for the recognition of different arm movements, artificial intelligence is implemented in Matlab®. The aim of the current experiment was to classify the processed EEG signals into two categories: left or right arm movement is executed. The movements are firstly executed physically for EEG signal evaluation. As the second step, the EEG signals resulting from imaginary "movements" are classified into the same category. For EEG signal acquisition an OpenBCI bundle is used, Fig. 1. For database construction each subject performed the following experiments: one minute with closed eyes; one minute with open eyes; two-minute run in which the subject opens and closes the left hand; two-minute run in which the subject opens and closes the right hand. The final dataset consisted in 100 recorded EEG signal sets.

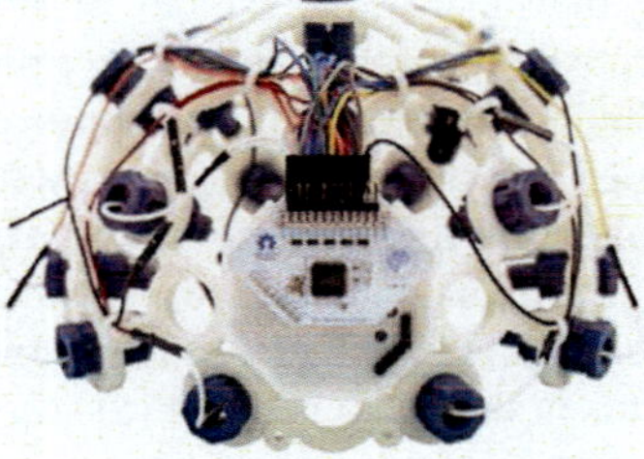

Fig. 1. The EEG signal acquisition equipment

One of the main issues of movement recognition from EEG signals are the artifacts. These are of two categories. Non-physiological artifacts originate from the medical device, the power supply, or the movement of the electrode leads. These artifacts can be removed from the EEG signal by applying suitable filtering. The elimination of frequency interferences from the electromagnetic field generated by the 50 or 60 Hz power lines superimposed on the EEG signal can be achieved with a narrow band filter, but not only the mentioned artifact is suppressed, but the signal generated by the brain activity is also affected. The second category, physiological artifacts have their source in different organs besides the brain: movements of the eyeballs such as blinking, muscle contraction, body movements in relation to the electrodes such as shaking of the head, heartbeat, arterial movements, sweating, teeth grinding, swallowing. The amplitude of the physiological artifacts is greater than that of the signals provided by the brain activity, which makes elimination more difficult [4]. For example, the movement of the eyeballs (also called electroocularographic information - EOG) produces a signal with the highest amplitude relative to signals associated with brain activity, and a visual method or automatic analysis must be used to remove the artifact. Eliminating heartbeat artifacts can be accomplished either by appropriately selecting a reference electrode so that potential differences can be measured only on the scalp, or by an automated analysis. Another example is the signal of an impulse caused by the contraction of a muscle (also called electromyographic information - EMG) that overlaps that of the spectrum of brain activity. In this case, a method to recover the correct signal using appropriate algorithms is needed [4]. In the present experiment, the EEGLAB software is used [8], with the Automated Artifact Rejection plugin. With this software the correction of electroocularographic (EOG) artifacts are realized by the Blind Source Separation (BSS) method. The used algorithm is the Second Order Blind Identification algorithm (SOBI), which uses a non-zero time delay auto correlation. The electromyography (EMG) artifacts are eliminated by Canonical Correlation Analysis (CCA), which attempts to recover the original signal sources by setting a time lag to ensure that each electrodes time source signals are related to each other. Independent Component Analysis (ICA) is also used to remove artifacts by removing the correlation of the data by a mixing matrix – in a similar way as the Principle Component Analysis (PCA) – using all order statistics.

The classification of EEG signals is the step in which useful information from the data set is converted into commands to be applied to a BCI system. EEG signals contain different types of waves with different frequencies and amplitudes and this large volume of information makes it difficult to make a decision in the classification stage. For the selection of useful information, the appropriate choice of a method for extracting the necessary and relevant features for the system and for the classification algorithm is needed. In the present work are used the neural network classifiers from machine learning. A Convolutional Neural Network (CNN) is implemented for binary images corresponding to the raw EEG signal, then a Long Short-Term Memory (LSTM)-type Recurrent Neural Network (RNN) is used for data sequences representing the processed EEG signal. The CNN consists of 2 convolution layers with ReLu activation function, 1 dropout layer, 2 fully connected layers, and a softmax function. The LSTM RNN consists of an input layer, 2 LSTM layers, 1 fully connected layer, and a softmax function.

Summarizing, in the present work the BCI system consists of the following components: data acquisition equipment, preprocessing, feature extraction, and classification of the extracted feature.

The performance analysis is realized based on the accuracy and confusion matrix. Accuracy shows how well the network was able to correctly predict the class the data belongs to and can be easily calculated by dividing the number of correct predictions by the total number of predictions. Its value is in the range [0, 1], where 0 is considered the worst accuracy and 1 is the best accuracy. The confusion matrix consists of a 2 × 2 table containing 4 outputs produced by the binary classifier. A binary classifier predicts all data instances in a test data set as positive or negative, which produces the following results:

- True Positive (TP): Correct positive prediction,
- False positive (FP): incorrect positive prediction,
- True negative (TN): correct negative prediction,
- False negative (FN): incorrect negative prediction.

Various measures such as precision, sensitivity, and specificity are derived from the confusion matrix:

$$Precision = \frac{TP}{TP + FP}$$

$$Sensitivity = \frac{TP}{TP + FN}$$

$$Specificity = \frac{TN}{TN + FP}$$

3 Results and Discussion

The acquired EEG signals and related channels for a subject can be viewed in EEGLAB software as in Fig. 2.

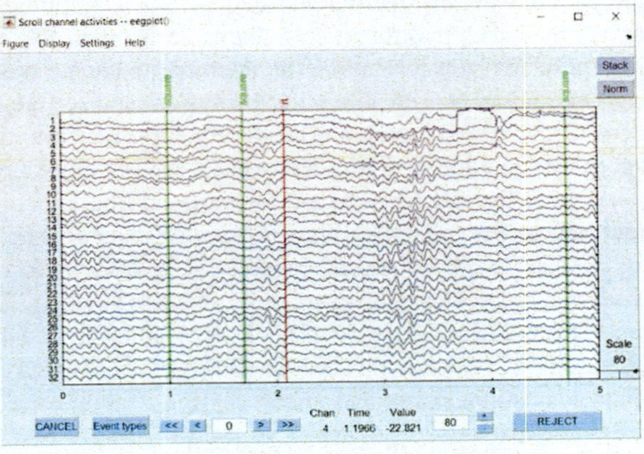

Fig. 2. The EEG signal plot in EEGLAB

An example of non-physiological artifacts removal is presented in Fig. 3. Subplot (a) presents the raw signal, while subplot (b) is the result after filtering. It can be observed a noticeable reduction of artifacts above 20 Hz and below 2.5 Hz.

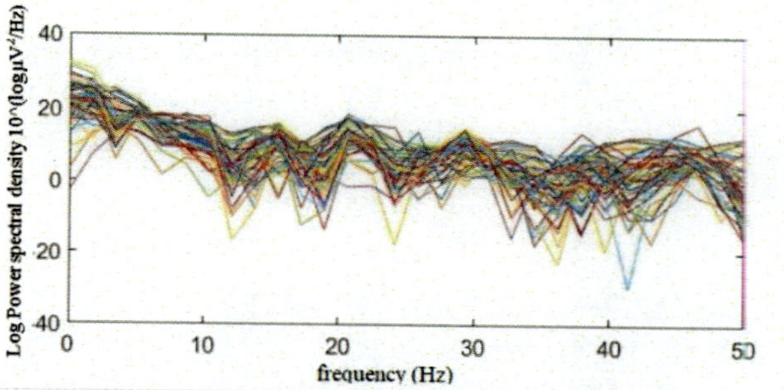

a)

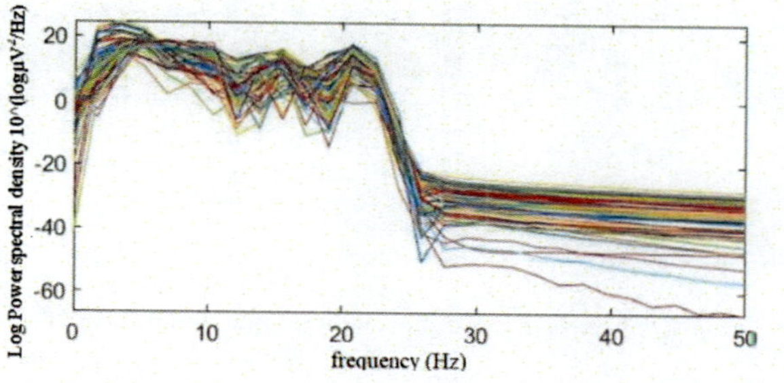

b)

Fig. 3. Signal power spectra before (a) and after (b) artifact removal

An example of EMG and EOG artifact removal is presented in Fig. 4. Subplot (a) presents the raw signal, while subplot (b) is the result after artifacts removal. It can be observed that the amplitudes of the EEG signal have an average of 50 μV with a maximum of 100 μV. The amplitude of an EOG signal is in the range of 50–200 μV and for EMG in the range of 20–200 μV [9]. In the example, the signal was reduced from about 180 to 60 μV.

An example of ICA applied to remove artifact is presented in Fig. 5.

The confusion matrix of the CNN shows 42.4% TP, 7.6% FP, 39.8% TN, and 10.3 FN. These leads to 84.8% precision, 80.45% sensitivity, and 83.96% specificity.The confusion matrix of the LSTM RNN reveals 45.3% TP, 4.9% FP, 41.8% TN, and 8% FN, meaning precision of 90.23%, sensitivity of 84.99%, and specificity of 89.5%.

The results show that the proposed models have the ability to distinguish EEG signals according to motor imaging, although EEG signals are very complex and noisy, and even when the same action for the same subject could manifest very differently in a series re-execution.

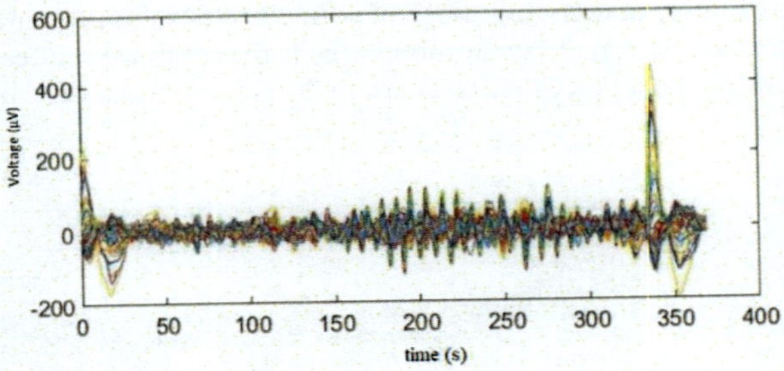

a.

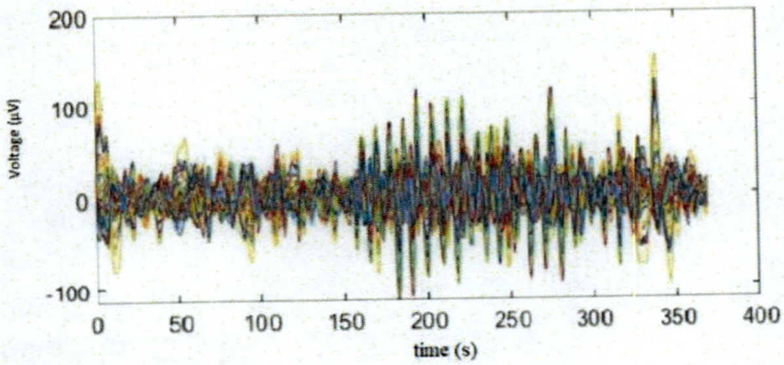

b.

Fig. 4. EEG signals with (a) and without (b) false artifacts

In terms of further development, the authors of this paper aim to physically realise an intelligent device that demonstrates the control abilities of a wheelchair using arm movements. The OpenBCI headset, capable of monitoring brain activity, will be used for this purpose. The information retrieved from it will be transmitted for analysis in the application developed and presented in this paper which will run on an ARM microcontroller. Using the GPIO ports of the microcontroller it will be possible to control the DC motors of the wheelchair, which will lead to the goal of physically controlling a wheelchair using hand movements.

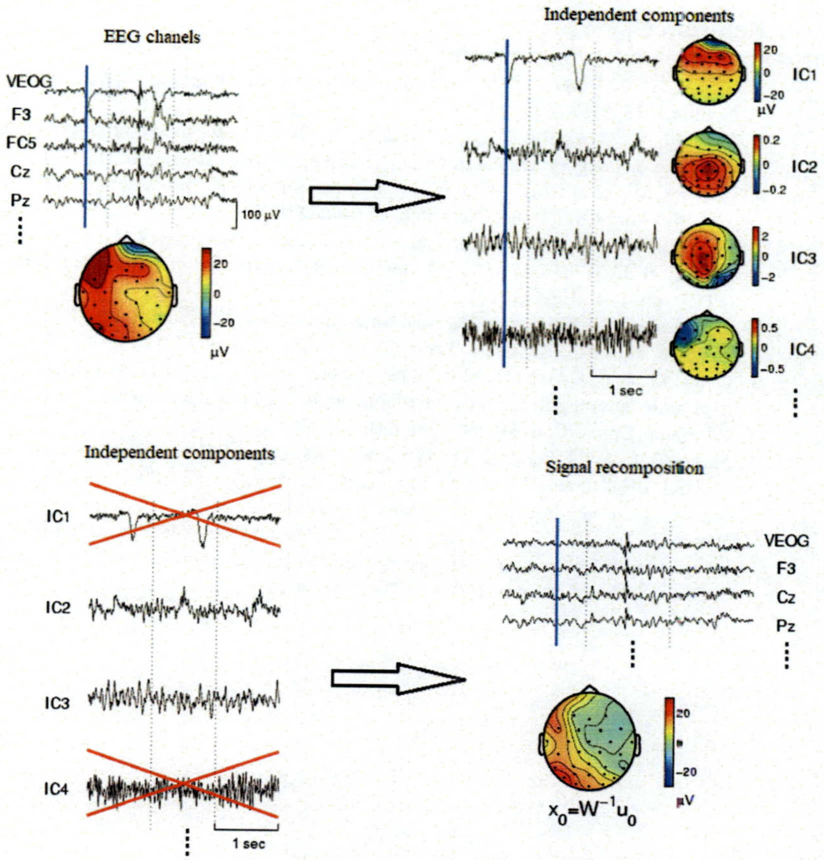

Fig. 5. Example of ICA used to remove artifacts

4 Conclusions

Although the results of 20 years of research into BCI technology have been encouraging, with various applications to improve the living standards of patients with neurological conditions, the results have not materialised in the form of standardised treatments that can be applied globally to all suffering patients. The present work tries to get closer to such a system by discussing the EEG signal processing and feature extraction for an arm movement. This research is only the first step in the final goal of a wheelchair control by EEG signal processing. The obtained great results confirm the possibility to design such a BCI system.

References

1. Saha, S., et al.: Progress in brain computer interface: challenges and opportunities. Front. Syst. Neurosci. **15**, 578875 (2021)
2. Padfield, N., Zabalza, J., Zhao, H., Masero, V., Ren, J.: EEG-based brain-computer interfaces using motor-imagery: techniques and challenges. Sensors **19**(6), 1423 (2019)
3. Cervera, M., et al.: Brain-computer interfaces for post-stroke motor rehabilitation: a meta-analysis. Ann. Clin. Transl. Neurol. **5**, 651–663 (2018)
4. Dulf, E.H., Berciu, A.G., Munteanu, R.A., Kovacs, L.: Advantages of prefilters in stroke diagnosis from EEG signals. In: 2021 International conference on e-Health and bioengineering (EHB), pp. 1–4. IEEE (2021)
5. Kobayashi, N., Nakagawa, M.: BCI-based control of electric wheelchair using fractal characteristics of EEG. IEE J. Trans. Electr. Electron. Eng. **13**, 1795–1803 (2018)
6. Onose, G., et al.: On the feasibility of using motor imagery EEG-based brain-computer interface in chronic tetraplegics for assistive robotic arm control: a clinical test and long-term post-trial follow-up. Spinal Cord **50**, 599–608 (2012)
7. Salguero, J., Avilás Sánchez, O., Mauledoux, M.: Design of a personal communication device, based in EEG signals. Int. J. Commun. Antenna Propag. (IRECAP) **7**, 88 (2017)
8. https://sccn.ucsd.edu/eeglab/index.php. Accessed May 2022
9. Wang, G., Teng, C., Li, K., Zhang, Z., Yan, X.: The removal of EOG artifacts from EEG signals using independent component analysis and multivariate empirical mode decomposition. IEEE J. Biomed. Health Inform. **20**(5), 1301–1308 (2015)

Virtual Instrument Used in the Analysis of Music Complex Influence on Emotions

Valentina M. Pomazan(✉)

Ovidius University, Bd. Mamaia 124, Constanta, România
vpomazan@univ-ovidius.ro

Abstract. The experience of listening to music can and has been objectified by research that has validated a certain probability of objectivity of the influence of music, of a musical sample, on human physiology and psyche. This opens the possibility of thinking a multifold understanding of music and its effects, with direct application in the therapeutic approach and in the emerging choices and customs in the new paradigm of reporting to external stimuli. Starting from recent research on the emotional reaction this work is constituted as a pilot study, which set out to identify correlations between two audio characteristics and a certain emotion evoked upon hearing it, as well as on certain medical parameters, representative for certain conditions. A Virtual Instrument to provide the carried energy in three frequency bands and the peak values of the frequency groups were considered and correlated with the emotions indicated by the patient. The results obtained, considered preliminary for this type of approach, show that there are undeniable positive or negative correlations between the energy carried by certain frequency bands, respectively the frequency peaks and the emotions identified, as the average of the values subjectively assigned by the sample of respondents.

Keywords: Virtual instrument · Correlation analysis · Music therapy

1 Introduction

1.1 Music and Emotions

Music is a vital and universal part of social life, regardless of culture. At the center of its cultural significance is the very well-documented ability of music to evoke subjective experiences, rich and full of meaning for the subject. The taxonomy of the experiences evoked by music is, however, insufficiently known, not being understood how these experiences are arranged in a semantic space and to what extent such a possible taxonomy of subjective experiences is maintained transculturally.

Therefore, emotional states, attitude determine the "way of things" at the physiological level. On this chain of coincidences, it seems natural to target those elements that can most easily, non-invasively, most effectively, emotional states, momentary and lasting attitude, to be able to modulate the functioning of the physical body.

Music is recognized as having modulatory valences for mental states, emotions, hence the transition to other somatic responses, likely to fortify, balance, harmonize the

S. Vlad and N. M. Roman (Eds.): MEDITECH 2022, IFMBE Proceedings 102, pp. 211–218, 2024.
https://doi.org/10.1007/978-3-031-51120-2_23

mind-body system and the processes of the physical body, therefore, achieving a state of well-being and health.

The question of which characteristics of a musical object locate a point in emotion space can be resolved with approaches at the intersection of musicology, psychology, and neuroscience. Transition, modulation, nuances, the rate at which their changes occur, the tempo of forms, all can influence the appearance and characteristics of emotional nuances. This study proposes the energy transported by a frequency interval and the frequency peaks as reference characteristics.

In everyday life, emotional responses can be extremely rapid and even precede cognitive analysis, which is understandable since stimuli have a biological and adaptive implication. Peretz [1] showed that 500 ms of music listening are sufficient to differentiate "happy" from "sad" music, and more recent research has lowered this limit to 250 ms. This means that the brain responds to music as quickly as to any biological stimulus (threat to life, presence of food, etc.). This response is enriched as the duration of the hearing increases and the characterization of emotions is more thorough.

1.2 Emotions and Health Conditions

There is an impressive body of research that unequivocally proves that music induces a multicomponent response, just as it does with non-aesthetically induced "utilitarian" emotions.

The generation of an emotion in the subcortical region of the brain (such as the amygdala) leads to the activation of the hypothalamus and the autonomic nervous system and the release of excitatory hormones such as noradrenaline and cortizol. Changes in the sympathetic nervous system associated with physiological arousal, such as increased heart rate and reduced skin conductance, are the most common peripheral indicators of emotion. Krumhansl [2] recorded subjective impressions and physiological effects (pulse, blood pressure, transit time and amplitude, respiration, conductance, and skin temperature) while subjects listened to music.

Changes in these measured parameters were associated with the emotional category of the music and were similar, although not identical to those observed for non-musical stimuli. Rickard [3] observed consistent, subjective, and physiological responses to music perceived by participants to have strong emotional impact. It turns out that the emotions evoked by music are "real" and objective, without being correlated with a primary need related to survival or other goals, as also pointed out by Scherer and Coutinho [4], who showed that music induces a certain type of primary aesthetic stimulus, an aesthetic emotion, driven by novelty and complexity rather than survival needs. It is possible for music to hijack the emotional system by sharing key aspects of stimuli correlated with goals or goals.

1.3 Sound Characteristics Influence on Emotion

One of the most systematic approaches to understanding the effect of the components of sound objects and musical characteristics has been made by Hughes and Fino [5], in an attempt to highlight the distinct, quantifiable aspects that make Mozart's music have the reported effects in the relief of epileptic seizures.

They converted the sound objects into waves, then studied the periodicity of the envelopes of the signal spectrum, for which they measured the relative amplitude as a function of time, for which, with a Fourier FFT analysis, they analyzed the periodicity of the signal. They found that the high periodicity, between 10–60 s of musical passages is noticed by the human brain and has beneficial correlating influences of the cerebral hemispheres. These musical structures were found in Mozart, J. S. Bach, especially. Signal analysis of the sound objects revealed the importance of power prevalence's of certain frequencies: G3 (196 Hz), C5 (523 Hz) and B5 (987 Hz). In contrast, Philip Glass's minimalist music and pop references, which do not exhibit this periodicity, did not influence spatial intelligence or the nature of epileptic seizures.

This paper presents the a sound analysis research objectives and setup, with the description of the research instruments and hypotheses, including the virtual instrument and a survey. The collected data were analyzed and correlated, results being presented in terms of graphical distribution of the valences, correlation graphs and correlations factors. Conclusions the conclusions discuss the research and its results in the context of a potential development of tools for the characterization of sound objects.

2 Research Method

2.1 Research Objectives and Setup

In this research, we considered that the energy conveyed by certain areas of the frequency spectrum is relevant, which, once determined, as the integral of the signal function, between the limits defined by the maximum and minimum of the frequencies practiced during the music play, can be correlated with the emotions induced upon hearing that music.

Research objectives are to identify the correlations between the characteristics of sound objects and certain emotion, conveyed by the audition.

Research targeted adult public, heterogenous in terms of age, education, musical education, traditions, and ethnicity. For this pilot study a sample of 35 persons were enrolled, 65% women, and 82% of urban provenience, 68% with high education and 36% possessing a postgraduate degree. 42% had at least 7 years of specific, musical education, in public education system.

The present study used two types of research instruments: a survey, structured in two items and a set of virtual instruments for signal analysis, built in LabView environment.

The first part of the survey collected general data, as age, gender, provenience, general education, musical education. The second item collected the responses regarding the emotions conveyed, their intensity and body dynamics associated with the respective emotions, on a 1 to 6 Lickert scale. Emotions are subjective experiences, short-term physiological responses. Therefore, a good strategy to bring them as close as possible to the area of objectivity is to accurately label them, as soon as the trigger was activated.

The emotions felt were to be chosen from a list of 25, encoded with a valence code: anger, sadness, melancholy, solitude, depressed, anxiety, nervousness, fright, fear, terror, serenity, joy, happiness, delight, amusement, sensuality, extasy, love, adoration, compassion, sacred love, surprise, shock, disgust, sound sorrow, regret

Since the musical characteristics of a music excerpt can vary in infinite combinations, for this study those excerpts were chosen in which there is as little variance of sound objects characteristics as possible, to be able to analyze the synergistic effect of sound objects distinct and detectable sound characteristics. Pieces were chosen from different genres, with binary or quaternary rhythm, with a pulsating rhythmic scheme, in which the main beats are marked in rhythmic schemes in which the beginning and end beats are marked, and the texture is homophonic; timbre, melody, tempo and dynamics are variable.

The means of research included a set of 6 sound objects, sequenced in a music file, excerpts from various musical pieces, from several genres. The median duration was 1.3 min, with fading on the last 10 s and 1 min and 30 s pause between consecutive sound objects. Because of extremely large variation of the musical elements combinations, the following elements were "fixed": binary time signatures, all are at the beginning in their parts, all have pulsatory beats and musical accents, all are sung by several instruments, in, basically, homophonic texture. Timbre, tempo, and dynamics are, among all, variable. An analysis of the sound objects was performed, with respect to the Beat, Higher Frequency Specter Energy (the median energy of higher pitches), Lower Frequency Specter Energy (the median energy of lowest pitches) and the correlation analysis between the occurrence of these characteristics and the emotions induced was performed.

Each participant received the electronic format of the sequenced sound objects and the printed survey, with the task to find a quiet period and space for the audition, listen each of them and immediately, fill in the conveyed emotion, its intensity and body dynamics associated. Body dynamics included any movement of any part of the body, induced/ appeared during the audition (including balance, beats, contractions, shivers, and tears). The responses were collected and built in a data base, along with the results of the sound analysis and musical characteristics. The field of emotion distribution was built for each sound object, using the median of the values collected.

2.2 The Virtual Instrument

For this work, a virtual instrument was designed in the Lab View programming environment, where the sound signal is analyzed, sampled in 3 frequency sectors: high, medium, and low, for which the instrument displays the carried energy. We believe that this indicator is a significant one, which, in an extended version of this study, can be joined to other signal characteristics, for a more thorough approach to the aspects that characterize a complex sound object.

The music samples were edited in the Reaper application, cut to the required length, with the same fading effect at the end.

The Virtual Instrument (Fig. 1) was built using LabView express tools for Signals Analysis for filtering and spectral measurements. The control panel (Fig. 2) was equipped with visuals for the waveform, power spectrum and respectively peaks values for the three frequency bands.

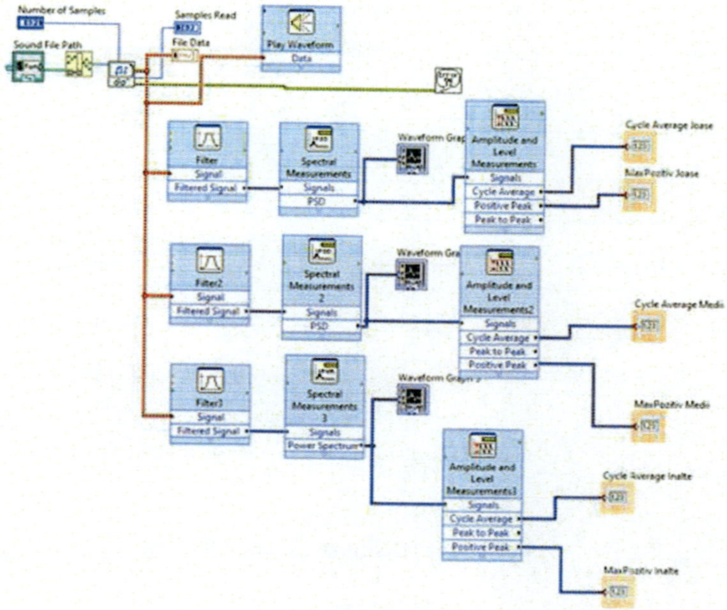

Fig. 1. The Virtual Instrument for three band frequency filter

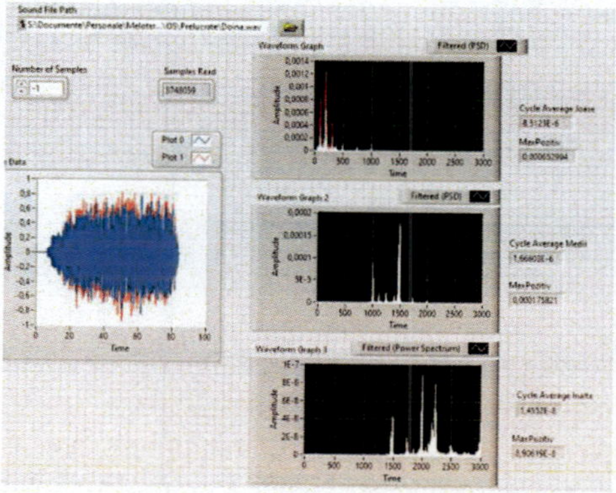

Fig. 2. The control panel and emotion distribution field for a music sample

3 Results

For each of the music piece, the representation of the intensity distribution (blue) of the identified emotions and the body dynamics associated with them (ochre) was made on a circular field (Fig. 3), while the emotions dynamics and intensity distribution is shown in Fig. 4.

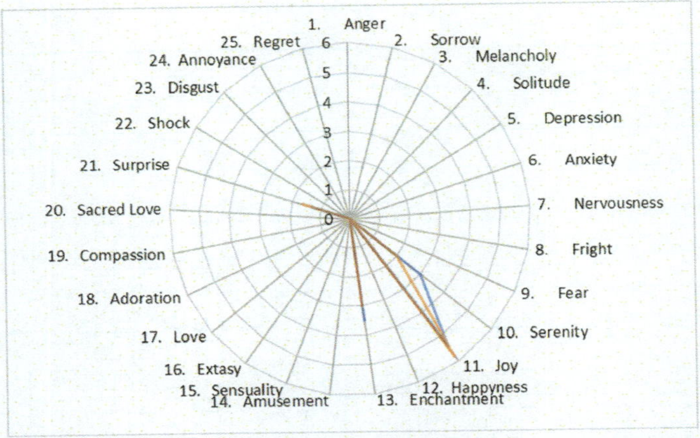

Fig. 3. The emotion distribution field for a music sample (Song from Maramureş)

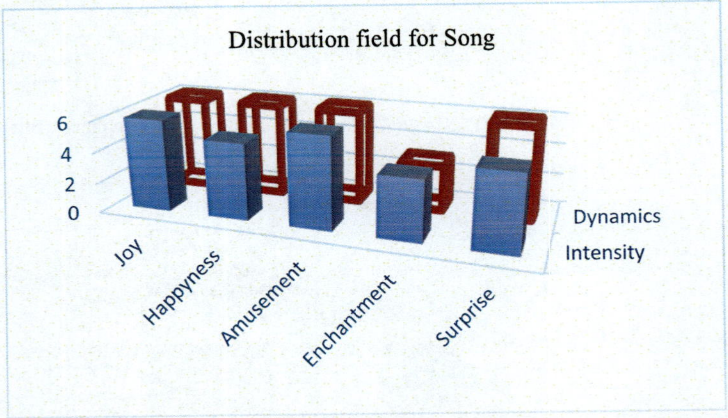

Fig. 4. The emotions dynamics and intesity for a music sample (Song from Maramureş)

Negative correlation is observed in emotions such as melancholy, loneliness, and the number of cycles of high frequencies, respectively with the peak values of high and medium frequencies, but a strong correlation with the number of cycles of medium and low frequencies, respectively the peaks of low frequencies.

Fun, as well as Happiness, appear to be highly correlated with the existence of high, medium frequency peaks and the number of cycles of low frequencies, but are inversely correlated with the persistence of high, medium frequencies and low frequency peaks. Following the analysis, on might be interested that Surprise is relatively correlated with the existence of high frequency peaks, not with the low ones.

Covariance shows a strong direct linear relationship between high frequency peaks and Energization, Happiness ($s = +45.39$) and an inverse linear relationship with Sacred

Love (s = −123.17). Revery and Solitude have noticeably higher frequencies (as noticed in pivot chart, Fig. 5, where revery scores are displayed against the sum of Maximum of High band frequencies). This frequency range is also strongly correlated with Fright, Nervousness, Fear, Sadness.

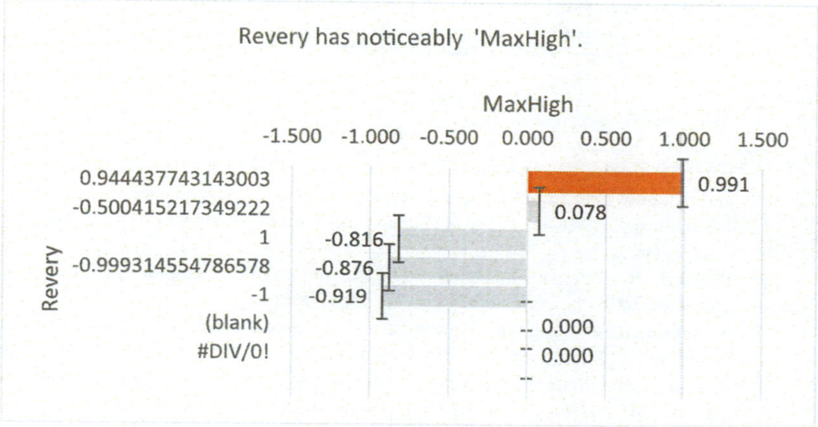

Fig. 5. The correlation of the revery emotion with the maximum of the high frequencies – covariance

Low frequency peaks an inverse linear relationship with Surprise (s = −45293.41), but directly linear with Delight (s = 22646.70), Loneliness (s = 129110 6), Sadness (s = 92986.4) and Energization (s = 83659.6). Nervousness does not appear to be correlated with low frequencies.

4 Conclusions

In the direction analyzed by Cowen, in 2020 [6], computer tools can be used to obtain refined analyzes of abundant data, which allow the integration of learning algorithms for the detection of multidimensional correlations.

A virtual tool was created in LabView to allow the analysis of sound samples and the graphical representation of waveforms, spectra and return values for the number of cycles of amplitude, frequency bands and peaks of frequency values. Correlation analysis was done on the data consisting of signal analysis values and emotion averages, identified on spot, after audition, by a lot of participants, for each music sample.

For some emotions, as Happiness, the relatively positive correlation with all aspects of frequencies suggests that there are elements or combinations of elements of sound characteristics that need to be studied, such as beat, timbre (spectral richness), etc.

The Virtual Instrument allowed some findings confirming results obtained or induced by other studies, such as the fact that Sadness, Melancholy are unlikely to be induced by high frequency peaks. It facilitates an objective analysis regarding how different combinations of musical features influence the nature of induced emotions.

The research perspectives opened by this study can aim at conclusions of sufficient generality and objectivity, which, based on the a priori analysis of a sound object, allow it to be placed in an emotional field, with a very good probability.

Such a study can enable the creation and use of complex virtual instruments that are generous in the variety of returned data. Thus, among the metadata of a piece of music, it will soon be possible to mention the nature of the emotion likely to be induced when listening to it, with the future aim to include its potential health benefits.

References

1. Peretz, I., Gagnon, L., Bouchard, B.: Music and emoţion: perceptual determinants, immediacy, and isolation after brain damage. Cognition **68**(2), 111–141 (1998)
2. Krumhansl, C.: Music: a link between cognition and emotion. Curr. Dir. Psychol. Sci. **11**(2), 45–50 (1997)
3. Rickard, N.: Intense emotional responses to music: a test of the physiological arousal hypothesis. Psychol. Music **32**(4), 371–388 (2004)
4. Scherer, K.R., Coutinho, E.: How music creates emotion: a multifactorial process approach. In: Cochrane, T., Fantini, B., Scherer, E. (eds.) Series in affective science. The emotional power of music: multidisciplinary perspectives on musical arousal, expression, and social control, pp. 121–145. Oxford University Press, Oxford (2013)
5. Hughes, J., Fino, J.: The Mozart effect: distinctive aspects of the music—a clue to brain coding. Clin. Electroencephalogr. **31**(2), 94–103 (2004)
6. Cowen, A.S., Xia, F., Sauter, D., Keltine, D.: What music makes us feel: at least 13 dimensions organize subjective experiences associated with music across different cultures. PNAS **117**(4), 1924–1934 (2020)

Abnormal Cardiac Condition Classification of ECG Using 3DCNN - A Novel Approach

Manu Raju(✉) and Ajin R. Nair

Department of Electronics and Communication Engineering, Bannari Amman Institute of Technology, Sathyamangalam, Tamilnadu 638401, India
{manuraju,ajinrnair}@bitsathy.ac.in

Abstract. The automated ECG data analysis identifies patients with cardiac problems, thereby ensuring accuracy, saving time and medical resources. This article presents a novel approach to the abnormal cardiac condition classification of ECG using 3DCNN. The classification is primarily based on three cardiac conditions: Sinus Rhythm, Abnormal Arrhythmia, and Congestive Heart Failure from the MIT-BIH arrhythmia database. The ECG signals are first converted to scalogram images using wavelet transform, and the scalogram images are then segmented and stacked to form a three-dimensional image. The scalogram conversion leverages the conventional filtering and feature extraction steps. The patch-wise approach focuses on the local patterns and extracts the subtle features relevant to the diseased and non-diseased conditions. The 3DCNN filters pose an advantage on 2DCNN by simultaneously learning representation from a few patches, thereby exploring the temporal properties of ECG. The extracted features from the filters are then classified using various classifiers, among which the Naive Bayes classifier performed the best, yielding the highest accuracy of 90.4%.

Keywords: 3DCNN · Abnormal ECG classification · CNN · CWT · Heart disease classification · Scalogram

1 Introduction

The most common health problem among young and older people is cardiovascular disease. So the early diagnosis and identification of cardiac-related diseases are necessary. The analysis and classification of ECG signals is a good solution for the early diagnosis of cardiovascular diseases. The ECG waveform of every human being is unique, and so it is even used as a biometric to identify individuals. However, the principal application of this electrical signal is to predict cardiac-related problems in individuals. A typically recorded ECG waveform or the NSR (Normal Sinus Rhythm) consisting of the five feature waves P, Q, R, S, and T is shown in Fig. 1, and the NSR characteristics are shown in Table 1. Here the P wave represents atrial contraction, the QRS complex represents the ventricular depolarisation just before ventricular contraction, and the T wave represents ventricular repolarisation. This is the expected ECG characteristic, but the ECG signals can have irregularity called Arrhythmia. Arrhythmia can be a single heartbeat or a series

S. Vlad and N. M. Roman (Eds.): MEDITECH 2022, IFMBE Proceedings 102, pp. 219–230, 2024.
https://doi.org/10.1007/978-3-031-51120-2_24

of irregular heartbeats. So this type of Abnormal Arrhythmia (ARR) classification of ECG is critical for early diagnosis of abnormal cardiac condition. Another significant heart problem is Congestive heart failure (CHF), which occurs when heart muscles cannot pump enough blood to the body. Heart failure can damage the liver or kidneys and pose other complications, including hypertension, heart valve problems, and cardiac arrest. Thus, analysing and predicting heart conditions based on NSR, ARR, and CHF from ECG data are crucial. Analysing an enormous amount of ECG data consumes much time and medical resources. This necessitates a fully automated classification of ECG signals to analyse various cardiac conditions.

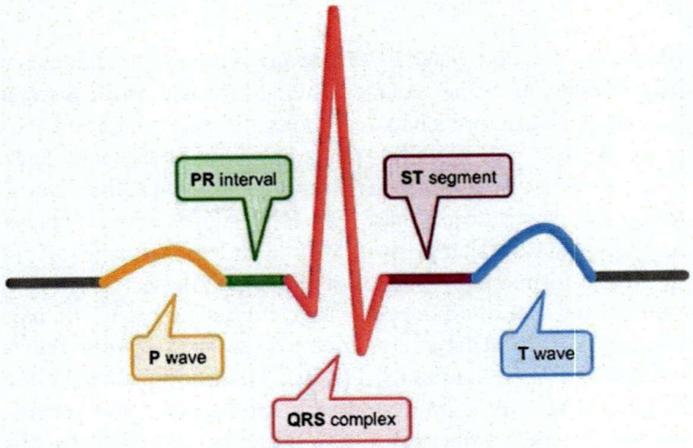

Fig. 1. Typical ECG signal.

Table 1. NSR characteristics

Metric	Value
Speed	60 and 100/min
Rhythm	Equal R-R and P-P distance
P Wave width	0.04 s–0.12 s
Amplitude	0.25 mV
PR distance	<0.20 s

The arrhythmia classification of ECG with a random forest classifier attained an accuracy of 98% [1]. The conventional feature extraction method from the ECG dataset requires pre-processing for noise removal, resulting in data loss and reduced performance. The classification of ECG using transfer learning-based CNN namely AlexNet, and GoogLeNet, showed results of 98.02% as mentioned in [2]. The extracted features of ECG fed to the SVM classifier obtained an accuracy of 85.58% in [3]. A combination of CNN with Extreme Learning Machine for ECG classification showed an accuracy of 97.50% [4]. An eight-layer CNN-based network used in [5] achieved 92.70% classification accuracy. A nine-layer CNN network for ECG classification attained an accuracy of 94.03% [6]. Also, the classification using deep learning and metaheuristics algorithms as given in [7–9] has attracted attention for the automated classification of bio-signals. The ECG classification based on one-dimensional CNN (Convolution Neural Network) is first explored in [10]. The method is used to classify five different arrhythmia signals based on extracted features using two convolution layers and one fully connected layer. Efforts to classify ECG using two-dimensional CNN are initially proposed in [11]. In 2DCNN, the input ECG signals are converted into two-dimensional scalograms or spectrogram images. Then various deep learning algorithms will be applied to these images along with ten-fold validation. This method gives better classification accuracy and avoids the conventional pre-processing of ECG signals. The diagnosis of Alzheimer's disease using MRI data with 3DCNN Features and Multilayer Perceptron was performed in [12, 13]. Here, the patch-based method focuses on local patterns and extracts subtle features relevant to the diseased and non-diseased conditions. The patches are stacked to form a three-dimensional image, and when 3DCNN techniques are applied to these images give good discriminating features relevant to the various cardiac conditions. Also, the temporal property of ECG is preserved, and computational complexity is reduced in the patch-based method. So here we propose a novel 3DCNN network for improved accuracy of heartbeats classification.

2 Methodology

This paper uses MIT-BIH Arrhythmia Database downloaded from Physio.Net. The data consists of 162 samples, of which 96 are ARR data, 30 CHF data, and 36 NSR data. The data set is 48 half-hour segments acquired by two-channel ambulatory ECG recordings from 47 subjects studied by BIH Arrhythmia Laboratory. The samples of segmented ECG signals of ARR, CHF, and NSR are shown in Fig. 2, and the 3DCNN-based process steps are depicted in Fig. 3.

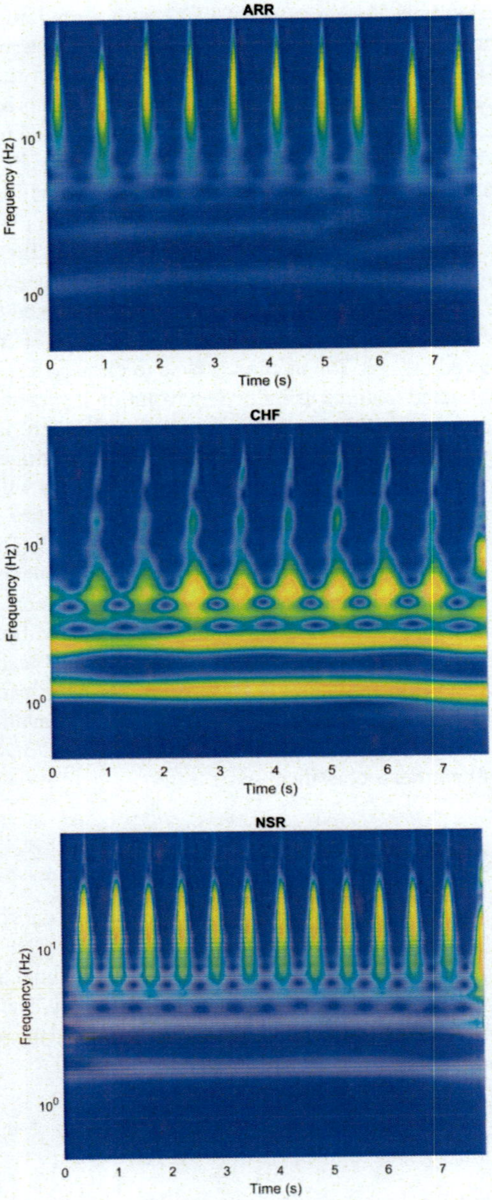

Fig. 2. Segmented ECG signals of different cardiac conditions.

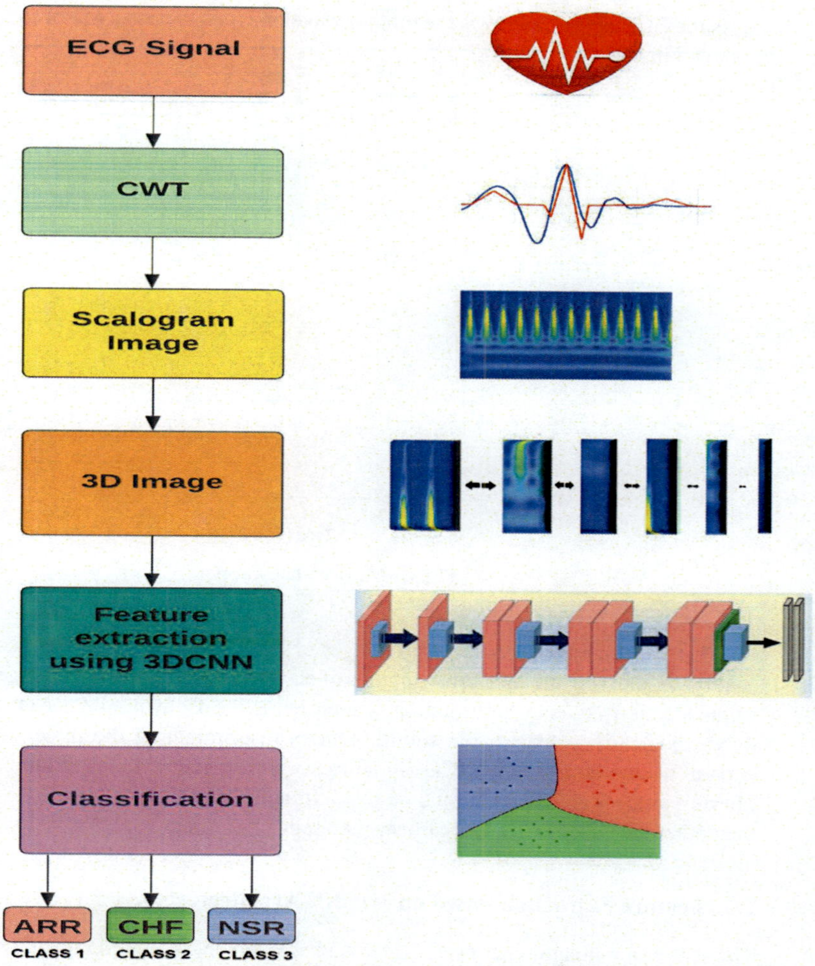

Fig. 3. 3DCNN based classification of ECG

2.1 Scalogram Creation

Scalogram is a time-frequency visual plot created using Continous Wavelet Transform(CWT) for multiscale signal analysis [14]. In this work, scalogram representation is made by correlating an ECG signal and a mother wavelet at different frequencies as given in (4).

$$CWT(x, y) = \frac{1}{\sqrt{x}} \int_{-\infty}^{+\infty} g(t) * \psi\left(\frac{t-y}{x}\right) dt \tag{1}$$

$$x \in R^{+} - 0, y \in R$$

g(t) is the ECG signal, and ψ is the mother wavelet. Here, we use a Mexican hat wavelet as shown in Fig. 4.

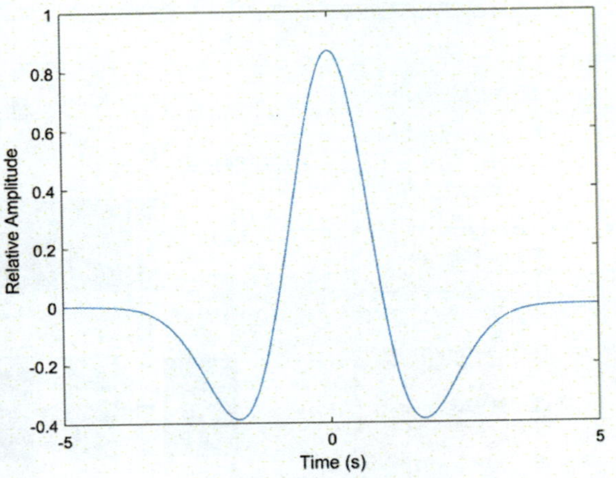

Fig. 4. Mexican hat wavelet.

The two-dimensional scalogram images of ARR, CHF, and NSR signals are generated by segmenting the first 1000 samples of each recorded signal. The images give each signal's time-frequency information, which helps the Convolutional Neural Network (CNN) [12, 15] to extract the subtle features discriminating the three signals. Conversion of one-dimensional ECG signal to scalogram image helps eliminate the noise filtering process and conventional feature extraction and feature selection steps, which may otherwise lead to the loss of beats and reduce accuracy.

2.2 Feature Extraction Based on 3DCNN Architecture

The scalogram images are of size 224 × 224 × 3, which, when fed into a 2DCNN architecture, can learn global features but not the local patterns relevant to disease conditions due to the large image size. To focus more on local patterns patch-based method is utilized to extract subtle features relevant to diseased conditions. We trained a 2DCNN architecture using patches by labelling all the patches with the same label of the whole image. But the performance is less because some patches are redundant for classification, and some are similar to other classes, leading to poor learning of the architecture. So we stacked the patches to form a three-dimensional image of size 32 × 32 × 147 by stacking 49 patches of size 32 × 32. A 3DCNN architecture is applied to the three-dimensional image to extract the features [16]. The features are provided to different classifiers to perform three-way classifications of ARR, CHF, and NSR. The architecture is a three-layered cascaded 3DCNN layer where each 3Dconvolutional layer is followed by a 3D max-pooling layer as shown in Fig. 5 to learn features hierarchically. The 3D

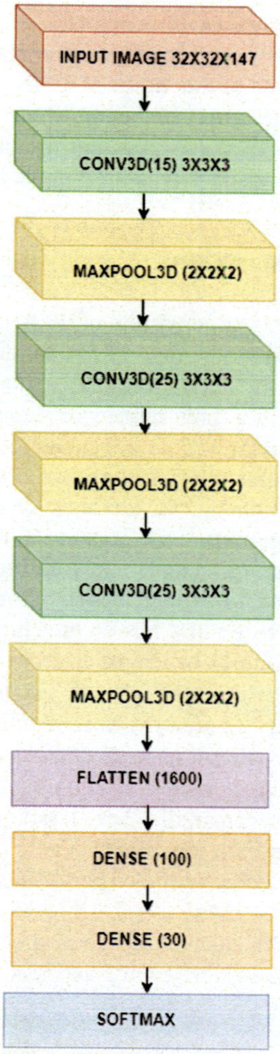

Fig. 5. 3DCNN architecture for feature extraction

convolutional operation is as shown below

$$X_{uv}^{z}(p, q, r) = \sum_{\delta p} \sum_{\delta q} \sum_{\delta r} F_{u}^{z-1}(p + \delta p, q + \delta q, r + \delta r) \times K_{uv}^{z}(\delta p, \delta q, \delta r) \quad (2)$$

p, q and r represents the pixel positions in the three-dimensional image. $K_{uv}^{z}(\delta p, \delta q, \delta r)$ represents the weights of kernel which links uth and vth feature map of $z - 1$ and zth layer, F_{u}^{z-1} is the uth feature map of the $z - 1$ layer, and δp, δq, δr represents the kernel sizes of p, q, r. $X_{uv}^{z}(p, q, r)$ represents convolution layer output. *Tanh* is applied as the activation function.

The architecture is trained with an input image size of $32 \times 32 \times 147$ to extract a feature size of 30 from the fully connected layer. The features are fed into different classifiers to check the performance of this novel 3DCNN-based method for ECG classification. Naive Bayes classifier, Support Vector Machine, Adaboost algorithm, Random forest and Simple Logistic Regression classifiers are used to classify ARR, CHF and NSR. The performance comparison is discussed in the next section.

3 Results and Discussion

A total of 162 ECG datasets consisting of 96 ARR, 30 CHF and 36 NSR are converted to scalogram images. With the help of the augmentation method, the total number of images is increased to 490. Each image is segmented into 49 patches of size 32×32 stacked together to form a three-dimensional data of size $32 \times 32 \times 147$. Patch-wise feature extraction always gives an advantage of focusing more on the local patterns and extract subtle features relevant to diseased and non-diseased conditions. 3DCNN filters learn representation by considering a few patches at a time, enabling them to consider the temporal properties of ECG signals. This makes 3DCCN more advantageous than 2DCNN in extracting features and classification. In this work, a 3DCNN-based architecture is proposed to extract features from the stacked volume of patches for classification. The proposed 3DCNN architecture is trained to 30 epochs with a batch size of 16 to extract features of length 30 from the dense layer. The hyperparameters were chosen based on grid search method. The training error became constant after 30 epochs. Among 30, only 14 features were significant and were taken for classification. Ten-fold cross-validation ensures proper classification without any biased conditions. The performance measures of different classifiers are shown in Table 2. The Naive Bayes classifier performs better than all other classifiers with 90.4 % accuracy. The features extracted are sparse and are low dimensional. The independent nature of the features enables Naive Bayes to come with such performance and sparsity to ease the computation of the classifier.

Performance metrics such as accuracy, precision, recall and F1 score are used to evaluate the performance of different classifiers. The equations are shown below.

$$Accuracy = \frac{TP + TN}{TP + FP + TN + FN} \tag{3}$$

$$Precision/TrueNegativeRate/Specificity = \frac{TP}{TP + FP} \tag{4}$$

$$Recall/TruePositiveRate/Sensitivity = \frac{TP}{TP + FN} \tag{5}$$

$$F1\ measure = \frac{2 \times Precision \times Recall}{Precision + Recall} \tag{6}$$

The recall value for ARR and NSR is 100 % for Naive Bayes, which shows the high sensitivity among all classifiers in predicting ARR patients correctly. In contrast, for SVM, the recall value for CHF and NSR is 100 %, which indicates the power of

Table 2. Performance of classifiers

Classifier	Class labels	Performance metrics			
		Precision	Recall	F1 measure	Accuracy (ternary classification)
SVM	ARR	1.000	0.679	0.809	89.79%
	CHF	0.789	1.000	0.882	
	NSR	0.957	1.000	0.978	
Naive Bayes	ARR	1.000	1.000	1.000	90.4%
	CHF	1.000	0.701	0.824	
	NSR	0.790	1.000	0.883	
Random Forest (RF)	ARR	1.000	0.776	0.874	83.2%
	CHF	1.000	0.701	0.824	
	NSR	0.683	1.000	0.812	
AdaBoost	ARR	1.000	0.500	0.737	77.14%
	CHF	1.000	0.701	0.824	
	NSR	0.612	1.000	0.760	
Logistic Regression	ARR	1.000	0.571	0.727	76.73%
	CHF	0.621	0.701	0.659	
	NSR	0.790	1.000	0.883	

the classifier to classify CHF patients correctly. When F1 measure and accuracy are considered Naive Bayes classifier performs well. So, we can use it with the 3DCNN-based method to develop a computer-aided detection system for ARR, CHF and NSR. The performance comparison is made in Table 3, where our method gives 90.4 % accuracy. The proposed method provides less accuracy than benchmark methods due to the unavailability of diverse datasets for the training of 3DCNN architecture. The maximum F1 measure obtained for ARR substantiates the reduced accuracy.

Table 3. Comparison of proposed model with existing models

References	Performance	Method	Class
Madan [17]	97.3%	2D-CNN-LSTM	ARR, CHF, NSR
Saeed [18]	99.2%	Slantlet transform, SVM	ARR, CHF, NSR
Cinar [19]	96.7%	Alexnet, SVM	ARR, CHF, NSR
Eltrass [20]	98.8%	CQ-NSGT,CWT,Alexnet	ARR, CHF, NSR
Olanrewaju [21]	98.7%	CWT,Alexnet	ARR, CHF, NSR
Kumari [22]	95.9%	DWT, SVM	ARR, CHF, NSR
Hussain [23]	AUC = 0.97%	SNN, KNN, Decision Tree	CHF
Nahak [24]	93.3%	Feature Fusion, SVM	ARR, CHF, NSR
Sandeep [25]	90.6%	CNN	ARR, CHF, NSR
Daqrouq [26]	90.6%	Wavelet Packet Transform, Feature Extraction	CHF, NSR
Isler [27]	96.4%	Multilayer Perceptron	CHF
Son [28]	90.6%	Rough Set, Logistic Regression	CHF
This paper	90.4%	3DCNN, Naive Bayes	ARR, CHF, NSR

4 Conclusion

A novel 3DCNN-based method for the classification of ARR, CHF and NSR is proposed in this work. Scalogram images divided into patches and stacked together to form a three-dimensional image helps to utilise the 3DCNN filters to extract subtle features relevant to cardiac conditions. The proposed method combined with the Naive Bayes classifier gives an accuracy of 90.4 %, which ensures the extraction of local and global features pertinent to the diseases. The Naive Bayes classifier is good for ARR classification, whereas the SVM is suitable for CHF classification. For ternary classification, Naive Bayes performs well compared to all other classifiers. In future, the work can be extended with other 3DCNN models trained with diverse datasets. Also, this method can be applied to different biomedical datasets.

Disclosure Statement

No potential conflict of interest was reported by the author(s).

References

1. Vimal, C., Sathish, B.: Random forest classifier based ECG arrhythmia classification. Int. J. Healthc. Inform. Syst. Inform. (IJHISI) **5**(2), 1–10 (2010)
2. Butt, F.S., et al.: Fall detection from electrocardiogram (ECG) signals and classification by deep transfer learning. Information **12**(2), 63 (2021)
3. Singh, N., Singh, P.: Cardiac arrhythmia classification using machine learning techniques. In: Engineering Vibration, Communication and Information Processing, pp. 469–480, Springer, Singapore (2019)
4. Zhou, S., Tan, B.: Electrocardiogram soft computing using hybrid deep learning CNN-ELM. Appl. Soft Comput. **86**, 105778 (2020)
5. Zubair, M., Kim, J., Yoon, C.: An automated ECG beat classification system using convolutional neural networks. In: 2016 6th International Conference on IT Convergence and Security (ICITCS), pp. 1–5. IEEE, Prague (2016). https://doi.org/10.1109/ICITCS.2016.7740310
6. Acharya, U.R., Oh, S.L., Hagiwara, Y., Tan, J.H., Adam, M., Gertych, A., et al.: A deep convolutional neural network model to classify heartbeats. Comp. Biol. Med. **89**, 389–396 (2017). https://doi.org/10.1016/j.compbiomed.2017.08.022
7. Prabhakar, S.K., Rajaguru, H., Lee, S.: A framework for Schizophrenia EEG signal classification with nature inspired optimization algorithms. IEEE Access **8**, 39875–39897 (2020). https://doi.org/10.1109/ACCESS.2020.2975848
8. Nair, A.R.: Analysis of energy harvesting in SWIPT using bio-inspired algorithms. Int. J. Electron. (2022)
9. Nair, A.R., Kirthiga, S., Jayakumar, M.: Estimation and compensation of IQ imbalance in SWIPT system. Int. J. Electron. Telecommun. **67**(4), 679–684 (2021)
10. Li, D., Zhang, J., Zhang, Q., Wei, X.: Classification of ECG signals based on 1D convolution neural network. In: 2017 IEEE 19th International Conference on e-Health Networking, Applications and Services (Healthcom), pp. 1–6 (2017). https://doi.org/10.1109/HealthCom.2017.8210784
11. Jun, T.J., et al.: ECG arrhythmia classification using a 2-D convolutional neural network. arXiv preprint arXiv:1804.06812 (2018)
12. Raju, M., Gopi, V.P., Anitha, V.S.: Multi-class classification of Alzheimer's disease using 3DCNN features and multilayer perceptron. In: 2021 Sixth International Conference on Wireless Communications, Signal Processing and Networking (WiSPNET), pp. 368–373 (2021). https://doi.org/10.1109/WiSPNET51692.2021.9419393
13. Raju, M., Gopi, V.P., Anitha, V.S., et al.: Multi-class diagnosis of Alzheimer's disease using cascaded three dimensional-convolutional neural network. Phys. Eng. Sci. Med. **43**, 1219–1228 (2020). https://doi.org/10.1007/s13246-020-00924
14. Wang, T., Lu, C., Sun, Y., Yang, M., Liu, C., Ou, C.: Automatic ECG classification using continuous wavelet transform and convolutional neural network. Entropy (Basel) **23**(1), 119 (2021)
15. Gao, J., Zhang, H., Lu, P., Wang, Z.: An effective LSTM recurrent network to detect arrhythmia on imbalanced ECG dataset. J. Healthc. Eng. **2019**, 6320651 (2019). https://doi.org/10.1155/2019/6320651
16. Atal, D.K., Singh, M.: Arrhythmia classification with ECG signals based on the optimization-enabled deep convolutional neural network. Comp. Methods Prog. Biomed. **196**, 105607 (2020). https://doi.org/10.1016/j.cmpb.2020.105607
17. Madan, P., et al.: A hybrid deep learning approach for ECG-based arrhythmia classification. Bioengineering **9**(4), 152 (2022)
18. Saeed, S.S., Yousif, R.Z.: A Slantlet based statistical features extraction for classification of normal, arrhythmia, and congestive heart failure in electrocardiogram. UHD J. Sci. Technol. **5**(1), 71–81 (2021)

19. Çınar, A., Tuncer, S.A.: Classification of normal sinus rhythm, abnormal arrhythmia and congestive heart failure ECG signals using LSTM and hybrid CNN-SVM deep neural networks. Comput. Methods Biomech. Biomed. Eng. **24**(2), 203–214 (2021)
20. Eltrass, A.S., Tayel, M.B., Ammar, A.I.: A new automated CNN deep learning approach for identification of ECG congestive heart failure and arrhythmia using constant-Q non-stationary Gabor transform. Biomed. Signal Process. Control **65**, 102326 (2021)
21. Olanrewaju, R.F., et al.: Classification of ECG signals for detection of arrhythmia and congestive heart failure based on continuous wavelet transform and deep neural networks. Indonesian J. Electr. Eng. Comput. Sci. (IJEECS) **12**(1), 1520–1528 (2021)
22. Kumari, C.U., et al.: Heart rhythm abnormality detection and classification using machine learning technique. In: 2020 4th International Conference on Trends in Electronics and Informatics (ICOEI), vol 48184, pp. 580–584 (2020)
23. Hussain, L., et al.: Detecting congestive heart failure by extracting multimodal features and employing machine learning techniques. Biomed. Res. Int. **2020**, 4281243 (2020)
24. Nahak, S., Saha, G.: A fusion based classification of normal, arrhythmia and congestive heart failure in ECG. In: 2020 National Conference on Communications (NCC) (2020)
25. Sandeep, K., Kora, P., Swaraja, K., Meenakshi, K., Pampana, L.K.: ECG classification using machine learning. Int. J. Recent Technol. Eng. (IJRTE). **8**(4), 2492–2494 (2019)
26. Daqrouq, K., Dobaie, A.: Wavelet based method for congestive heart failure recognition by three confirmation functions. Comput. Math. Methods Med. **2016**, 7359516 (2016)
27. Isler, Y.: Discrimination of systolic and diastolic dysfunctions using multi-layer perceptron in heart rate variability analysis. Comput. Biol. Med. **76**, 113–119 (2016)
28. Son, C.S., Kim, Y.N., Kim, H.S., Park, H.S., Kim, M.S.: Decision-making model for early diagnosis of congestive heart failure using rough set and decision tree approaches. J. Biomed. Informat. **45**(5), 999–1008 (2012)

Detection of Respiratory Disorder and Performance Analysis from PPG Signals

Harikumar Rajaguru[1], M. Kalaiyarasi[2], B. Santhosh[3](✉), and A. Senthamil Selvi[3]

[1] ECE, Bannari Amman Institute of Technology, Sathyamangalam, Erode, Tamilnadu, India
[2] EIE, Bannari Amman Institute of Technology, Sathyamangalam, Erode, Tamilnadu, India
[3] BME, Bannari Amman Institute of Technology, Sathyamangalam, Erode, Tamilnadu, India
santhoshbojaraju1@gmail.com

Abstract. Diseases related to respiration are the most common disorders in India and around the world. There are several techniques for the initial diagnosis of respiratory disorders. One of the methods to find respiratory disease is calculating the PCO_2 level in the blood. Capnography is the measurement of the partial pressure of CO_2 (carbon-dioxide) in the respiratory gases during inhalation and exhalation. It is a non-invasive measurement of PCO_2. Through capnography, information about airway management on alveolar ventilation and pulmonary perfusion can be found. In this paper, various kinds of respiratory disorders are found using classifiers and the performance of classifiers is analyzed. Dimensionality reduction techniques based on Expectation Maximization (EM) and Fast Fourier Transform (FFT) are used. Classifiers such as Linear Regression (LR), Non Linear Regression (NLR), Bayesian Linear Discriminant Classification (BLDC), Logistic regression (LSR), PSO (Particle swarm optimization), KNN (K-Nearest Neighbor) and a hybrid classifier KNN-NLR This paper discusses about seven classifiers, and it provides an effective method for diagnosis. The PSO Classifier gave the highest accuracy of 90.2439% with a low error rate of 9.7609% for both EM and FFT.

Keywords: PPG · Capnography · Respiratory disorder · Non Linear Regression · KNN

1 Introduction

Respiratory diseases are common in India and globally. Over a quarter of Indians have respiratory disorders. Asthma, COPD, lung cancer, pneumonia, apnea, and lung cancer are common in India. Physical exams, chemical, endoscopic, immunological, and genomic techniques can detect respiratory disorders [1]. Photoplethysmography (PPG) monitors oxygen saturation by detecting light passing through the skin or reflected back. The PPG uses a light-emitting diode as a source and a light-dependent resistor as a detector [2].

S. Vlad and N. M. Roman (Eds.): MEDITECH 2022, IFMBE Proceedings 102, pp. 231–242, 2024.
https://doi.org/10.1007/978-3-031-51120-2_25

2 Related Works

Harikumar Rajaguru et al. analysed the performance of the classifiers for PPG signals using NLR and EM classifiers with an accuracy of 89.1% [1]. Sannasi et al. did their work on non-linear models with extreme machine learning techniques [3]. Ganesan et al. have done the performance analysis of KNN classifiers with various metrics methods [4]. Sunil et al. used the Expectation Maximization technique to optimize the data to get better results [5]. Prabhakar and Rajaguru investigated the use of expectation maximization and non linear regression classifiers for epilepsy detection [6]. Harikumar et al. observed 83.45% by using a Bayesian Linear discriminant classifier in Breast Cancer Classification [7].

3 Materials and Methods

3.1 Dataset

The Photoplethysmography (PPG) signal is the input used by the proposed system. The information sample length acquired from the PPG signal is 1,44,000, with 720 segments overall, because the PPG signal dataset was sampled at a rate of 300 Hz. Each segment comprises 200 samples separated by equal intervals [8]. The real data set taken from PPG sensor were used for the testing purpose.

3.2 Methodology

The PPG dataset consists of around 144,000 data points from 41 with normal 41 with respiratory conditions. In this article dimensionality reduction and feature extraction techniques used to reduce the complex data to processable data with the dimensionality reduction techniques like Fast Fourier Transform and Expectation Maximization.

The statistical parameters are analysed classified by Linear Regression, Non Linear Regression, Bayesian Linear Discriminant Classifier, KNN, Logistic Regression, KNN-NLR and PSO. The methodology is described in the following flowchart (Fig. 1).

4 Dimensionality Reduction

Dimensionality reduction means transforming high-dimensional data into a lower-dimensional representation. The reduced representation's dimensionality should match the data's. Information is intrinsically dimensional because its properties can be described with a few parameters. In the last decade, many nonlinear dimensionality reduction methods have been proposed [9]. This paper analyses expectation maximization and FFT. Real-world data, such as fMRI scans, audio signals, bio signals, digital photos, etc., are very dimensional [10]. To process real-world data effectively, one must reduce its dimensionality. Dimensionality reduction reduces high-dimensional data to low-dimensional, meaningful data. Non-linear methods are better for difficult artificial jobs [11]. A query of time series is denoted by X = x1,...,xn, while the set of time series that make up the database is denoted by Y = Y1,..., YK. That each sequence

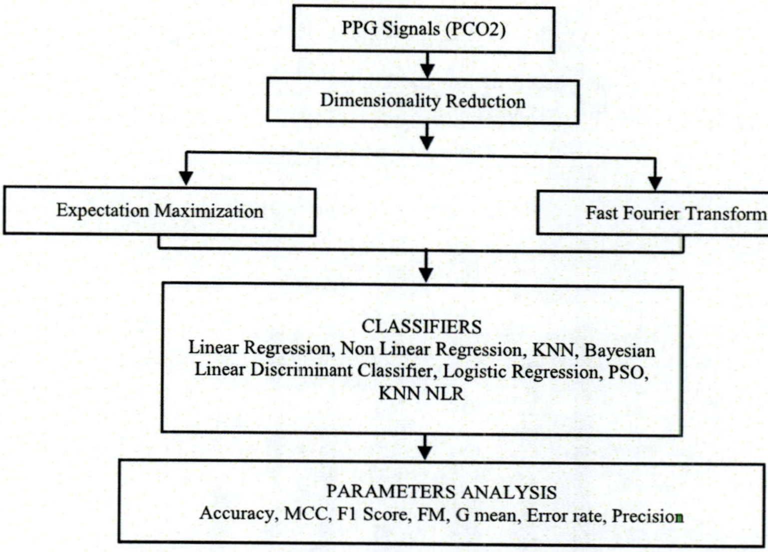

Fig.1. Methodology of classification and detection

in Y is n units long without sacrificing generality. Let N denote the converted space's dimensionality. (1 £N £) n For the sake of simplicity, let N be a factor of n. Although it is not a prerequisite of our method, it does make notation easier. A vector X x, xN 1 = represents the time series X of length n in N space. An element of X can be calculated with the given equation.

$$\overline{x}_i = \frac{N}{n} \sum_{j=\frac{n}{N}(i-1)+1}^{\frac{n}{N}i} x_j. \tag{1}$$

4.1 Expectation Maximization

Signal processing involves calculating probability distribution function parameters. Signal-in-noise mean calculation is a common estimation problem. Because data access is difficult and some data is missing, estimation is difficult. The problem is sorted by the Expectation Maximization Algorithm. EM estimates parameters with maximum likelihood when mapping many underlying data sets to observed data [5]. Signal processing members who understand estimation theory can use the algorithm. The histogram shows the graphical representation of respiratory and normal data of the respiratory disorder detection dataset as shown in Fig. 2. When the distribution of the internal complete data is exponential, and the expectation maximization algorithm can be used in equations as E-step compute (Eq. 2) and M-step compute (Eq. 3)

$$t^{[k+1]} = E[t(x), \theta^{[k]} \tag{2}$$

$$\theta^{[k+1]} = argmaxc(\theta)^T t^{[k+1]} - \log a(\theta) \tag{3}$$

There will be a need to use the common statement of expectation maximization algorithm as in Eqs. (4) and (5):

$$Q(\theta|\theta^{[k]}) = E[\log f(x|\theta)|y, \theta^{[k]}] \tag{4}$$

$$\theta^{[k+1]} = argmaxQ(\theta|\theta^{[k]} \tag{5}$$

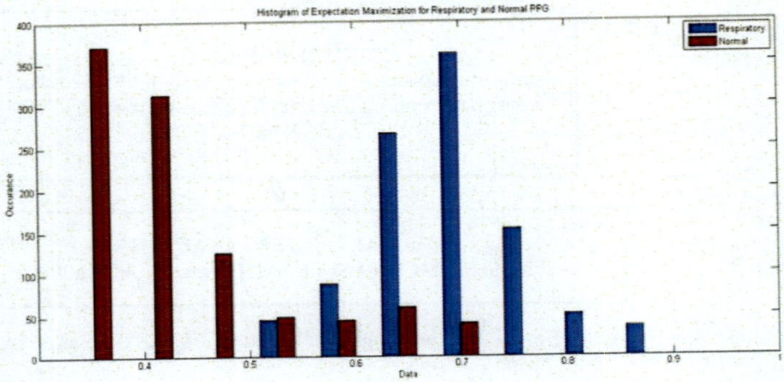

Fig. 2. Histogram of expectation maximization for respiratory and normal PPG

Mathematically, the very difficult part of the Expectation Maximization (EM) Algorithm is E-Step. This is also the very difficult computational step for the general expectation maximization algorithm [6]. The expectation should be calculated all over the values of unnoticed variables. In many other algorithms that will be applied, e.g., gradient descent.

4.2 Fast Fourier Transform

FFT uses computer-simulated filters and spectrum analysis. The FFT simplifies non-practical problems. Inefficient FFT forms Two procedures reorder row-column indexes. FFT dominates. [2N] complex input and output [9] allocation DFT to FFT is a short process. The basic FFT formulas are radix-2 or radix-4, although other radix-r forms can be found for

$$X(K) = \sum X(n) W_N nK \tag{6}$$

FFT uses power spectrum analysis and computer-simulated filters. FFT solves non-practical problems quickly. Two FFT forms are inefficient. Two procedures permute row and column index orders. FFT divides-and-conquers. [2N] is required for complex input and output. Short transforms and recombinations create FFT from DFT. In most cases, FFT is stated and programmed as a complex number operation. Directly using the complex DFT would be costly due to duplicate storage and computation. The scatterplot shows the relationship between the respiratory and normal data for respiratory disorders (Fig. 3).

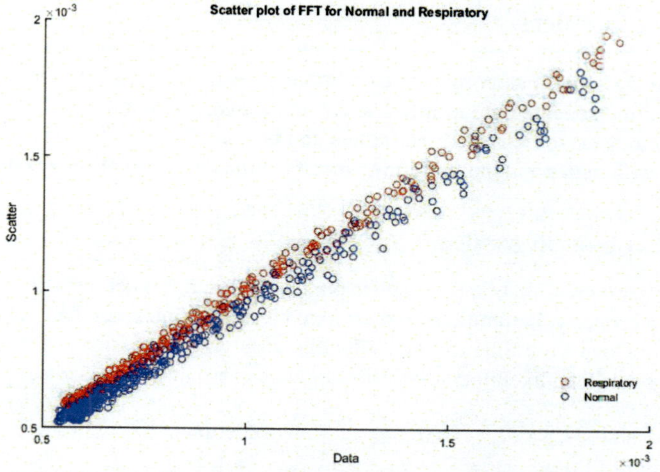

Fig. 3. Scatter plot of Fast Fourier Transform for respiratory and normal PPG

4.3 Statistical Analysis

The statistical features are calculated using the formulas.

Table 1. Statistical features of Fast Fourier Transform and Expectation Maximization for respiratory and normal PPG signals

Parameters	Fast Fourier Transform		Expectation Maximization	
	Respiratory	Normal	Respiratory	Normal
Mean	15.27872	9.151494	1.04587	0.2331
Variance	16430.02	6468.757	0.009226	0.003922
Skewness	20.91144	21.44294	−0.0024	1.149449
Kurtosis	512.4674	524.5614	0.49512	0.639042
Pearson CC	0.999648	0.998776	0.049857	0.516037
CCA	0.790433		0.73066	

The Table 1 shows the results of statistical parameters obtained for the respiratory and normal data for both Expectation Maximization and Fast Fourier Transform feature extraction techniques. Skewness is based on the symmetry of the data distribution. The Pearson correlation coefficient explains the relationship between two continuous data sets. Canonical Correlation Analysis gives the association between the two sets of data. Here, the data in both EM and FFT have a correlation.

5 Classifiers

The classifiers categorize the data into classes or clusters in order to predict or find the required specific output. Inference on the statistical parameters shows the non-linearity in the data, so non-linear classifiers can be used. The continuous training of data ends up with better and more accurate results in the detection of the respiratory disorder.

5.1 Linear Regression

Linear regression is appropriate to predict continuous outcomes, like predicting the value of a property. Its predicted output may be any complex number, varying from negative to positive from time to time. Whereas supplying regression is for classification issues that predict a likelihood that varies between zero and one. The Eq. (7) has the shape

$$A = c + dB \tag{7}$$

where A is the variable quantity and B is the experimental variable, 'd' is the slope of the road, and 'c' is the y-intercept. This method measures sample-to-class distance. Same-class subspace measurement. Linear regression and an unknown class sample can calculate the reconstruction error for each class. This linear regression determines x and y's linear relationship. Linear regression predicts class data with a constant slope.

5.2 Non Linear Regression

Two variables become nonlinear (i.e., dependent and independent variables). Linear regression is outperformed. Regression assumes linear data. Curvy data trends require nonlinear regression. Performance is analysed by applying the residue price to the non-linear equation [3]. The criterion variable in nonlinear regression depends on 1 or more independent variables. Nonlinear regression combines model parameters nonlinearly based on one or more independent variables. If the variable y (Eq. 8) is a measured variable, X is a predictor variable, and thus the deviation is represented by

$$y = \alpha_0 + \alpha_1 X_{i1} + \alpha_2 X_{i2} + \cdots + \alpha_{p-1} X_{i,p-i} + \varepsilon_i. \tag{8}$$

5.3 Bayesian Linear Discriminant

Discriminant investigation is used in generative modelling to measure the within-class thickness of X given the lesson name. Bayes' equation combines the earlier (unconditioned) likelihood of classes with Y's back likelihood. The Bayes hypothesis relates the likelihood of X being in each lesson to the likelihood of X's input in each course [7]. For ease, there should be 1 input variable, which is X. BDA stands for Bayes discriminant analysis, and is a classification method supporting linear discriminant analysis ideas [12]. Thomas Bayes' formula uses the bound criteria to create each class of discriminant function.

5.4 KNN Classifier

The abbreviation of KNN is "K-Nearest Neighbor". It is a kind of supervised machine learning. The formula will be used to solve each classification and regression downside statement [13]. The number of nearest neighbors to a replacement for an unknown variable that should be foreseen or classified is denoted by the image 'K'. KNN works with the distances between a question and each of the examples within the knowledge base. Then, they choose the desired variety of examples (K) highest to the question, then vote for the most frequent label (in the case of classification) or average the labels [4]. The k-nearest neighbors (KNN) rule is an easy-to-implement kind of supervised machine learning rule that may be used to resolve regression and classification problems. The Minkowski distance is the most popular option. The Eq. (9) is as follows:

$$distance(x, z) = (dr = 1|xrzr|p)1/p). \tag{9}$$

5.5 Logistic Regression

In statistics, the model is applied to the chance of a win/lose, pass/fail, healthy/sick, or alive/dead category or event. This will be extended to the models of many categories, such as determinants, cats, dogs, lions, etc. A logistic regression is a rule for categorising observations [14]. Regression transforms output mistreatment, allowing sigmoid to produce a chance value. Logistic Regression is an algorithm. Given free variables, it won't predict a binary outcome (1/0, Yes/No, True/False). You can also consider supplying regression to be a subset of regression when the end result variable is categorical [15]. It predicts the likelihood of an event by using a logistic function.

5.6 PSO

PSO is abbreviated as "Particle swarm optimization." The PSO classifier is useful for optimizing non-linear functions. There are two main component methodologies. There are two different forms of component methodologies. There are more familiar PSO, which are artificial life (A-LIFE), fish schooling, bird flocking, and swimming theory. Particle swarm optimization is a very simple concept, and its paradigms are implemented in just a very few lines of computer code. PSO uses simple mathematical operators; it is also very cheap regarding memory requirements and speed. In past testing experiments, the use of PSO to be very helpful in various types of problems is found. It is derived as Eqs. (10) and (11).

$$v_i = Wv_i + c_1r_1\left(P_{best,i} - x_i\right) + c_2r_2\left(g_{best,i} - x_i\right) \tag{10}$$

$$x_i = x_i + v_i \tag{11}$$

i = the velocity of the ith particle. $P_{best,i}$ = Personal Best of the Ith Particle. Xi = Ith particle's position. r1 and r2 are random numbers. Gbest stands for global test. c_1 and c_2 are acceleration coefficients. W = Inertia weight. Still, there is much research remaining which is to be conducted on this concept and the paradigm. PSO uses the concept of fitness as an evolutionary paradigm.

5.7 KNN NLR

A hybrid classifier uses two different algorithms or methods to derive the best output out of it. This classification method is based on local apologies, where computations are deferred until after function evaluation. Normalizing the training data can improve the algorithm's accuracy dramatically when features show different physical units that come in vastly different scales because this algorithm is based on distance for classification. Data written in nonlinear form can be described with nonlinear regression, a statistical technique. Regression models that are nonlinear are normally assumed to be parametric, in the sense that they are described as equations with nonlinear coefficients.

6 Results and Discussion

A confusion matrix is the specific table that visualizes the performance of algorithms. The confusion matrix gives the results of four kinds: true positive (TP), true negative (TN), false positive (FP), and false negative (FN). Various parameters such as accuracy, Mathews correlation coefficient (MCC), F1 Score, Fowlkes-Mallows (FM), error rate, G mean, and precision are analyzed using the classifiers. The stopping criteria for all the classifiers is MSE (Mean Squared Error). It is the average squared difference between actual values and obtained values (Eq. 12). The following Table 2 shows the confusion matrix and MSE of FFT and EM.

$$\frac{1}{n}\sum_{i=1}^{n}(Y_i - \widehat{Y_i})^2 \tag{12}$$

n–Number of data points
Y_i–Observed values
$\widehat{Y_i}$–Predicted values.

Table 2. Confusion matrix and MSE of Fast Fourier Transform and Expectation Maximization

Classifiers	Fast Fourier Transform					Expectation Maximization				
	TP	TN	FP	FN	MSE	TP	TN	FP	FN	MSE
LR	12	12	9	8	6.82E-05	13	13	8	7	5.19E-05
NLR	13	12	9	7	6.85E-05	12	18	3	8	3.43E-05
BLDC	11	16	5	9	5.59E-05	11	12	9	9	8.26E-05
KNN	11	17	4	9	4.65E-05	12	14	7	8	5.71E-05
Log. Reg	14	11	10	6	1.04E-04	15	12	9	5	7.16E-05
PSO	18	19	2	2	2.21E-06	18	19	2	2	1.44E-06
KNN NLR	16	15	6	4	1.06E-05	17	16	5	3	7.38E-06

The PSO classifier has the lowest mean square error in both the dimensionality reduction techniques. Though the logistic regression has the lowest mean square value in FFT, it has the highest MSE in the EM technique. Also, the other classifiers have drastic changes in MSE in both the feature extraction techniques. The analysis on performance of FFT and EM are done and the results are shown in the table 3.

Table 3. Performance analysis of Fast Fourier Transform and Expectation Maximization

Classifiers		Accuracy	F1 score	MCC	FM	G mean	Error rate	Precision
LR	EM	63.41	63.41	0.26	0.63	63.43	36.58	61.90
	FFT	58.53	58.53	0.17	0.58	58.55	41.46	57.14
NLR	EM	73.17	63.57	0.47	0.69	74.42	26.82	80
	FFT	60.97	61.90	0.22	0.61	61.09	39.02	59.09
BLDC	EM	56.09	55	0.12	0.55	56.06	43.90	55
	FFT	65.85	61.11	0.31	0.61	66.33	34.14	68.75
KNN	EM	63.41	61.53	0.26	0.61	63.39	36.58	63.15
	FFT	68.29	62.85	0.37	0.63	69.24	31.70	73.33
Log Reg	EM	65.85	68.18	0.32	0.68	66.42	34.14	62.5
	FFT	60.97	63.63	0.22	0.63	61.43	39.02	58.33
PSO	EM	90.24	90	0.80	0.9	90.23	9.75	90
	FFT	90.24	90	0.80	0.9	90.23	9.75	90
KNN NLR	EM	80.48	80.95	0.61	0.81	80.66	19.51	77.27
	FFT	75.60	76.19	0.51	0.76	75.77	24.39	72.72

PSO classifiers outperform with 90.243 accuracy compared with other classifiers with 90.237 of G mean, 9.756 as an error rate, and precision using both FFT and EM extraction techniques. Linear regression has shown the linearity in the parameters in both the extractions. The FM values of all the classifiers lie between 0.6 and 0.9 and are similar in FFT and EM for each of the classifiers. The precision of KNN in FFT is almost similar to that of KNN NLR in FFT. All the parameters have their best result in the Particle Swarm Optimization (PSO) classifier. PSO has given better accuracy with a low error rate.

The accuracy chart (see Fig. 4) shows the performance of classifiers under Fast Fourier Transform and Expectation Maximization extraction techniques. There is a non-linearity and overlap in the respiratory and normal data, which results in non-linear outputs. The results show that the PSO classifier outperforms with the best accuracy.

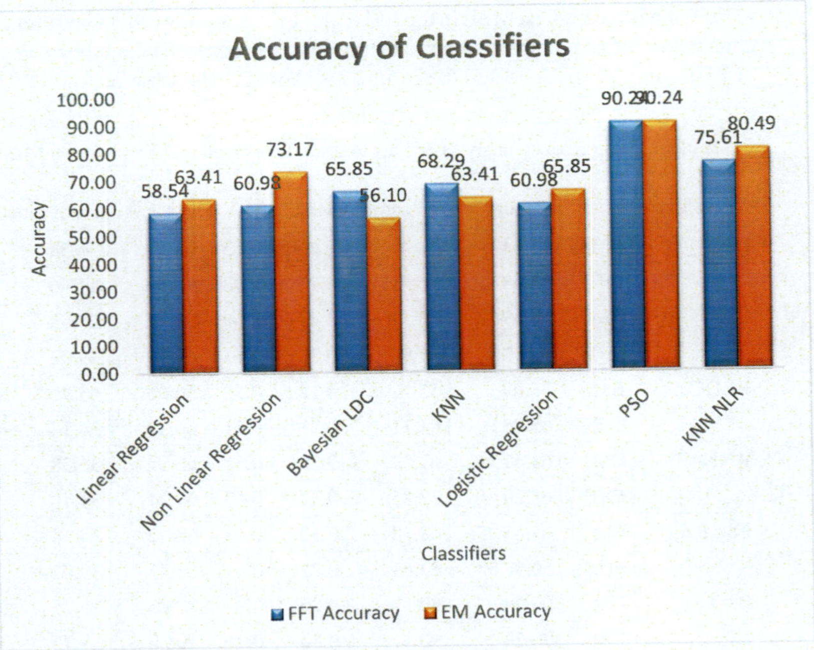

Fig. 4. Accuracy chart for Classifiers in FFT and EM

7 Conclusion

The statistical features are extracted using seven classifiers. Out of seven classifiers, particle swarm optimization has given the most accurate result of 90.2439% and with a low error rate of 9.7561% for both FFT and EM, when compared to the remaining classifiers. The Linear Regression classifier gives the lowest accuracy of 58.5365% and the highest error rate of 41.4634% for FFT. The Bayesian Linear Discriminant classifier gives the lowest accuracy of 56.0975% and the highest error rate of 43.9024% for EM. From the obtained data, a wide range of respiratory disorders can be detected. Thus, the PSO classifier provides the more accurate results. Here, the performance analysis is done for the classifiers to predict the presence of respiratory disorders in the given dataset. Furthermore, deep learning and metaheuristic techniques can be applied and prediction of specific respiratory disorders can be done.

Conflict of Interest. The authors declare that they have no conflicts of interest.

References

1. Rajaguru, H., Karthikamani, R.: Performance analysis of classifiers in detection of respiratory disorder through capnography. In: 2021 Smart Technologies, Communication and Robotics (STCR), pp. 1–4 (2021). https://doi.org/10.1109/STCR51658.2021.9588820
2. Allen, J.: Photoplethysmography and its application in clinical physiological measurement. Physiol. Meas. **28**(3), 1–39 (2007). https://doi.org/10.1088/0967-3334/28/3/R01
3. Sannasi Chakravarthy, S.R., Rajaguru, H.: Detection and classification of microcalcification from digital mammograms with firefly algorithm, extreme learning machine and non-linear regression models: a comparison. Int. J. Imaging Syst. Technol. 1–21 (2019). https://doi.org/10.1002/ima.22364
4. Ganesan, K., Rajaguru, H.: Performance analysis of KNN classifier with various distance metrics method for MRI images. In: Wang, J., Reddy, G., Prasad, V., Reddy, V. (eds.) Soft Computing and Signal Processing. Advances in Intelligent Systems and Computing, vol. 900. Springer, Singapore. (2019). https://doi.org/10.1007/978-981-13-3600-3_64
5. Prabhakar, S.K., Rajaguru, H.: Comparison of fuzzy output optimization with expectation maximization algorithm and its modification for epilepsy classification. In: Guru, D., Vasudev, T., Chethan, H., Kumar, Y. (eds.) Proceedings of International Conference on Cognition and Recognition. Lecture Notes in Networks and Systems, vol. 14. Springer, Singapore (2018). https://doi.org/10.1007/978-981-10-5146-3_25
6. Setoodeh, P., Habibi, S., Haykin, S.: Expectation maximization. In: Nonlinear Filters: Theory and Applications, pp.185–201. Wiley (2022). https://doi.org/10.1002/9781119078166.ch10
7. Rajaguru, H., Kumar Prabhakar, S.: Bayesian linear discriminant analysis for breast cancer classification. In: 2017 2nd International Conference on Communication and Electronics Systems (ICCES), pp. 266–269 (2017).https://doi.org/10.1109/CESYS.2017.8321279
8. Karlen, W., Turner, M., Cook, E., Dumont, G.A., Ansermino, J.M.: CapnoBase: signal database and tools to collect, share and annotate respiratory signals. In: Annual Meeting of the Society for Technology in Anesthesia (STA) Conference, 25 (2010)
9. Reddy, G.T., et al.: Analysis of dimensionality reduction techniques on big data. IEEE Access **8**, 54776–54788 (2020). https://doi.org/10.1109/ACCESS.2020.2980942
10. Ray, P., Reddy, S.S., Banerjee, T.: Various dimension reduction techniques for high dimensional data analysis: a review. Artif. Intell. Rev. **54**, 3473–3515 (2021). https://doi.org/10.1007/s10462-020-09928-0
11. Jia, W., Sun, M., Lian, J., et al.: Feature dimensionality reduction: a review. Complex Intell. Syst. **8**, 2663–2693 (2022). https://doi.org/10.1007/s40747-021-00637-x
12. Marini, F., Walczak, B.: Particle swarm optimization (PSO). A tutorial. Chemometr. Intell. Lab. Syst. **149**, Part B, 153–165 (2015). ISSN 0169-7439, https://doi.org/10.1016/j.chemolab.2015.08.020
13. Uddin, S., Haque, I., Lu, H., et al.: Comparative performance analysis of K-nearest neighbour (KNN) algorithm and its different variants for disease prediction. Sci. Rep. **12**, 6256 (2022). https://doi.org/10.1038/s41598-022-10358-x
14. Huang, F.L.: Alternatives to logistic regression models in experimental studies. J. Exp. Educ. **90**(1), 213–228 (2022). https://doi.org/10.1080/00220973.2019.1699769
15. Putri Wibowo, V.V., Rustam, Z., Laeli, A.R., Sa'id, A.A.: Logistic regression and logistic regression-genetic algorithm for classification of liver cancer data. In: 2021 International Conference on Decision Aid Sciences and Application (DASA), pp. 244–248 (2021). https://doi.org/10.1109/DASA53625.2021.9682242

16. Panda, N.R.: A review on logistic regression in medical research. Natl. J. Commun. Med. [Internet]. 2022 Apr. 30 [cited 2022 Oct. 14]; **13**(4), 265–270
17. Hemachandira, V.S., Viswanathan, R.; A framework on performance analysis of mathematical model-based classifiers in detection of epileptic seizure from EEG signals with efficient feature selection. J. Healthc. Eng. **2022**, Article ID 7654666, 12 p. (2022). https://doi.org/10.1155/2022/7654666

A Dual-BRAM Solution for BTSx Instructions on FPGA Processors

Cristian Ignat, Paul Faragó(✉), Mihaela Cîrlugea, and Sorin Hintea

Technical University of Cluj-Napoca, Cluj-Napoca, Romania
paul.farago@bel.utcluj.ro

Abstract. Processing time is very important in biomedical equipment and affects decision taking, result interpretation or calculus for a variety of targeted applications: ECG, PPG or SpO_2. To answer the need for rapid medical application prototyping, we present a solution to optimize instruction execution on FPGA processors. The targeted applications account for multiple input signal acquisition in a scenario of body worn sensors. This work addresses the implementation of bit/byte-oriented register operations, reducing the operating time of the processor by simultaneously reading and writing from/in the memory block. During customary execution, bit/byte test skip instructions introduce a one clock-cycle delay. This paper proposes a dual-instruction memory solution, implemented using block RAM modules, to eliminate the respective execution delay. The proposed solution enables the simultaneous retrieval of two instructions which would follow the execution path, regardless whether the skip decision has been taken or not. The VHDL implementation of the proposed solution was simulated in Vivado and was validated on an Artix7 35T and a Kintex Ultrascale+ FPGA respectively.

Keywords: Biomedical equipment · Biomedical signal processing · FPGA processor · BTX instruction

1 Introduction

The electronic biomedical applications that are based on biosignals, like cortical mapping, neuromuscular problems, study of sleep, detection of seizure, ischemia detection etc., represent an important part of the medical life today. Instrumentations that measure and monitor these signals are important to be fast and precise [1]. The microcontrollers used are important to be low cost but efficient, linking the hardware with the software. Usually, it needs to have high processing power, a flexible oscillator structure and other important performances [1]. Fast signal processing is always a priority, in particular in medical applications or medical devices, on one hand because the human health is on stake, the patient's and medical staff's safety and, on the other hand, one has to assure that the medical equipment is working properly, are not outdated and thus tested in various maintenance programs, like for instance, presented in [2, 3]. In quality control tests, training processes, service and monitoring of the medical equipment, various analyzers and simulators are used, like arrhythmia simulators, frequency electrosurgical analyzers,

S. Vlad and N. M. Roman (Eds.): MEDITECH 2022, IFMBE Proceedings 102, pp. 243–253, 2024.
https://doi.org/10.1007/978-3-031-51120-2_26

blood pressure simulators etc., where signal precision, speed and acquisition are most important, proving the reliability, usability and quality of the equipment. Determining the breakdown time is also important for companies providing medical devices, while they also take care about calibration and testing, especially for high-tech medical devices [4]. Another example of bidirectional data transfer that allows a fast processing and response is presented in [5], where an instrumentation system was created for safe line-powered bio-potential measurements, successfully used for ECG, EMG or EEG. Other applications that require a fast response of the circuits are presented in an electronic application used for the driver's safety, from monitoring the driver's vigilance to the management of the "in-car health" [6]. The signal monitoring in ECG must be accurate, person-specific and in real-time, so that effective systems are necessary to identify the high-risk patients for prioritizing in hospital treatments [7]. FPGA board machines can be used, as in [8], for biosignal recording and processing systems in case they must perform in real-time robust machine learning analyses for accelerating these systems, increasing the rate of data transmitted, allowing thus machine learning operations to be performed in parallel with tasks regarding the data processing [9].

2 FPGA Microprocessor Prototyping

Field programmable gate arrays (FPGA) are a powerful platform for microprocessor (μP) prototyping and testing [10]. In this framework, we have previously proposed and validated a novel μP architecture, developed around the Harvard architecture and a pipeline implemented with two block RAM (BRAM) memory modules [11]. Microprocessors execute 5 main classes of instructions: bit-oriented file register operations, byte-oriented file register operations, control operations, literal operations and data memory & program memory operations [12, 13]. Out of these classes, bit- and byte-orientated instructions are those instructions which affect bits of bytes of data respectively [13, 14].

Bit or byte test skip (BTSx) is a collection of uP instructions, with x standing for E, C, S, R, L and G respectively, as listed in Table 1. These instructions determine a skip over the next instruction if the condition denoted by x is fulfilled. As such, the BTSx instructions can implement the conditional instructions from programming languages, e.g. if…else…, and loops, e.g. for and while. Thus, it is important for microprocessors, as well as microcontrollers, to implement this class of instructions.

BTSx instructions require a specific execution procedure. Since the BTSx skip decision is taken based on a comparison result, the BTSx instruction can only be executed only after data memory access, which introduces an execution delay. In order to overcome the execution delay, this paper proposes a novel hardware solution for the execution of BTSx instructions in a single clock cycle. The proposed solution is based on a dual-BRAM architecture. The advantage of the proposed solution is twofold. On one hand, the dual-BRAM architecture enables the simultaneous retrieval of two instructions. On the other hand, the employment of BRAM enables the simultaneous writing and reading of the same memory module.

Table 1. BTSx instruction set for the processor previously proposed in [11].

Address	Instruction	Remarks
0x30	BTSSL	Bit test skip set literal
0x31	BTSS	Bit test skip set
0x32	BTSCL	Bit test skip Clear literal
0x33	BTSC	Bit test skip Clear
0x34	BTSEL	Bit test skip Equal literal
0x35	BTSE	Bit test skip Equal
0x36	BTSNL	Bit test skip if Not equal literal
0x37	BTSN	Bit test skip if Not equal
0x38	BTSLL	Byte test skip if lower literal
0x39	BTSL	Byte test skip if lower
0x3A	BTSGL	Byte test skip if greater literal
0x3B	BTSG	Byte test skip if greater

3 Execution of BTSx Instructions

Consider for exemplification the pipeline of the successive execution of two common instructions, as illustrated in Fig. 1.

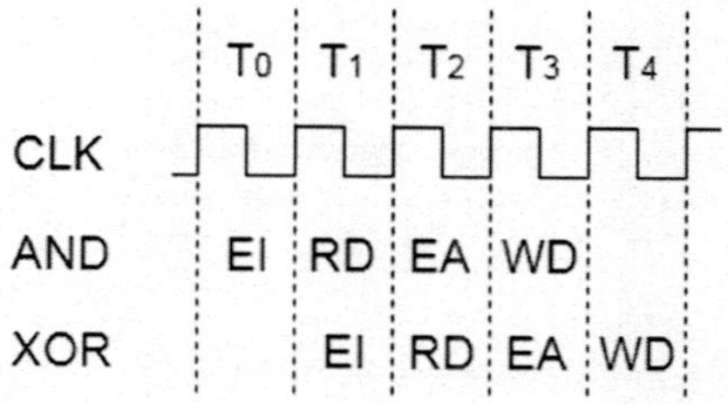

Fig. 1. Common instruction execution pipeline.

Now, consider replacing the AND instruction with the BTSE instruction, as illustrated in the pipeline from Fig. 2. Assuming the current instruction is

$$\text{BTSE addr1 addr2} \tag{1}$$

the Program Counter (PC) will generate a skip over the next instruction if the data from addr1 is equal to the data from addr2, otherwise the instructions follow normal execution. The decision whether this skip takes place or not can only be taken after the data has been retrieved from the indicated memory addresses, namely after the T0 → T1 rising edge. As such, the BTSE instruction could be executed earliest at T1.

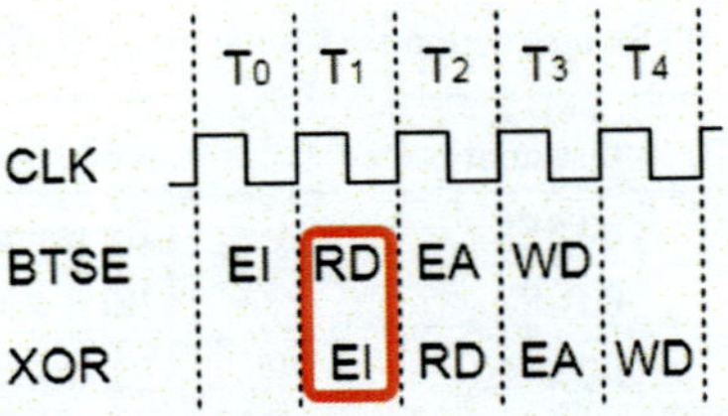

Fig. 2. BTSE instruction execution pipeline.

At T1, the execution of Read Data (RD) for the BTSx instruction is performed in parallel with the execution of Extract Instruction (EI) for the XOR instruction. Considering that EI from the second command is already executed, the BTSE testing doesn't make sense anymore, because the instruction from the immediate next address is already in execution.

Two solutions are applicable to overcome this issue. The first solution assumes the introduction of a one clock cycle delay before extracting the next instruction. Specifically, this solution assumes that, as soon as a BTSx current instruction was identified, the Instruction Enable (i_EN) signal of the instruction memory will be set to LOW for one clock period to avoid the extraction of the next instruction, as illustrated in the pipeline from Fig. 3. Accordingly, once a BTSx instruction was identified at T0, the PC is inhibited for one clock cycle during T1 where the i_EN signal is LOW.

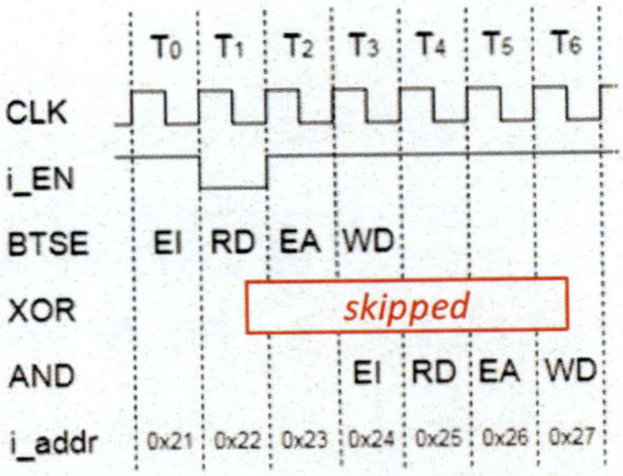

Fig. 3. BTSE instruction execution pipeline with the one clock-cycle invalidation of the instruction memory

The second solution assumes to inhibit the writing of the data memory. As such, the Write Data Memory (WDM) signal is set to LOW during the BTSx instruction, and in case equality was tested, during the following XOR instruction as well, as illustrated in the pipeline from Fig. 4.

The FPGA implementation of the memory read/write invalidation solutions is straightforward. The drawback is that it introduces a supplementary clock cycle, i.e. execution of BTSx instructions occupies two clock periods.

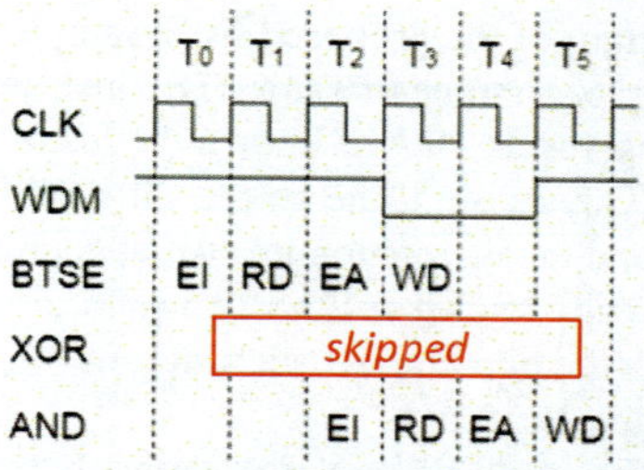

Fig. 4. BTSE instruction execution pipeline with the two clock-cycle invalidation of the data memory

4 Proposed FPGA Implementation

The solution proposed per to eliminate the supplementary clock cycle during BTSx execution is to deploy two instruction memories, in an approach similar to the one we previously proposed in [11]. The block diagram of the dual instruction memory solution for the one-clock cycle execution of the BTSx instructions is depicted in Fig. 5. Both memory blocks are dual port memories, with port A used only for writing into the instruction memory. The two memories will always provide the instructions from successive addresses ADDR_i and ADDR_i + 1.

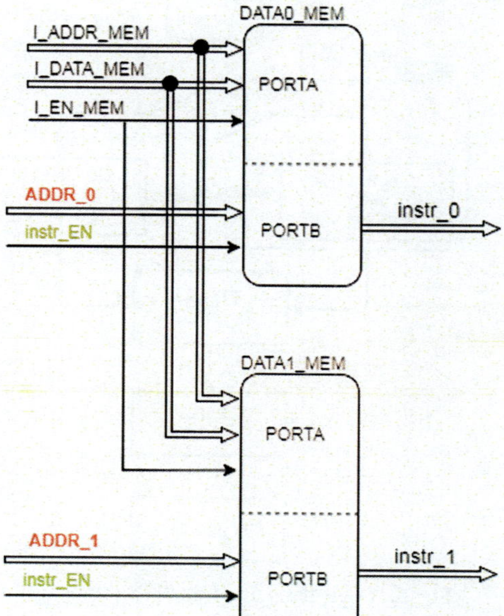

Fig. 5. Block diagram of the proposed BTSx execution hardware

The logic diagram of the proposed FPGA implementation of the BTSx instruction is illustrated in Fig. 6. Assume that the BTSx instruction is located at a generic address addr = A. If the test result is FALSE, then the instruction located at address A + 1 will be executed next. Otherwise, if the test result is TRUE, then the instruction at address A + 1 is skipped and the instruction located at address A + 2 will be executed next. As illustrated, it is already known at time T1 which of the two commands will be selected for routing through the pipeline. As such, at time T2, the data necessary for the selected instruction is already extracted.

According to the proposed implementation, both instructions from addresses A + 1 and A + 2 respectively will be read **during the same clock cycle**, namely T1 in Fig. 7. Moreover, as illustrated in Fig. 7, the instructions from addresses A + 1 and A + 2 are extracted from the instruction memory simultaneously with reading the data memory for the BTSx instruction from address A. As a matter of fact, all necessary elements required to decide which of the two instructions fed into the pipeline after BTSx, is available at T1 for going through the pipeline. Consequently, the one clock cycle delay described previously is unnecessary for the proper execution of BTSx in the proposed implementation.

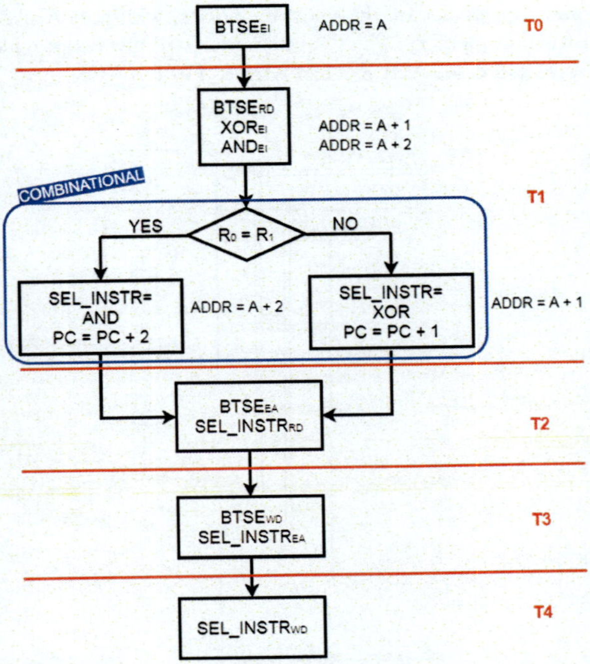

Fig. 6. Logic diagram of the BTSx implementation on FPGA

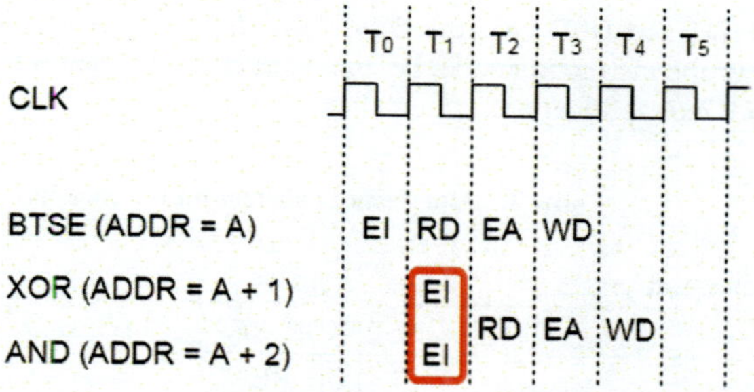

Fig. 7. Proposed BTSE instruction execution pipeline

5 BTSx Instruction Test Results

The proposed solution for the execution of BTSx instructions was implemented in VHDL and simulated in Vivado. Practical tests, carried out on an Artix7 35T and a Kintex Ultrascale+ FPGA respectively, validate the proposed solution.

An assembler (ASM) code compiler, developed in VBScript, was used to translate the ASM code into machine code for FPGA testing. The ASM code to test the proposed BTSx implementation is shown in Fig. 8, along with the data memory addresses on the left and the machine code instructions on the right.

```
    to_init:

001     XOR_RES = 0xF4              00F40114
002     OR_RES = 0x44               00440214
003     A = 0xA5                    00A50314
004     B = 0x28                    00280414

005     JP to_infinite_loop         00060021

    to_infinite_loop:

006     BTSE XOR_RES OR_RES         02010035
007         R = A XOR B             0403050C
008     R = A AND B                 04030510

009     XOR_RES = A XOR B           0403010C
00A     OR_RES = A OR B             04030208

00B     A = A ADDL 0x0D             0D030301
00C     B = B ADDL 0x02             02040401

00D     JP to_infinite_loop         00060021
```

Fig. 8. BTS instruction ASM test code

As illustrated in Fig. 8, the format of an instruction is the following:

$$0xD1D1D0D0AdrAdrOpOp \quad (2)$$

where D1D1 and D0D0 are the data, AdrAdr is the result address and OpOp is the operator or the instruction code, i.e. the instruction that needs to be executed. Consider Table 2 for exemplification.

Table 2. Data memory content for the code in Fig. 8.

Data memory address	Variable	Value
0x01	XOR_RES	0xF4
0x02	OR_RES	0x44
0x03	A	0xA5
0x04	B	0x28

The ASM code from Fig. 8 is executed as follows: PC (signal pc_q) indicates the instructions memorya address. At the next clock cycle, the instruction is extracted from the instruction memory from the indicated address. This is visible in the signal diagram when pc_q is 0x06, which indicates that the next extracted instruction is “0x02010035” corresponding to BTSE. Consider Fig. 9 for correlation.

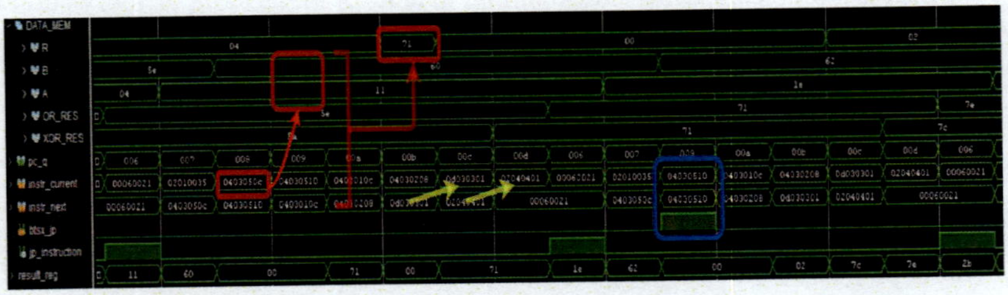

Fig. 9. BTSE instruction simulation result for the test code in Fig. 8.

The instructions are executed in the ALU as follows: The equality check is performed for OR_RES and XOR_RES, as prescribed by the BTSE instruction. In case of equality, as indicated with blue in Fig. 9, the code execution skips address 0x07. After this, the ALU reports to the PC via the signal ‘btsx_jp’ that a skip took place. Thus, when the next instruction arrives, the PC will update the address with a delay of one clock cycle. This happens because flip-flops are used and the update can be made only during the next clock period.

To be noticed that, when the skip occures due to the BTSE, the pc_q which provides the address of the next instruction misses the instruction from 0x08. In reality, the skip takes place over instruction 0x07, which can be confirmed following the results obtained in the data memory. Although the PC reports the instruction execution order to be 0x06, 0x07, 0x09, thus skipping over 0x08, indicated with blue in Fig. 9, one can notice that the current instruction is overwritten with the next instruction. This phenomenon takes place only when the skip occurs, and consequently, the instructions are executed sequentially as prescribed.

In the case that the BTSE does not result in a skip, indicated with red in Fig. 9, the instructions are executed sequentially, namely: 0x06, 0x07, 0x08, 0x09,..., 0x0D. Next, a jump occurs back to address 0x06, indicated with yellow in Fig. 9, because of the command "JP to_infinite_loop" instruction.

The red rectangles actually indicate the execution of the instruction from 0x07, i.e. the one which is skipped when btsx_jp is a logical '1'. The instruction is extracted from the instructions memory. During the next clock cycle, the data is extracted from the data memory and anly afterwards is the command executed. After that, during the next clock cycle, the result is written in the memory into the address 0x05, this being the location for variable R, which stores the result of the XOR and AND operation between operands A and B.

Processor operation is illustrated in Fig. 10, which plots the instruction addresses captured during processor execution using the Integrated Logic Analyzer (ILA) available from Xilinx. The test code assumes an infinite loop following the code listed in Table 3.

As such, Fig. 10 illustrates the waveforms of the signals internal to the FPGA during operation, namely *instr_selected* for the instruction which is to be executed and which is chosen from either *instruction* of *next_instruction* based on the BTSx condition. Figure 10 validates the proposed FPGA implementation of the BTSx instruction set.

Table 3. Test code for the BTSEL instruction.

Instruction address	Machine code	ASMcode
0x01	00030114	a = 0x03
0x02	00040214	b = 0x21
0x03	00340314	c = 0x34
0x04	01020201	b = b ADD 0x01
0x05	08020034	BTSEL b 0x08
0x06	02010103	a = a SUBL 0x02
0x07	00040021	JP 0x04

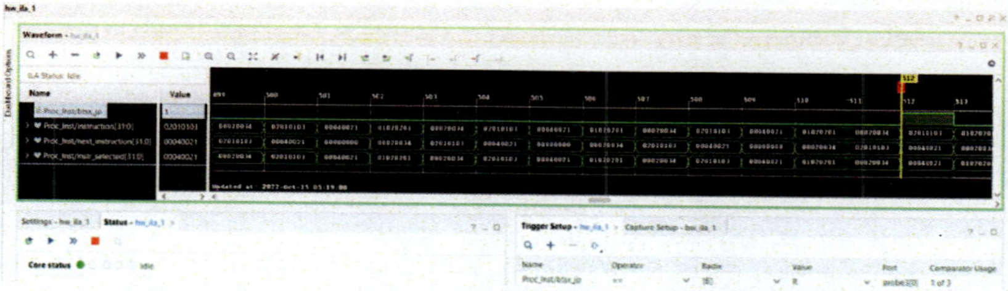

Fig. 10. Instruction addresses during the executin of the BTSEL instruction.

6 Conclusion

This paper proposed a novel solution to execute BTSx instructions in a single clock cycle considering the dual-BRAM architecture for the purposed processor. The advantage of the solution is two-fold. First, the dual-BRAM architecture enables the simultaneous retrieval of two pieces of data during process execution. Second, the employment of BRAM blocks enables the simultaneous writing and reading of the data memory. As such, the proposed solution overcomes the delay issues in the customary execution of BTSx instructions.

The proposed solution for BTSx execution was implemented in VHDL, the design was simulated in Vivado, and was validated practically on an Artix7 35T and a Kintex Ultrascale + FPGA respectively.

Practical validation of the proposed solution was carried out with a 60 MHz FPGA clock frequency. For comparison to other processor solutions of BTSx instructions we prefer to consider the number of clock cycles required for execution.

Other processors execute test skip instructions in multiple clock cycles. For exemplification, the PIC24FJ128GA204 datasheet [15] reports on 2 or 3 clock cycles provided the test condition was met. As another example, the PIC16F18325 datasheet [16] reports on 2 clock cycles provided the test condition was met. For both cases, one cycle execution only happens if the skip doesn't take place.

Another aspect which must be accounted for is that the two microcontrollers don't execute instructions in every clock cycle. For exemplification, the PIC24 reports on 16 MIPS operation @ 32 MHz, meaning that the instructions are executed at half the clock frequency.

Similar results are reported for the Atmel family, see Ref. [17].

From this point of view, the proposed FPGA implementation of the BTSx instruction set exhibits an operation speed of a fixed one clock cycle.

Because the processing time is critical in biomedical applications and equipment, considering decisions, result interpretation or calculus, for devices used for ECG, PPG or SpO_2, this paper presents an optimization of the FPGA processor time that can be efficient in case of signal acquisition from body worn sensors. The present work is an important step towards machine-learning analysis systems, offering a solution to answer the need for rapid prototyping and use in medical equipment.

References

1. Ajani, A.S., Alade O.M., Ajani, O.S., Alabi, O.J.: Development of ha mobile multimodal biosignal instrument for simultaneous measurement and analysis of four clinically relevant biosignals, obtained from both normal and pathological subjects. Int. J. Biosens. Bioelectron. **4**(3), 148–157 (2018). Author, F., Author, S.: Title of a proceedings paper. In: Editor, F., Editor, S. (eds.) CONFERENCE 2016. LNCS, vol. 9999, pp. 1–13. Springer, Heidelberg (2016)
2. Corciova, C., Fuior, R., Andritoi, D., Luca, C.: Assessment of medical equipment maintenance management. In: Operations Management, pp.1–15. Intechopen Publisher (2022)
3. Ghasemi, M., Mazaheri, E., Hadian, M., Karimi, S.: Evaluation of medical equipment management in educational hospitals in Isfahan. J. Educ. Health Promotion **11**(3) (2022). http://www.jehp.net

4. Hamel, B.S.: Breakdown time analysis in the effort to maximize medical equipment productivity in hospital. In: Proceedings Muhammadiyah International Public Healthcare and Medicine Conference, Faculty of Public Health, Jakarta, vol.1, no.1 (2021)
5. Piipponen, K.V.T., Sepponen, R., Eskelinen, P.: A biosignal instrumentation system using capacitive coupling for power and signal isolation. In: IEEE Transactions on Biomedical Engineering, vol.54, no. 10, pp. 1822–1828 (2007)
6. Heuer, S., Chamadiya, B., Gharbi, A., Wagner, M.: Unobtrusive in-vehicle biosignal instrumentation for advanced driver assistance and active safety. In: IEEE EMBS Conference on Biomedical Engineering and Sciences (2010)
7. Kiranyaz, S., Ince, T., Chowdury, M.E.D., Gabbouj, M.: Biosignal time-series analysis. In: Deep Learning for Robot Perception and Cognition, pp. 491–539. Academic Press, Elsevier Inc. (2022)
8. Li, H., Wang, J., Zhao, S., Tian, F., Yang, J., Sawan, M.: Real-time biosignal recording and machine-learning analysis system. In: IEEE 4th International Conference on Artificial Intelligence Circuits and Systems (AICAS), pp. 427–430 (2022)
9. Dillen, A., Steckelmacher, D., Efthymiadis, K.: Deep learning for bio-signal control: insights from basic to real-time methods with recommendations. J. Neural Eng. **19**(1) (2022)
10. Roth, C.H., Kurian, J., Jr.: Digital Systems Design Using VHDL, 2nd edn. Cengage Learning (2008)
11. Ignat, C., Faragó, P., Hintea, S.: FPGA implementation of a novel dual—BRAM processor architecture. In: 2020 43rd International Conference on Telecommunications and Signal Processing (TSP), pp. 124–128 (2020)
12. ***, PIC18Fxxx Instruction Set. http://technology.niagarac.on.ca/staff/mboldin/18F_Instruction_Set/. Accessed 10 May 2022
13. ***, PIC16F84A—Instruction Set. https://www.circuitstoday.com/pic16f84a-instruction-set. Accessed 10 May 2022
14. ***, Byte Orientated Instructions. http://www.pcbheaven.com/picpages/Byte_Orientated_Instructions/. Accessed 10 May 2022
15. ***, PIC24FJ128GA204 FAMILY. https://ww1.microchip.com/downloads/en/DeviceDoc/30010038c.pdf. Accessed 15 Oct. 2022
16. ***, PIC16(L)F18325/18345. http://ww1.microchip.com/downloads/en/devicedoc/40001795e.pdf. Accessed 15 Oct. 2022
17. ***, AVR Instruction Set Manual. http://ww1.microchip.com/downloads/en/devicedoc/atmel-0856-avr-instruction-set-manual.pdf. Accessed 15 Oct. 2022

Author Index

S. Vlad and N. M. Roman (Eds.): MEDITECH 2022, IFMBE Proceedings 102, pp. 255–256, 2024.
https://doi.org/10.1007/978-3-031-51120-2